The Handbook of Forensic Mental Health in Africa

The Handbook of Forensic Mental Health in Africa traces the history of forensic mental health in Africa, discussing the importance of considering cultural differences when implementing Western-validated practices on the continent while establishing state-of-the-art assessment and treatment of justice-involved persons.

Experts in the field of forensic mental health throughout Africa explore the current state of forensic mental health policy and service provision, as well as the unique ethical challenges which have arisen with the recent growth of interest in the field. The African and international research literature on violence risk assessment, competency to stand trial, malingering assessment, Not Guilty by Reason of Insanity (NGRI) evaluations, report writing as an expert witness and mental health legislation in the context of forensic practice are explored throughout. Finally, future directions for forensic mental health in Africa are discussed for juvenile, female and elderly offenders.

This text is ideal for mental health, criminal justice and legal professionals working in clinical, research and policy contexts.

Adegboyega Ogunwale, LLM, FWACP, is a chief consultant psychiatrist at the Neuropsychiatric Hospital, Aro, Abeokuta, Nigeria. His research has focused on general adult psychiatry, abnormal homicide, mental health services in prison and mental health legislation. He was awarded the Rafaelsen Young Investigator's Award of the International College of Neuropsychopharmacology in 2011 and the UK Chevening Scholarship in 2017.

Adegboyega Ogunlesi, MBBS, FWACP, FRCPsych, is a retired provost and chief medical director at the Neuropsychiatric Hospital, Aro, Abeokuta, Nigeria. He has published 39 scientific articles and book chapters, and he is a Fellow of the Royal College of Psychiatrists (UK), the National Postgraduate Medical College of Nigeria and the West African College of Physicians.

Stephane M. Shepherd, PhD, is an associate professor of forensic psychology at the Centre for Forensic Behavioural Science, Australia. His research explores cross-cultural issues at the intersection of the criminal justice system and psychology. He has received numerous regional and international awards including a Fulbright Scholarship, the 2019 American Psychology-Law Saleem Shah Early Career Award and the 2016 IAFMHS Christopher Webster Young Scholar of the Year, and was recently named as an Australian ABC 2020 top 5 researcher under 40.

Katrina I. Serpa, MSc, is the training consultant for Multi-Health Systems Inc.'s Public Safety Division and the program director for the Global Institute of Forensic Research, Canada. She specializes in providing cutting-edge curriculum development and training solutions to mental health, correctional and legal professionals working in both general care and forensic settings around the world. She completed her graduate studies in forensic psychology at Maastricht University, Netherlands.

Jay P. Singh, PhD, is a Fulbright scholar, clinical associate in the Department of Psychiatry at the University of Pennsylvania, USA, and visiting scholar in the Institute of Criminology at the University of Cambridge, UK. He completed his graduate doctoral studies in psychiatry at the University of Oxford, UK, and clinical psychology at Universität Konstanz, Germany.

The Handbook of Forensic Mental Health in Africa

Edited by
Adegboyega Ogunwale,
Adegboyega Ogunlesi,
Stephane M. Shepherd,
Katrina I. Serpa,
and Jay P. Singh

Routledge
Taylor & Francis Group
LONDON AND NEW YORK

First published 2021
by Routledge
2 Park Square, Milton Park, Abingdon, Oxon OX14 4RN

and by Routledge
605 Third Avenue, New York, NY 10158

Routledge is an imprint of the Taylor & Francis Group, an informa business

British Library Cataloguing-in-Publication Data
A catalogue record for this book is available from the British Library

Library of Congress Cataloging-in-Publication Data
Names: Ogunwale, Adegboyega, editor.
Title: The handbook of forensic mental health in Africa/edited by Adegboyega Ogunwale [and four others].
Description: Milton Park, Abingdon, Oxon; New York, NY: Routledge, 2021. | Includes bibliographical references and index.
Identifiers: LCCN 2021000436 (print) | LCCN 2021000437 (ebook) | ISBN 9780367456108 (hardback) | ISBN 9780367456078 (paperback) | ISBN 9781003024354 (ebook)
Subjects: LCSH: Forensic psychology--Africa. | Forensic psychiatry--Africa. | Mental health services--Africa.
Classification: LCC RA1148 .H353 2021 (print) | LCC RA1148 (ebook) | DDC 614/.15096--dc23
LC record available at https://lccn.loc.gov/2021000436
LC ebook record available at https://lccn.loc.gov/2021000437

ISBN: 978-0-367-45610-8 (hbk)
ISBN: 978-0-367-45607-8 (pbk)
ISBN: 978-1-003-02435-4 (ebk)

Typeset in Baskerville
by MPS Limited, Dehradun

Contents

Affiliations of Contributing Authors

Name: Nafisa Abdulla
Designation: Chief Occupational Therapist; Forensics
Institution: Valkenberg Psychiatric Hospital, Cape Town, South Africa

Name: Dr. Jibril O. Abdulmalik
Designation: Senior Lecturer, Consultant Psychiatrist & Founder, Asido Foundation
Institution: Department of Psychiatry, College of Medicine, University of Ibadan, Oyo State, Nigeria

Name: Dr. Gbonjubola Abiri
Designation: Consultant Psychiatrist and Medical Director
Institution: Tranquil and Quest Behavioural Health, Igbo-Efon, Lekki, Lagos, Nigeria

Name: Dr. Samuel Adjorlolo
Designation: Senior Lecturer
Institution: Department of Mental Health Nursing School of Nursing and Midwifery, Ghana

Name: Dr. Aishatu Yusha'u Armiya'u
Designation: Consultant Forensic Psychiatrist
Institution: Jos University Teaching Hospital, Nigeria

Name: Dr. Olayinka Atilola
Designation: Senior Lecturer, Department of Behavioural Medicine, Lagos State University, Ojo, Lagos Nigeria & Honorary Consultant in Child and Adolescent Psychiatrist, Lagos State University Teaching Hospital, Ikeja Lagos, Nigeria
Institution: Lagos State University, Ojo, Lagos Nigeria Lagos State University Teaching Hospital, Ikeja Lagos, Nigeria

Name: Dr. Olamiji Abiodun Badru
Designation: Consultant Psychiatrist
Institution: Federal Medical Center, Abeokuta, Department of Mental Health and Behavioral Medicine, Nigeria

Name: Dr. Kofi E. Boakye
Designation: Senior Lecturer, School of Social Sciences, Anglia Ruskin University, Cambridge, UK and Affiliate Fellow, Institute of Criminology, University of Cambridge, UK
Institution: School of Humanities and Social Sciences, Anglia Ruskin University, Cambridge, UK

Name: Dr. Majekodunmi Oluyinka Emmanuel
Designation: Chief Consultant Psychiatrist
Institution: Department of Clinical Services, Neuropychiatric Hospital, Aro, Abeokuta, Ogun State, Nigeria

Name: Madri Engelbrecht
Designation: Occupational Therapist and Director
Institution: Altitude Supported Employment (Pty) Ltd., Wynberg, South Africa

Name: Dr. Michael Elnemais Fawzy
Designation: Consultant Psychiatrist
Institution: Al Abbassia Mental Health Hospital, Cairo, and Technical Advisor at the Technical Office of Egyptian Minister of Health, Egypt

Name: Zerina Hajwani
Desgination: Occupational Therapist and Director
Institution: Altitude Supported Employment (Pty), Ltd., Wynberg, South Africa

Name: Dr. Yusuf Jika
Designation: Professor
Institution: Department of Psychiatry, Ahmadu Bello University Teaching Hospital, Shika-Zaria, Nigeria

Name: Dr. Mary Ozioma Madu
Designation: Specialty Resident in Forensic Psychiatry
Institution: Victorian Institute of Forensic Mental Health, Victoria, Australia

Name: Theoca Moodley
Designation: Occupational Therapist; Forensics
Institution: Valkenberg Psychiatric Hospital, Cape Town, South Africa

Name: Dr. David Ndegwa
Designation: Consultant Forensic Psychiatrist
Institution: South London and Maudsley NHS Foundation Trust, UK

Name: Dr. Fakorede Omokehinde Olubunmi
Designation: Consultant Psychiatrist
Institution: Federal Medical Centre, Idi-Aba, Abeokuta, Ogun State, Nigeria

Name: Dr. Shubulade Smith
Designation: Consultant Psychiatrist; Clinical Senior lecturer
Institution: South London and Maudsley NHS Foundation Trust; Institute of Psychiatry, Psychology and Neuroscience, King's College, London, UK

Name: Dr. Olanrewaju Sodeinde
Designation: Assistant Director, Clinical Psychology
Institution: Neuropsychiatric Hospital, Aro, Abeokuta, Ogun State, Nigeria

Name: Dr. Oladipo Sowunmi
Designation: Consultant Emergency Psychiatrist
Institution: Neuro-Psychiatric Hospital, Aro, Nigeria

Name: Professor Gail Whiteford
Designation: Strategic Professor/Conjoint Chair of Allied Health and Community Wellbeing
Institution: Charles Sturt University & MNCLHD, NSW, Australia

Foreword

Shubulade Smith CBE

Africa is no different to anywhere else in the world; the World Health Organization estimates that one in four people have a mental health problem. Likewise, in Africa, there are people with mental health problems who fall foul of the criminal justice system and others who may behave violently because of their mental health problem. It is estimated that 55% of the prison population has a mental disorder. In many African countries, mental health services are chronically poorly resourced and thus mental health system infrastructure is not robust or is non-existent. The numbers of trained psychiatrists in Africa vary by country from about 1000 in Egypt, 320 in South Africa, 280 in Nigeria, to only 4 psychiatrists in Malawi. Contrast this with the UK where there are nearly 12,000 psychiatrists.

In such circumstances, how can offenders with mental health problems receive the effective and compassionate care they require? Clearly there has to be reliance on non-psychiatrically trained practitioners in many instances. In several other situations, the call of duty would fall on non-forensically qualified psychiatrists. However, we know that without any guidance, even the most conscientious of practitioners will sometimes get it wrong. That's where this book comes in. It provides the practitioner working with people in forensic settings or with people with forensic issues, the tools with which to improve their practice.

Patients, their carers and the services in which they are need to know that the practitioners providing care are competent and knowledgeable and can provide care even in the most straitened of circumstances. This book contains a truly comprehensive and wide-ranging overview and discussion of forensic mental health in Africa. The authors outline the history of forensic mental health in Africa and discuss how best to provide clinical services as well as ethics and ensuring that these are embedded into care delivery. They highlight violence risk assessment issues and cultural sensitivity in forensic mental health care. There are sections on how to recognize a malingerer using an evidence-based approach in addition to those on understanding competence to stand trial and psychiatric defences, providing reliable expert witness testimony in an impartial fashion and writing court reports. Finally, the authors finish with a review of specialist areas with advice for practitioners about how best to manage patients across the age spectrum and what to do with female patients.

This book will increase the confidence of any practitioner in providing more effective and reliable care to people in forensic settings. Not only will this book be invaluable to practitioners working at the interface of the criminal justice system and mental health, but for all those working in mental health in jurisdictions where resources are limited. This includes individuals practicing in many countries beyond the African continent. For those working in high-income countries, this book will be invaluable for improving cross-cultural understanding. Finally, the massive diversity that exists within the African continent is something that African practitioners will be very used to. The authors have provided Western practitioners with essential learning and food for thought about how to work with diverse population groups in a way that will support them to better provide equitable services in their own jurisdictions. This is a first – the first book of forensic mental health based on the African experience, for Africans, by Africans. I feel sure it will not be the last.

Part I

Introduction

1 The history of forensic mental health in Africa

Adegboyega Ogunlesi and Adegboyega Ogunwale

Introduction

Mental health and by extension, forensic mental health, had been confined to the back burner in many Sub-Saharan African countries for various reasons. Njenga (2006) articulated some of these reasons in the *World Psychiatry* medical journal. Not much has changed since then. The problems include widespread preternatural beliefs about mental disorder in deeply cultural African societies, stigma, and low budgeting for health generally (subliminally for mental health). Others include the focus on urban or peri-urban non-decentralized, stand-alone, often-neglected mental health facilities ("orphan units") where the dignity of clients is accorded little respect, as well as absence of modern legislative framework to replace obsolete laws which basically reflected colonial mental health practices in the 18th and 19th centuries respectively. Many African countries were colonized by European powers during those periods (e.g., South Africa by the Dutch and British at various times, Kenya by the British, and Rwanda by Belgium, among others). As such, mental health care approaches in those colonized countries simply mirrored the existent realities within European civilization in those earlier centuries. Equally, the legal framework for mental health services in the colonized countries were modeled after the laws that were in force within the colonial governments themselves. As to be expected, forensic mental health services evolved hand-in-hand with "general" mental health services in most African countries based on this critical interaction between "medical" services related to mental health care and legal aspects of the assessment/treatment as well as custody of the mentally ill. With time, the legal structures or arrangements lagged behind the medical care. Thus, forensic mental health as a structured sub-unit of the overall mental health services suffered a retardation in its evolutionary progress and became shrouded in "mystery and confusion" Njenga (2006) as it became left behind by those fields of psychiatry considered more clinically oriented.

Along this evolutionary trajectory, South Africa provides the most robust history of forensic mental health development in the regional blocks described in this chapter. Gillis (2012) has provided a comprehensive history spanning over five centuries of psychiatry in South Africa since the arrival of the first settlers from Europe in the Cape of Good Hope in 1652. He described three phases viz: the era of restraint, the psychiatric hospital stage, and the modern era when mental health services have become fully developed.

Outpatient clinics as well as legislation providing for community service provision in areas linked with some psychiatric hospitals emerged in the mid-1970s. The first South African academic training leading to the diploma in psychological medicine commenced in 1949. A more comprehensive fellowship program of the Faculty of Psychiatry (later changed to the College of Psychiatry) emerged in 1961. Formal forensic psychiatry practice currently takes place in about seven specially designated hospitals, with about ten psychiatrists having a dedicated commitment to the practice in this field (Ogunlesi, Ogunwale, De Wet, Roos, & Kaliski, 2012). The manpower in this subspecialty should improve in the near future, especially with the emergence of a training program (diploma in forensic psychiatry) by the College of Psychiatrists in South Africa.

In the Eastern Cape, forensic mental health services are provided by the Komani Hospital (Queenstown Mental Hospital) and the Fort England hospital in Grahamstown. Others offering formal forensic facilities in other provinces include Valkenberg Hospital, Lentegeur Hospital and Alexandria Hospital in Cape Town. The Weskoppies Hospital in Pretoria and the Oranje Hospital in Bloemfontein also engage in the delivery of forensic mental health services. Generally speaking, the Eastern Cape is under-resourced with regard to mental health when compared with the Western region (Sukeri et al., 2016).

In the arena of mental health legislation, the first unified legislation was introduced in 1916 (Mental Disorder and Defective Persons Act) and expectedly, emphasized seclusion and restraint in its care approach. Since then, various revisions have occurred to this Act, leading to the most recent Mental Health Care Act 17 of 2002, which replaced the penultimate Mental Health Act of 1973, and is established on the ten basic principles set out by the WHO guiding mental health care law (WHO, 1996). The latest act aligns the country to current global trends, shifting from institutional care to community care, integrating mental health into Primary Health Care and it protects the rights of patients. The history of mental health service development in South Africa would be incomplete without a cursory mention of the influence of the apartheid regime on service provision prior to the dissolution of apartheid in 1994. During this era, service provision for the mentally ill was essentially hospital based and was segregated along racial lines (De Kock & Pillay, 2017), with the inequities in service delivery being predominant in the homelands (Sukeri et al., 2016).

Botswana, an upper middle-income country (World Bank, 2015) with a population of about 2 million people (Statistics Botswana, 2011) has 0.29 psychiatrists and 0.37 psychologists per 100,000 people respectively. It has only one psychiatric hospital in Lobatse with 300 beds, located 80 km from its capital, Gabrone. The Sbrana psychiatric hospital is a stand-alone public hospital with teaching and forensic facilities. There are five psychiatric units in general hospitals across the country (Sidandi et al., 2011; Maphisa, 2019). The Mental Disorders Act of 1969 is the primary legislation focusing on mental health in the country and is self-rated to score four out of five on compliance with human rights covenants. The ongoing efforts at updating the Act are expected to address the perceived shortcomings.

In Kenya, the Mathari Hospital in Nairobi which was previously an isolation center for infectious diseases in the 19th century before it became a lunatic Asylum in 1910 is the largest psychiatric hospital in East Africa. It provides 70% of all the psychiatric beds in Kenya (Ibrahim, 2014). A CNN documentary on Mental Health in Kenya titled "Locked up and forgotten" (Mckenzie, 2011) revealed overcrowding, underfunding, and human rights abuse of patients in this major mental health facility. As a result of this publicized palpable neglect of the mentally ill, a Mental Health Amendment Bill 2018 was passed by the senate in July 2019.

Rwanda, a small country in Central Africa, belongs to the East African block. With a population of about 12 million (2017) (Eytan et al., 2018), it had ten psychiatrists in the entire country as at October 2017 (Eytan et al., 2018), superintending over the two main structures providing specialized care in mental health viz, the Ndera Psychiatric Hospital (foremost psychiatric hospital with a bed capacity of 300 and located in the capital city of Kigali) and the psychological counseling center. A dedicated mental health legislation is not available in the country, but in 2019, a proposal to introduce one was put forward. Legal provisions concerning mental health care are covered in some of the other laws (e.g., general health legislation, disability, welfare, etc.). Eytan et al. (2018) in a study aimed at assessing the practices and needs for improvement in the field of forensic psychiatry in Rwanda, conducted a one-week visit in 2017 and interviewed key stakeholders at decision-making levels in the departments of health, justice and security. Three areas of development and improvement in service delivery were identified:

1. A need for a clearer, updated legislative framework.
2. The need to close the gaps created by the absence of a secured unit, thus leading to a compromise of the quality of care for the forensic patients nursed on general psychiatric wards and the security of the other patients and staff.
3. Gaps in supervision and training in forensic mental health needed to be closed through international collaboration.

With these improvements in place, they envisaged that Rwanda could become in the next few years a leading light to illuminate other African countries in the subspecialty of forensic psychiatry.

Eytan et al. (2018) identified four major developmental stages of the Rwandan psychiatric system. The pre-colonial era (emphasized traditional therapies for mental health care) while the colonial stage saw the inputs of Western psychiatry. During the post-independence stage which commenced in 1962, the foremost psychiatric hospital (Ndera) was constructed. The post-genocide period commenced after the 1994 massacre, and saw a rise in the number of mental health professionals (ten psychiatrists as at October 2017).

For Uganda, the situation is similar, as mental health services are generally skewed to the urban areas proximal to the capital, while the majority of those living in the rural areas have little access to mental health care. Mental health service delivery is grossly underfunded, with only about 1% of the health expenditure channeled to mental health. Per 100,000 population, there were 1.83 beds in mental hospitals, 1.4 beds in community based psychiatric in-patient units and 0.42 beds in forensic facilities. The total personnel working in mental health facilities were 310 (1.13 per 100,000 population). Only 0.8% of the medical doctors and 4% of the nurses had a specialized training in psychiatry (Kigozi et al., 2010).

The Ugandan mental health legislation (The Mental Treatment Act of 1964), which provided no guarantee for the rights of the stigmatized mentally ill, was replaced with the Mental Health Bill 2014, which provides a more humane template for the mentally ill, in terms of rights protection and provision of treatment facilities at Primary Health Care Centers, among others (World Economic Forum, 2019). The history of forensic psychiatry in West Africa may, arguably, be traced to the colonial societies that emerged from the mid-19th century onwards. Prior to 1951, there were no African psychiatrists on the continent (Forster, 1962). The earliest forensic mental health practice could be said to have been stimulated by the Lunacy Asylum Order, Cap 70 of the Gold Coast (modern-day Ghana), which was passed in 1888 (Asare, 2012; Ogunlesi et al., 2012).

By the governor's order, the old High Court in Victoriaborg was converted into the first lunatic asylum in the Gold Coast (Forster, 1962). The order essentially made provisions for the custodial care of mentally ill patients, which was basically imprisonment given the absence of effective treatment for mental disorders at the time. Within 16 years, the number of inmates had surpassed 100 and a few years later, a purpose-built asylum was built on the outskirts of Accra. Patients in this new facility were looked after by a visiting doctor who was also in charge of the prisons. In a primitive but quite ingenuous means of achieving some form of forensic psychiatric rehabilitation, the "criminal lunatics" were saddled with the responsibility of preparing the meals of other patients under the nurses' supervision (Forster, 1962). Currently, there are three mental health hospitals in the country with a total of 1322 beds. There are 79 dedicated forensic beds across the three hospitals and in 2011, there were 148 forensic admissions to the country's mental health hospitals (World Health Organization, 2011).

In terms of mental health legislation, Ghana succeeded in updating its 1972 mental health law (Mental Health Decree NRCD 30) into the Mental Health Act (2012) and set the pace for mental health law reform for many West African countries. Nonetheless, a number of interesting commentaries have highlighted the post-adoption implementation challenges of the new legislation (Doku, Wusu-Takyi, & Awakame, 2012; Walker, 2015; Walker & Osei, 2017).

In Nigeria, the history of forensic psychiatric services dates back to the establishment of asylums in Calabar and Yaba by 1907 (Ladapo et al., 2008; Ogunlesi et al., 2012; Ogunlesi & Ogunwale, 2018). The Lantoro "lunatic asylum" was established in 1944 under the Laws of Nigeria (1948b). In addition to these three asylums in the south of the country, some native authorities in the north were equally empowered by law to set up asylums as well (Laws of Nigeria, 1948b). Some designated prison cells in selected prisons all over the country were also deemed asylums (Ogunlesi & Ogunwale, 2018).

The Lantoro asylum was specifically established to receive mentally ill soldiers returning from the Second World War. However, its remit began to cover mentally ill offenders who were found "Not Guilty By Reason of Insanity" (NGBRI) (Laws of the Federation of Nigeria, 2004) over time. To provide a contextualized history, it is important to note that since the earliest versions of criminal legislation in the country, legal insanity had been determined on the basis of the insanity plea, the success of which could result in the NGBRI verdict. The insanity plea is an adaptation of M'Naghten's rules achieved by adding a volitional prong ("capacity to control voluntary action") as well as a broader definition of mental disorder (Laws of Nigeria, 1948a; Rex v Omoni, 1949; Yeo, 2008).

The Lantoro asylum continued to function as an administrative prison/psychiatric asylum in the 1960s and 1970s when Tola Asuni (later professor of psychiatry) supervised its rudimentary forensic services and also conducted research embracing criminology and mental health (Asuni, 1962, 1969; Oyebode, 2011). He extended mental health services to the federal prison in Abeokuta at the time as well. By 1972, only three psychiatrists were handling all court referrals for psychiatric evaluation at the Aro Hospital for nervous diseases (now Federal Neuropsychiatric Hospital, Aro, Abeokuta) established as an offshoot of the Lantoro Asylum in 1954 (Asuni, 1969; Bienen, 1974). Sometime in the late 1970s, Freda Schoenberg, an expatriate consultant psychiatrist took over the service from Asuni and she ran it until 1983 when she was succeeded by one of the authors (Adegboyega Ogunlesi), a UK-trained Nigerian psychiatrist. He was in charge of the unit until 2009. Since that period, leadership of the service has been provided by two consultant psychiatrists with subspecialty interest in forensic psychiatry. Along with developments at the Neuropsychiatric Hospital Aro, several other forensic psychiatric services began to evolve in other parts of the country. Similar to the service at Aro, these services in stand-alone specialist hospitals and university departments of psychiatry as well as some state psychiatric hospitals were developed by general psychiatrists with special interest in law and psychiatry. Service evaluation data suggest that there are 22 forensic in-patient beds in the country with close to 70% of forensic patients spending more than 10 years in hospitals (World Health Organization, 2006c).

With regard to mental health legislation, the country has a law that is over a century old (Laws of Nigeria, 1948b) although one of the states within the federation (Lagos) succeeded in passing a new law in January 2019 (Lagos State Mental Health Law, 2018). Nevertheless, there is currently a national mental health bill before the Nigerian senate which has already passed through a second reading and public hearing. Hopes are high among mental health professionals that this new bill will be eventually enacted.

In North Africa, the history of forensic psychiatry is hardly separable from that of forensic medicine in general that is deeply rooted in Egyptian civilization

(Kharoshah, Zaki, Galeb, Moulana, & Elsebaay, 2011; Wecht, 2005). The first psychiatric unit was established in Kalaoon Hospital in Cairo in the 14th century and Egypt was the first North African country to have mental health legislation in 1944 (El Hamaoui, Moussaoui, & Okasha, 2009; Okasha, 2004). As of 1983, the Khankah Hospital was the only psychiatric facility in Egypt that had a special ward for mentally abnormal offenders (Soothill et al., 1983). Currently, mentally ill offenders are assessed and treated at the Abassia Hospital in Cairo or the El-Khankah Hospital in Kalyobia. By 2006, there was a total of 725 forensic in-patient beds in Egypt (World Health Organization, 2006a).

In Morocco, the early days of forensic psychiatry showed that only the Berrechid Hospital and the Tit Mellil housed mentally ill offenders. Both facilities were built in 1920, with the Berrechid Hospital being the first to commence operations as a general psychiatric unit (World Health Organization, 2006b). The current situation is slightly different, with all psychiatric facilities in the country providing beds for mentally ill offenders who unfortunately remain incarcerated within them for prolonged periods (El Hamaoui et al., 2009). Regional psychiatric hospitals with smaller bed capacities have been established in Marrakech, Oujda, Fès, Tangiers, Tétouan and Meknès (World Health Organization, 2006b). In both Tunisia and Algeria, only one hospital each received mentally disordered offenders for several decades until a regionalization of services took place (El Hamaoui et al., 2009).

Regarding mental health legislation, Egypt appears to have the most recent law enacted in 2009 with a clear focus on access to mental health services and protection of the human rights of patients. In Morocco, mental health law is still largely represented by the *Dahir* enacted in 1959. Obviously old, there have been interesting arguments to the effect that it still aims at the prevention of mental illnesses and the protection of patients' rights in the context of care (El Hamaoui et al., 2009). Algerian legislations were enacted in 1985 and 2004, respectively.

Conclusion

This historical review demonstrates that the practice of forensic mental health within Africa dates back to the late 19th century. Since then, forensic mental health services have evolved, although most are still largely rudimentary with daunting challenges. Very few centers are actively engaged in forensic mental health practice and a limited number of specialists characterize such. Equally, there exists a dearth or total absence of specialists serving in correctional facilities. This is largely fueled by the absence of structured training programs for forensic mental health. Practitioners in the subspecialty need to actively engage with a view to addressing the problems which should improve access to care for mentally ill offenders. The need to update mental health legislation, develop appropriate, culturally relevant risk assessment protocols where necessary and recruit additional multidisciplinary personnel into forensic mental health practices is clearly urgent.

References

Asare, J. B. (2012). Comment: A historical survey of psychiatric practice in Ghana. *Ghana Medical Journal, 46*(3), 114–115.

Asuni, T. (1962). Suicide in Western Nigeria. *British Medical Journal, 2*(5312), 1091–1097. https://doi.org/10.1136/bmj.2.5312.1091

Asuni, T. (1969). Homicide in Western Nigeria. *British Journal of Psychiatry, 115*(527), 1105–1113. https://doi.org/10.1192/bjp.115.527.1105

Bienen, L. (1974). Criminal homicide in Western Nigeria 1966-1972. *Journal of African Law, 18*(1), 57–78. doi:10.1017/S0021855300012699.

De Kock, J., & Pillay, B. (2017). A situation analysis of psychiatrists in South Africa's rural primary health care settings. *African Journal of Primary Health Care & Family Medicine, 9*(1), a1335. https://doi.org/10.4102/phcfm.9:1.1335

Doku, V. C. K., Wusu-Takyi, A., & Awakame, J. (2012). Implementing the Mental Health Act in Ghana: Any challenges ahead? *Ghana Medical Journal, 46*(4), 241–250.

El Hamaoui, Y., Moussaoui, D., & Okasha, T. (2009). Forensic psychiatry in North Africa. *Current Opinion in Psychiatry, 22*, 507–510.

Eytan, A., Ngirababyeyi, A., Nkubili, C., & Mahoro, P. N. (2018). Forensic psychiatry in Rwanda. *Global Health Action, 11*(1), 1509933.

Forster, E. B. (1962). A historical survey of psychiatric practice in Ghana. *Ghana Medical Journal*, (September), 25–29.

Gillis, S. (2012). The historical development of psychiatry in South Africa since 1652. *South African Journal of Psychiatry, 18*(3), 78–82. 10.4102/sajpsychiatry.v18i3.355.

Ibrahim, M. (2014). Mental health in Kenya: not yet Uhuru. *Disability and the Global South, 1*(2), 393–400.

Kharoshah, M. A. A., Zaki, M. K., Galeb, S. S., Moulana, A. A. R., & Elsebaay, E. A. (2011). Origin and development of forensic medicine in Egypt. *Journal of Forensic and Legal Medicine, 18*(1), 10–13. https://doi.org/10.1016/j.jflm.2010.11.009

Kigozi, F., Ssebunnya, J., Kizza, D., Cooper, S., & Ndyanabangi, S. (2010). An overview of Uganda's mental health care system: results from an assessment using the world health organization's assessment instrument for mental health systems (WHO-AIMS). *International Journal of Mental Health Systems, 4*, 1–9.

Ladapo, H., Aina, O., Lawal, R., Adebiyi, O., Olomu, S., & Aina, R. (2008). Long stay patients in a psychiatric hospital in Lagos, Nigeria. *African Journal of Psychiatry, 11*, 128–132.

Lagos State Mental Health Law (2018). Ikeja: Lagos State Government.

Laws of the Federation of Nigeria (2004). *Criminal Procedure Act CAP.* Federal Ministry of Justice, C41.

Laws of Nigeria. (1948a). *Criminal code act, CAP. 77. Vol. II.* Lagos: Government Printer.

Laws of Nigeria. (1948b). *Lunacy Ordinance, Vol. IV, CAP. 121.* Lagos: Government Printer.

McKenzie, D. (2011). Kenya's mentally ill locked up and forgotten (online). *CNN World Untold Stories.* http://www.cnn.com/2011/world/africa/02/25/kenya.forgotten

Njenga, F. (2006). Forensic psychiatry: The African experience. *World Psychiatry, 5*(2), 97.

Ogunlesi, A., & Ogunwale, A. (2018). Correctional psychiatry in Nigeria: Dynamics of mental healthcare in the most restrictive alternative. *British Journal of Psychiatry International, 15*(2), 35–38. https://doi.org/10.1192/bji.2017.13

Ogunlesi, A., Ogunwale, A., De Wet, P., Roos, L., & Kaliski, S. (2012). Forensic psychiatry in Africa: Prospects and challenges. *African Journal of Psychiatry, 15*, 3–7. https://doi.org/10.4314/ajpsy.v15i1.1

Okasha, A. (2004). Focus on psychiatry in Egypt. *British Journal of Psychiatry, 185*(3), 266–272. https://doi.org/10.1192/bjp.185.3.266

Oyebode, F. (2011). Tolani Asuni: Formerly professor of Psychiatry, University of Ibadan, Nigeria. *The Psychiatrist, 35*(12), 478. https://doi.org/doi:10.1192/pb.bp.111.037440

Rex v Omoni. (1949). *12 W.A.C.A 511-513.*

Sidandi, P, Opondo, P, & Tidimane, S. (2011). Mental health in Botswana. *British Journal of Psychiatry International, 8*(3), 66–68. 10.1192/S1749367600002605.

Soothill, K. L., Adserballe, H., Bernheim, J., Dasananjali, T., Harding, T. W., Thomaz, T., Reinhold, F., & Ghali, H. (1983). Psychiatric reports requested by the courts in six countries. *Medicine, Science and the Law, 23*(4), 231–241. https://doi.org/10.1177/002580248302300402

Statistics Botswana (2011). Population and Housing Census. https://www.statsbots.org.bw/sites/default/files/publications/population%20and%20Housing%20census%202011pdf

Sukeri, K., Betancourt, O., Emsley, R, Nagdee, M, & Erlacher, H. (2016). Forensic mental health services: Current service provision and planning for a prison mental health service in the Eastern Cape. *South African Journal of Psychiatry, 22*(1), a787.

Walker, G. H. (2015). Ghana mental health Act 846 2012: A qualitative study of the challenges and priorities for implementation. *Ghana Medical Journal, 49*(4), 266–274.

Walker, G. H., & Osei, A. (2017). Mental health law in Ghana. *BJPsych International, 14*(2), 38–39.

Wecht, C. H. (2005). The history of legal medicine. *The Journal of the American Academy of Psychiatry and the Law, 33*(2), 7.

World Bank (2015). Botswana-systematic country diagnostic. http://documents.worldbank.org/curated/en/489431468029502 82/Botswana-systematic-country-diagnostic

World Economic Forum (2019). World economic forum on Africa. www.weforum.org>agenda>2019/08>>uganda-mental-health-stigma

World Health Organisation (1996). Mental health care law: Ten basic principles. Geneva: World Health Organization, Division of Mental Health and Prevention of Substance Abuse. https://www.who.int/mental_health/media/en/75.pdf

World Health Organization. (2006a). *WHO-AIMS report on mental health system in Egypt*, Cairo, Egypt: WHO and Ministry of Health.

World Health Organization. (2006b). *WHO-AIMS report on mental health system in Morocco*, Rabat, Morocco: WHO and Ministry of Health. https://www.who.int/mental_health/evidence/morocco_who_aims_report.pdf?ua=1

World Health Organization. (2006c). *WHO-AIMS report on mental health system in Nigeria*, Nigeria: WHO and Ministry of Health. https://www.who.int/mental_health/evidence/nigeria_who_aims_report.pdf?ua=1

World Health Organization. (2011). *WHO-AIMS report on mental health system in Ghana*, Republic of Ghana: WHO and Ministry of Health. https://www.who.int/mental_health/who_aims_country_reports/ghana_who_aims_report.pdf?ua=1

Yeo, S. (2008). The insanity defence in the criminal laws of the commonwealth of nations. *Singapore Journal of Legal Studies*, 241–263.

2 Cross-cultural sensitivity in forensic mental health care

Adegboyega Ogunwale, David Ndegwa, and Stephane Shepherd

Introduction

Culture refers to a set of behavioral norms, practices and beliefs shared by a group of individuals within a defined population. It differs slightly from "ethnicity" which implies a shared origin, language, history and other cultural factors (Hicks, 2004). A consideration of an individual's cultural background is important in a clinical context. Culture can shape behavior (what is expected, typical deviant, taboo), how we communicate (convey pain and stress, regulate emotions), what health models we subscribe to (individualized explanations vs holistic models) and help-seeking behaviors (first point of call, how we interact with professionals, family involvement and stigma). Cultural dynamics can also impact how we interact cross-culturally as well as how we interpret and manage behaviors. The role of spirituality as being central to the human experience in non-Western cultures has also been advanced (Fernando, Ndegwa, & Wilson, 1998). As such, learning about the practices and idiosyncrasies of different cultural groups gives professionals an improved ability to engage with multi-cultural clientele.

The impact of culture on forensic mental health practice is understudied. This is even more so in societies such as those found in Africa and many other developing parts of the world. The lack of advancement in this aspect of practice could be due to the fledgling nature of the forensic mental health field itself in Africa. As noted in other chapters of this volume, forensic mental health systems are nascent, if at all existing, in large parts of the continent and so formalized cross-cultural best practice has yet to materialize. These considerations will require some attention given the cultural heterogeneity of African societies. For example, Nigeria has more than 250 ethnic nationalities (Lasebikan, 2016). In other countries like South Africa, they are both multi-ethnic and multi-racial which can lead to cross-cultural tension. Indeed, structural changes in South Africa over the last 30 years have led to fluctuations in power dynamics and inequalities in health care (Coovadia, Jewkes, Barron, Sanders, & McIntyre, 2009; Das-Munshi et al., 2016) which may play out in multi-racial forensic consultations. Furthermore, with migration of Africans within Africa, there is an emerging form of "national" rather than "ethnic" minority status within various African countries with the attendant deprivations of minority status that hold significant implications for involvement in the criminal justice system as well as for access to and availability of mental health services within that environment (Hartwell, 2001).

A further issue is the predominance of Western-style approaches to forensic mental health within the continent and how these methods generalize to African populations. A growing body of literature asserts that clinical approaches (i.e., risk assessment instruments, diagnostic tools and clinical interaction styles) have been developed on Western populations and worldviews and may not be applicable to diverse sub-groups, minoritized populations and non-Western cultures (Shepherd & Lewis-Fernandez, 2016).

Hicks (2004) identified eight critical issues that could constitute a "cultural framework" within forensic mental health care in Africa, namely: diagnosis, dangerousness assessment, involuntary commitment, competency, criminal matters, children-related issues, tort cases and the expert witness role. Within this context, aspects of cultural sensitivity such as cultural competence (scientific mindedness, dynamic sizing, specific cultural expertise), cultural validity of clinical/forensic assessments, "idioms" of distress, culture-bound syndromes in relation to offending behavior as well as rituals of communication will be explored. This chapter will focus on aspects of cultural sensitivity in forensic mental health, with some consideration of Hicks' framework. Figure 2.1 presents a schematic diagram illustrating this expanded framework.

What is cultural competence?

A basic definition of cultural competence is the possession of the cultural knowledge and skills of a particular culture aimed at delivering effective interventions to members of that culture (Sue, 1998). It is regarded as comprising three basic skills: (i) scientific mindedness, (ii) dynamic sizing and (iii) culture-specific expertise (Hicks, 2004; Sue, 1998). Scientific mindedness refers to the clinician's capacity to formulate hypotheses rather than draw hasty or premature conclusions about the status of individuals from varied cultural backgrounds. It also involves developing creative ways of testing these "hypotheses" and basing action on acquired data. Scientific mindedness helps the clinician to avoid the "myth of sameness." By forming hypotheses around cultural meanings attached to psychopathology, more valid clinical inferences may be drawn.

Dynamic sizing is related to the ability of the clinician to recognize "when to generalize and be inclusive" as well as "when to individualize and be exclusive" (Sue, 1998). Without dynamic sizing, stereotypes emerge (explicitly as well as implicitly) to color the clinician's view of the individual patient such that the individual's attitudes are attributed to the group's characteristics. Culture-specific expertise on the part of the practitioner involves having good knowledge and understanding of one's worldview as well as having specific knowledge about the cultural groups with whom one is working. It also centers on the clinician's proficiency in the use of culturally based interventions in addition to the ability to develop and use culturally appropriate strategies. While these three domains are quite

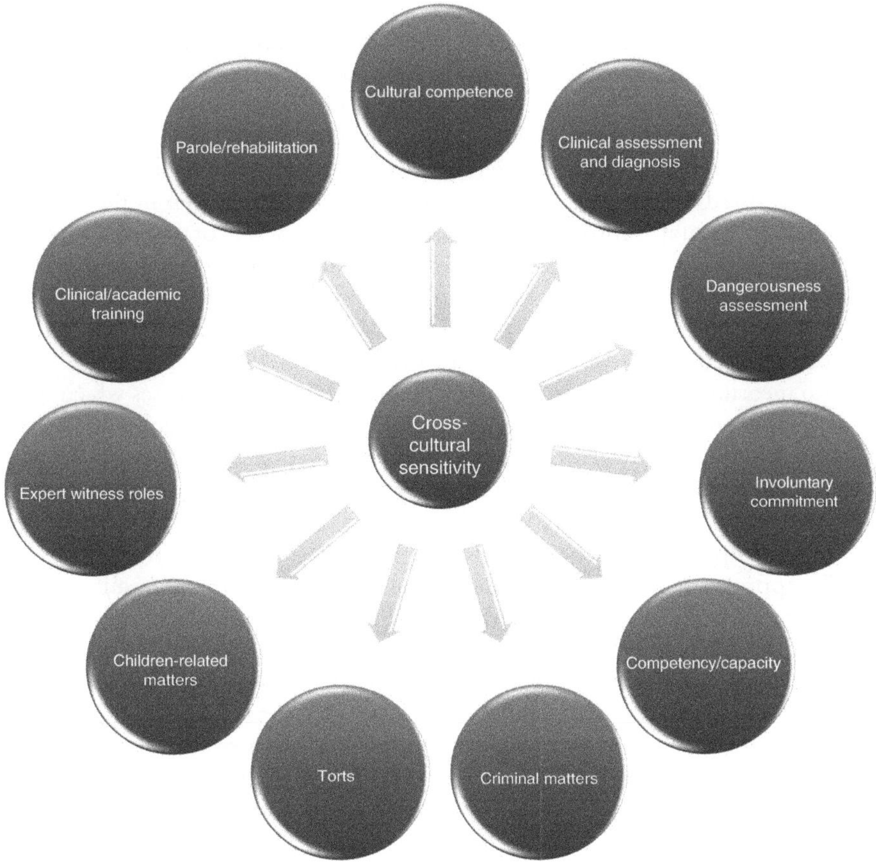

Figure 2.1 A framework for understanding cross-cultural sensitivity in forensic mental health.

important in achieving cultural competence, it has been argued that clinicians vary in the extent to which they possess each skill. Cultural competence is crucial to the successful navigation of different culture-laden aspects of forensic assessment and intervention as we shall see in the succeeding aspects of this chapter.

Clinical assessment and diagnosis

Forensic opinions are founded upon valid and thorough clinical assessments. These opinions are based on assessment and diagnosis and can affect the offense a person is charged with or whether the person would be charged at all. For instance, the presence of mental disorder at arrest may trigger a diversion approach or determine how the trial is conducted and what disposal is available post-conviction.

Cultural biases in clinical assessments

Yet, these assessments may be open to cross-cultural biases. Within this context, four types of biases affecting cross-cultural diagnosis have been identified: cross-cultural construct bias, cross-cultural item bias, cross-cultural method bias and cross-cultural clinical judgment bias (Mikton & Grounds, 2007). Cross-cultural construct bias refers to cultural differences in the construct of behavior/conduct being measured or assessed. A good example of such bias is seen in the African construct of mental disorder as being of a spiritual origin or supernatural intervention, which is in contrast to Western biomedical conceptualizations of health (Fabrega, 1991; Gureje, Lasebikan, Ephraim-Oluwanuga, Olley, & Kola, 2005; Iheanacho et al., 2016; Lasebikan, 2016; Sheikh, Adekeye, Olisah, & Mohammed, 2015). Cross-cultural item bias refers to the specific items being used to measure the construct while the method bias relates to biases which may arise in the process of administering tests or measures. Cross-cultural clinical judgment bias results from cultural values affecting clinical judgment in certain cases. Indeed, it has been argued that psychiatric diagnoses are interpretations of interpretations (Kleinman, 1996). In this sense, it is contended that the patient's report of symptoms is an interpretation of subjective experience framed in culturally appropriate words, feelings and images that capture the reality of the symptoms. It is this subjective interpretation that the clinician attempts to convert into an objective interpretation that may equally be loaded with the clinician's cultural tendencies. An illustration of this could be seen in the distinction between an offender's over-valued ideas and delusions based on culturally framed content. Whereas a psychiatrist with a Western orientation might be quick to determine that an acute awareness of the preternatural influence of witches on a patient is a delusion of persecution, the African psychiatrist who is more culturally informed could regard it as an overvalued idea. An overvalued idea has been more recently referred to as "extreme overvalued belief" and may be defined as: "*… one that is shared by others in a person's cultural, religious, or subcultural group. The belief is often relished, amplified, and defended by the possessor of the belief and should be differentiated from an obsession or a delusion … The individual has an intense emotional commitment to the belief and may carry out violent behaviour in its service*" (Rahman, Meloy, & Bauer, 2019, p. 2; Rahman et al., 2020).[1]

It is fitting to note that cross-cultural biases may not only feature overt, conscious forms, which could suggest intentional discrimination or institutional racism, but may manifest as implicit bias that represents stereotypes capable of affecting our understanding, actions and decisions unconsciously (Kerner et al., 2020).

Culture and prevalence of mental disorders

Given the role of cultural factors in diagnosis, research from Western populations suggest that there could be racial disparities in the prevalence rate of mental disorders. African Americans, Latino/Hispanic Americans and BAME populations are found to be diagnosed with psychotic disorders at higher rates than White Americans/Europeans (Cohen & Marino, 2013; Halvorsrud, Nazroo, Otis, Hadjukova, & Bhui, 2019; Schwartz & Blankenship, 2014). Disparities in psychotic disorder diagnoses have been attributed to clinical misdiagnosis and social/environmental explanations (Halvorsrud et al., 2019; Schwartz & Blankenship, 2014). Psychopathy appear to generalize cross-culturally (Latzman et al., 2015; Sullivan, Abramowitz, Lopez, & Kosson, 2006) and levels of this disorder have been found to be similar for both black and white Americans (Skeem, Edens, Camp, & Colwell, 2004). Similarly, African American adolescents are more likely than whites to be diagnosed with conduct and psychotic disorders (Schwartz & Blankenship, 2014). A recent study in South Africa found that there were higher risks of common mental disorders and Posttraumatic Stress Disorder (PTSD) among blacks and adolescents of color compared with whites (Das-Munshi et al., 2016).

Etic and Emic approaches to clinical assessments

Practitioners can take two positions in the clinical assessment of mental disorders. One can identify the presence of a mental disorder by using what is currently in the international classification of diseases – version 10 (World Health Organization, 1992) without citing cultural limitations. This culture-blind approach is likely to be the stance taken by Western-trained practitioners working in African countries or similar developing nations when they conduct mental health assessments for forensic purposes. This has been referred to as an "etic perspective" (Fabrega, 1991) defined as the observing scientist's conceptualization of mental disorder.

The second position is attempting to examine the validity of diagnoses within a cultural perspective. In this position, issues of cross-cultural validity should be based on extensive ethnographic study of what the emic concepts of psychopathology are. The emic perspective refers to local cultural criteria for determining whether a behavioral manifestation constitutes mental disorder or not (Fabrega, 1991). This task of appreciating the emic view point while espousing a seemingly "global" etic diagnostic standard would be necessary to avoid concepts of illness or disorder developed in other cultures being applied uncritically to a particular African group under consideration.

Culture-bound syndromes in forensic context

These cultural considerations are most profoundly represented in what has been termed "idioms of distress" (i.e., cultural manifestation or presentation of mental symptoms which may or may not be necessarily pathological) (Jacob, 2019; Keys, Kaiser, Kohrt, Khoury, & Brewster, 2012; Kidron & Kirmayer, 2019; Nichter, 2010). The key implication of these "idioms" is the extent of their difference from what may be regarded as the "axioms" of illness (i.e., "universally" accepted criteria for the diagnosis of mental disorders). A similar concept, "culture bound syndromes" refers to a pattern of symptoms recognized as a disorder within a cultural group. For example, the culture-bound syndrome "Amok" has been cited as a likely underpinning for mass murders in Malaysian experience (Hempel, Levine, Reid Meloy, & Westermeyer, 2000; Pal, 1997), while "dhat" has been regarded as a psychopathological explanation for rape in some cultures (Sarkar, 2013). The syndrome of "spirit possession" has been implicated in crimes in settings such as Nigeria, South Africa and Zimbabwe. Here, two culture-bound syndromes – "amafufunyana" and "ukuthwasa" serve as explanations for abnormal behavior according to Xhosa traditional healers. The Ndebele people of Zimbabwe attribute such behavior to possession by ancestral spirits ("amadhlozi") or witchcraft ("mthakati") (Menezes, Oyebode, & Haque, 2009). These experiences may involve irresistible impulses or made affect/volition imposed upon the sufferer by external forces against which they may demonstrate no control resulting in violent conduct including homicide.

Cultural formulation in clinical assessments

The DSM-5 Cultural Formulation interview (Lewis-Fernandez et al., 2014) and other resources (Aggarwal, 2012; Barber-Rioja & Rosenfeld, 2018) comprise a list of questions that enable clinicians probe such cultural rationalizations for behaviors. Some of these supplementary questions may assist clinicians in identifying cultural perceptions of illness (i.e., How would you describe your issue to your community? What does your family/community think is causing your problem?). Kleinman and Benson (2006) propose a cultural formulation different from that in DSM-5. In theirs, the first step is to ask about ethnic identity. The second step is to identify what is at stake in the assessment and consequent decisions. The third is to elicit the illness narrative and the fourth is describing the relevant psychosocial stressors. The fifth is defining influence of culture on clinical relationships and the sixth involves examining the problems of a cultural competency approach.

Other cultural factors relevant to clinical assessments

Another pertinent question is whether meaning could be lost in translation. It is important that where translators are involved in the clinical interview, clinicians should be familiar with current best practice in the use of translators. In an African context, other factors such as the age, gender, neutrality, dialectical variations and language expertise of the translator as well as their relationship to the patient are important in the selection of the translator. To ensure that that the interview material is available for back translation or interpretation and for review by other investigators, it may be useful to have a form of contemporaneous recording.

Furthermore, when the indigenous meanings and perspectives of psychopathology are available, the clinician might want to compare them with their own or Etic concepts from their training or practice. This latter consideration is vital for court reports in which the mental health professional has to answer legal questions based on medical opinion typically framed from an Etic perspective.

Social desirability is likewise important in deeply cultural societies as found in Africa in which communitarian ethos and paternalism are prominent ideologies. The defendant may not want to present themselves in a negative light to the interviewer, who is typically a psychiatrist frequently regarded as an "authority" figure in their social sphere and whose opinion might not be called to serious question in a patently paternalistic cultural framework. Thus, it is possible that in forensic settings, social desirability bias on the part of the defendant may lead to the systematic under-reporting of mental health–related symptoms as well as previous or current offending behaviors (Fisher, 1993). This may perhaps lead to inconsistencies in the forensic formulation of the current offense as well as inaccuracies in the estimation of risks of future offending. In other instances, the revelation of personal information may be associated with social shame that may impede communication during the interview process (Perlin & McClain, 2009) and result in imprecisions in the forensic formulation.

In a similar vein, the impact of stigma in relation to mental disorders may give rise to minimization of psychiatric symptoms or presentation of symptoms among offenders in African societies. It may be preferable to be seen as someone who offended "by mistake" than to be tagged as being of unsound mind. A genetic attribution to the mental disorder may further worsen the stigma (Matshabane, 2019) because future generations may be regarded as tainted as well. In another dimension, there have been arguments that symptom minimization may follow a mind-body dualism perspective in which Africans and Asians have been observed to under-report psychological symptoms of depression while emphasizing the somatic complaints that accompany it ("psychologizers" vs "somatizers") although this distinction is not always tenable along cultural lines (Kirmayer & Young, 1998).

Another salient forensic as well as clinical assessment consideration is malingering, the presence or absence of which may impact the legal outcome of a defendant. Attempts at structured assessments of malingering have centered largely on Western samples and insufficient information exists with regard to non-Western populations, including Africans. Where malingering assessment scales developed in one culture are applied without validation to a defendant from another culture, it may lead to inaccurate measurements and potentially, a miscarriage of justice. Thus, less culture-biased, non-verbal assessment scales for such measurements have been suggested (Weiss & Rosenfeld, 2010). However, such scales are not entirely culture-neutral, as they could have been constructed based on images relevant to one culture while being irrelevant or differently perceived in another.

At the level of treatment, where there is a close relationship or similarity between the Emic and Etic viewpoints, there is likely to be good therapeutic alliance, compliance with agreed treatments and better engagement with services. On this basis, it would be helpful for African practitioners to interrogate offender-patients' perception of the role of religion and spirituality in treatment and rehabilitation given that research has demonstrated that there is a cultural preference for spiritual and religious explanations for the etiology of mental disorders among Africans. Sensitivity to such cultural tendencies will further bridge the gap between the Emic and Etic perspectives, thereby strengthening treatment engagement and, perhaps, improving outcomes.

In clinical research where research tools developed in cultures other than that under study are being considered, it is important to ensure that the various types of equivalence – linguistic, conceptual, scale and norm – are known. Although these assessments of equivalence can be complex and time-consuming, they are essential to ensure validity and reliability particularly in epidemiological studies of mental disorders. They are also important in ensuring the validity of expert opinion within the context of the legal process.

Culture and antisocial personality

Antisocial personality disorder warrants attention as it is defined in culturally relative terms in both the ICD 10 and DSM-IV. There are also intra-cultural issues of diagnostic bias as well (Mikton & Grounds, 2007). It had been observed in the UK that Caucasians were 2.6 times more likely to receive a diagnosis of antisocial personality disorder and 2.8 times more likely to be diagnosed with any personality disorder compared with Afro-Caribbean patients (Mikton & Grounds, 2007). The systematic under-diagnosis of personality disorder among Afro-Caribbeans is thought to result from cross-cultural diagnostic bias and has significant implication in terms of entry into forensic secure services or the criminal justice system. This racial disparity may play out in a similar way within multi-racial African societies (e.g., South Africa), although data appears to be lacking at the moment. Within single-race multi-ethnic settings, it is likely that its manifestation could be along an "ethnic majority versus ethnic minority" line or social class based and may be so subtle as not to be noticeable as such.

Engaging with cultural issues in practice

In providing a common-sense guide to navigating the interaction dynamics between culture and clinical assessment as well as diagnosis, Duncan (1990) had described an eight-stage process of engagement as shown in Box 1. Similarly, Weiss and Rosenfeld (2012) have provided a number of helpful suggestions on how a forensic practitioner ought to engage with cross-cultural issues. They stress the need for the examiner to consider their own level of cultural competence before accepting an assessment referral and the importance of gauging the degree of acculturation of an evaluee when from another culture. They highlight the importance of considering the validity and reliability of scales developed in one culture when they are to be used with an evaluee from another culture. Where interpreters are used, they must be objective, well trained and able to provide the verbatim translation of the evaluee's responses and for translations. They advise that they should be in advance rather than ad-hoc.

Box 1

1. Problem definition.
2. Clear focus on identified problem and circumstances.
3. Data collection.
4. Determination of the context of the problem being examined.
5. Diagnostic statement that avoids cultural stereotypes or bias.
6. Familiarity (on the part of the evaluator and the evaluee) with the process and the underlying assumptions.
7. Value placed by the society on the process of assessment as well as contact with mental health services and the law.
8. Impact of communication and language.

Dangerousness assessment

"Dangerousness" is a socio-legal construct (Adshead, 2003; Eastman, Adshead, Fox, Latham, & Whyte, 2012; Szasz, 2003). Research suggests that clinicians tend to over-predict inpatient violence by non-Caucasian patients and under-predicting it among Caucasians, although there is no proof that inpatient violence rates differ by ethnic status (Hicks, 2004). In an older study that evaluated "race thinking" as opposed to "ideological racism" among British psychiatrists, it was demonstrated that black Caribbean patients were rated as being more violent than whites and more suitable for criminal justice system intervention (Lewis, Croft-Jeffreys, & David, 1990). Young black males and Hispanics of all ages – essentially ethnic minorities – were found to receive harsher punishments for crimes committed in a US study (Steffensmeier, Painter-Davis, & Ulmer, 2017). Conversely, Kerner et al. (2020) found no racial differences in dangerousness levels (proxied by admission rates) between patients identifying as black compared with Caucasians. Similarly, racial disparities in the rates of involuntary admission in the UK have been observed to be better explained by higher rates of mental illness, heightened risk and poorer social support rather than ethnicity (Gajwani, Parsons, Birchwood, & Singh, 2016). Thus, it appears more balanced to consider dangerousness as being more implicitly connected with deeper psychosocial factors that may be associated in some way with minority ethnic status rather than to draw a direct link between ethnicity and dangerousness.

To a large extent, the political culture might have predetermined what the dangerousness associated with a particular conduct is and this determination does not appear static. It may be influenced by economics, personalities of politicians, spirituality, religion and political ideologies. These political or cultural positions may be so powerful in the operation of a criminal justice system that they reduce the usefulness of psychiatric knowledge in the social construction of dangerousness.

Research has demonstrated that lack of insight is significant in dangerousness assessment and could be culturally influenced. A study found that African-American men with severe mental illness were less likely to perceive themselves as being mentally ill compared with white American males, white females or African-American females. Additionally, African-American men and women were less likely to offer a biomedical illness perspective while being more likely to provide religious or spiritual interpretations compared with white men and women (Millet, Sullivan, Schwebel, & Myers, 1996) similar to what had been reported in other non-western cultures (Nathan, Wylie, & Marsella, 2001). Perhaps arising from lack of insight, it has also been articulated that persons from ethnic minority groups may be less willing to accept mental health diagnoses from clinicians who belong to majority groups as they may misconstrue such diagnoses as professional validation of social labeling resulting from persistent marginalization (Hicks, 2004).

It is also critical to examine the role of cultural factors in the estimation of violence risk. Shepherd (2016) has highlighted some of these to include, among others, perceived racism, cultural engagement, intergenerational trauma (e.g., apartheid in South Africa and ethnic hegemony in many others), religion and spirituality, communal support/family support, stigmatization and cultural identity. While it has been argued that there appears to be a uniformity of violence risk factors across cultures (Andrews & Bonta, 2010; Grieger & Hosser, 2014; Gutierrez, Wilson, Rugge, & Bonta, 2013; van Horn, Eisenberg, Souverein, & Kraanen, 2018), it is nevertheless crucial to validate Western-derived risk assessment instruments in African populations in order to establish the predictive accuracy of such risk assessment tools prior to constructing medico-legal opinions upon them. It is also important to regularly consider the effect of cultural issues on clinical interaction dynamics when risk formulations are being constructed especially when structured professional judgment approaches to risk assessment are adopted (Shepherd, 2014).

Similarly, the assessment of dangerousness using tools which are developed in other cultures alien to traditional African societies in which they are used requires not only an understanding of concepts of equivalence as mentioned earlier but also an awareness of information-processing biases that are found in decision-making tasks (Fernando, Ndegwa, & Wilson, 1998). It is important that assessors avoid bringing in pre-conceived notions of the client based on their supposed ethno-culture and instead allow the client to identify the extent to which they are engaged with a culture group and hold particular belief systems associated with that group. Every client possesses a personal culture which will include intersectional aspects of their life beyond their ethno-culture (i.e., vocational, neighborhood, religious, sexual, political, culture). As such, a clinician should consider all relevant aspects of a patient's life and conduct the assessment in a genial, open-minded and non-judgmental fashion without fixating on their ethno-culture unless salient. Another cogent observation is that the strengths (or protective factors) which are identified as relevant in risk reduction in one culture may not be perceived as strengths in a different culture where perhaps that type of activity does not exist or is modified, or has little bearing on desistance. Additionally, institutional or community surveillance as well as treatment or after-care services vary by country and might be absent in poorly resourced countries. As such, the relevance of each of the items on a risk assessment tool (especially those on Structured Professional Judgment tools) could be ascertained through regional community peer review (Shepherd & Willis-Esqueda, 2017).

The assessment of dangerousness should also include the risk of harm to self. Cultural differences exist with regard to suicide and attempted suicide (Hjelmeland et al., 2008). Suicide rates vary by country with low and middle-income countries being responsible for about 79% of all suicides globally (World Health Organization, 2019). While many countries have decriminalized attempted suicide, it remains a crime in many African jurisdictions (e.g., section 327, Criminal Code Act, Laws of the Federation of Nigeria, 2004a) and is heavily stigmatized (Hjelmeland et al., 2008). Thus, contemporary acts suggestive of suicide attempts may attract criminal justice responses rather than mental health service interventions in such settings. Awareness of such possibilities may impair honest disclosures, thereby affecting the accuracy of the risk assessment process and amplifying the likelihood of completed suicide.

Involuntary commitment

Involuntary commitment is largely driven by considerations of public safety as well as the well-being of those with mental illnesses (Deshpande, Kaur, Zaky, & Loza, 2013; Moosa & Jeenah, 2008). Thus, it cannot be far removed from societal contemplations on dangerousness or violence whether directed at self or others (Alem, Jacobsson, Lynöe, Kohn, & Kullgren, 2002; Szabo, Kohn, Gordon, & Hart, 2000). The use and duration of involuntary hospitalization are not only determined by clinical factors but cultural perspectives on the dangerousness of the mentally ill as well (Binder, 1999). Data on involuntary hospitalization/treatment is not readily available in Africa and reviews suggest that its institutional framework is still developing in many parts of the continent (Igbinowanhia & Akanni, 2019; Moosa & Jeenah, 2008). Existing literature from South Africa indicates a rate of 12.8/100,000 population, which is similar to France (11/100,000) and below the UK rate (48/100,000) (Moosa & Jeenah, 2010). In a recent South African study, certain socio-cultural factors were implicated in recurrent involuntary hospitalization, including being male, black, young, unemployed and belonging to a low-income area (Marufu, 2019).

Furthermore, family involvement in instigating involuntary hospitalization has been observed in southern and eastern Africa, although this may not necessarily be determinative of the final clinical decision to hospitalize involuntarily (Alem et al., 2002; Szabo et al., 2000). Linguistic diversity has also been implicated in a non-African analysis as being associated with compulsory treatment albeit in a community context (Kisely & Xiao, 2018). If this reasoning is extended to multi-ethnic multilingual African societies, it is also possible that language barriers may also play a part in driving involuntary hospitalization decisions in some cases.

In societies that are not fully democratic, as may be found in some African countries (e.g., those under military rule or dictatorships), involuntary hospitalization powers may be exercised by state authorities with little or no protection from abuse of such powers offered to the mentally ill.

Competency/capacity

Cultural constructs of mental disorders determine the societal view of competency/capacity. Where mental illness is regarded as a "global," "all-or-none" affectation of the mind, capacity is presumptively regarded as entirely lacking in the mentally ill. Be that as it may, three fundamental approaches to competency/capacity have been identified in the literature (Law Commission, 1995). These are the status, outcome and functional approaches. The basic principle of the status approach is that a patient with a mental disorder is *ipso facto* deprived of "all contractual capacity," thereby obviating the need for an objective assessment of task-specific competence. This is obviously not supportive of autonomy and fails to recognize the task-specific as well as time-bound nature of capacity.

The outcome approach focuses on the content of the final decision of the individual (decisional outcome) and according to the Law Commission, "it penalises individuality and demands conformity at the expense of personal autonomy." In two English cases, *Re C and Re T*, the court took the view that the content of a decision even if irrational, unknown or non-existent was not determinative of incapacity. Thus, common law does not toe the line of the outcome approach.

The functional approach assesses whether an individual at a given time when a specific decision is to be made is able to understand its nature and effects. In practice, it recognizes both partial and fluctuating capacity, thereby ensuring that persons who should otherwise be competent are not misclassified as being incompetent. In its favor, it endorses individual autonomy and departs from an "all or none" construct of capacity, which is not pragmatic. It also supports the use of fairly defined standards for testing specific cognitive domains related to decision making.

In light of the above, it would seem that the status and outcome approaches are anti-autonomy and negatively paternalistic in orientation. Nevertheless, it had been observed that an outcome approach could be preferable for physicians who might portray a tendency to find patients agreeing with their recommendations as being competent and those dissenting as lacking capacity (Law Commission, 1995). On the other hand, perhaps the most prominent argument in favor of the outcome approach in particular is the fact that the doctor better "understands" or "appreciates" the treatment information provided. Thus, it may be more self-serving (even if not entirely autonomy-enabling) to agree with the "better" position. It may equally be advanced that an outcome approach (in scenarios where treatment refusal may lead to death) would permit considerations for the sanctity of life to prevail over autonomy which is the default mode of the medical profession (World Medical Association, 1948). This approach makes clinical practice more ethically balanced and easily justifiable from the physician's perspective in such ethical quandaries.

While it seems that the Western position seems to have shifted toward the recognition of individualistic autonomy even over the sanctity of life, on the contrary, communitarian ethics and paternalism seem to predominate in African settings and the sanctity of human life is virtually sacrosanct. These ethos are underpinned by religious beliefs, power dynamics and implicit trust in communal existence. Autonomy is likely to be framed in a group-focused manner rather than an individualistic libertarian form. Within this context, it would seem most culturally appropriate for other family members to make decisions for the mentally ill member while following a laid-down hierarchy of decision makers. The role of family members in instigating involuntary treatment for mental disorder has been highlighted in Africa (Szabo et al., 2000). Additionally, the power dynamics in a patently paternalistic culture would drive the physician who is regarded as "knowing best" to easily disregard the wishes of a patient/offender who is arriving at what appears to be irrational treatment decisions. These seemingly irrational decisions may arise from factors such as linguistic diversity in multi-ethnic societies (Kisely & Xiao, 2018) as well as fear of stigma related to mental illness and its treatment, which is prominent among Africans (Iheanacho et al., 2016; Stefan, 1996).

Other forensic issues relevant to capacity such as fitness to plead may equally be affected by language barriers and lack of education (Hicks, 2004). The use of advance directives may be less culturally appropriate in African settings where faith in God and the afterlife may preclude the need to take the future into one's own hands. Additionally, the cultural need for family involvement in decision making may obviate the need for the individual to take decisions about his/her future (Dupree, 2000).

Criminal matters

Culture and offending behavior

It is important to mention that apart from clinical diagnosis, an ethnographic approach would also be useful in understanding the indigenous concepts of offending which includes explanatory models, causation, seriousness and best ways of addressing offending or conflict. In eliciting offense narratives, it would be important to also look at narratives like identity, masculinity and discrimination (on the basis of race, ethnicity, class, religion, political ideology, economic class, gender, disability, etc.). These are areas that are important in the assessment of risk and in formulating treatment interventions. These offense narratives in the clinical/assessment context may clash with national policy and views of crime. The differences between the two need to be identified. As an illustration, a person from some nomadic tribes might not regard taking someone else's cattle as stealing but simply a way of returning animals to their original owners. Another example is deliberate self-harm/attempted suicide within the context of major depressive illness occurring in a country in which attempted suicide is a crime.

Furthermore, culturally determined expectations may influence the behavior of the person who is accused of an offense and what they might say in an interview. In addition, culture and politics are important in the definition of what constitutes an offense as well as how the offenses are investigated, prosecuted and punished. The explanations for these definitions can be very selective and can depend on the convenience of public sentiments and ideologies at a given time. Forensic practitioners need to always be aware of the effect of their opinions on the lives of the persons who come in contact with the law.

Cultural defenses

The question of "cultural defenses" also arises. The assumption here is that human beings will think and conduct themselves in line with cultural patterns in which they developed. Renteln has argued that influence of cultural tendencies should be an integral part of what is termed "individualized justice" and should not be seen differently from taking other factors such as gender, age, childhood adversity and mental state into legal considerations (Renteln, 2005). Time-honored legal traditions such as right to fair trial, freedom of religion and equality under the law are in support of cultural defenses. Additionally, international law provides for the protection of the right to culture (United Nations, 1966; article 27) and by extension, the right to inject such considerations into one's defense in a litigation. One of such defenses in traditional African societies is the framing of the insanity defense in terms of specific delusions relating to "voodoo," witchcraft, juju and other forms of negative spiritual influences (Aremu, 1980; Dumin, 2006; Nzimande, 2016; Rentein, 2005). The existing case law in this respect within Nigerian jurisdictions (Ani v State, 2002; Arum v State, 1980; Konkomba v Queen, 1952) suggests that such defenses based on culturally framed delusions have never been successful (Ogunwale, Ogunlesi, & Majekodunmi, 2011). This perhaps implies that in spite of the cultural validity of such legal excuses, they are not taken lightly in law nor are they afforded an unduly low admissibility threshold which might be quickly prone to abuse. Moreover, it has been argued that the judicial interpretation of the specific delusions that come under the highlighted cultural defenses appears to be quite restrictive in some jurisdictions compared with the broader interpretations given to the insanity plea more generally (Ogunwale & Oluwaranti, 2020). In ensuring appropriate use and preventing abuse of the cultural defense, a three-pronged test has been advanced to assess its veracity as follows: (i) Is the litigant a member of the ethnic group? (ii) Does the group have such a tradition? (iii) Was the litigant influenced by the tradition when he/she acted? (Renteln, 2005).

Children-related issues

Cultural factors are important in the assessment of children within the family context. The key issues in child assessment include child abuse, child custody and the termination of parental rights especially in the context of divorce and adoption. Cultural practices may affect parenting capacity, particularly when such practices are viewed from a different cultural perspective. For example, the dominant contemporary Western view of child rearing condemns corporal punishment even when it is not explicitly criminalized. Virtually all African countries have ratified the UN Convention on the Rights of the Child and subscribe to its moral underpinnings of respect for the dignity of the child (African Charter on the Rights and Welfare of the Child, 1990; Gose, 2002). However, evidence abounds that many African jurisdictions still consider corporal punishment as a legitimate approach to child discipline, although there are those who have adopted the Western approach (Denis & Frances, 2014). In the Nigerian Criminal Code Act, for instance, "a blow or other force, not in any case extending to a wound or grievous harm" may be justified for the purpose of correcting a child (below 16 years) as long as the child is capable of understanding the purpose for which the punishment is inflicted (Laws of the Federation of Nigeria, 2004a; section 295). In Ghana, section 41 of the Criminal Offences Act (1960) as well as article 13(2) of the Children's Act (1998) have been reported to allow "justifiable" and "reasonable" corporal punishment of children (Law and Development Associates, 2018). Given the caveats raised in such laws, drawing the line between legitimate punishment and abuse is crucial and can only be justly achieved by a culturally competent expert witness on the basis of cultural relativity. Moreover, under the African Charter on the Rights and Welfare of the Child (1990; article 31), children have an obligation to respect their parents, superiors and elders within the context of strengthening African traditions. Although this has been regarded as imposing a duty to unquestioning obedience on children which may be abused, it is in reality based on moral suasion rather than legal enforceability (Gose, 2002). While overall the global shift is toward the non-use of corporal punishment in the discipline of children, this paradigm change must take into account long-held religious and cultural ideals which underpin the use of corporal punishment in the first place.

Child custody and parental rights appear interwoven in communal settings that typify African civilization. The communitarian and paternalistic ethos of African societies demand that these issues be considered on a pluralistic basis rather than the paramountcy of the "welfare" or "best interests" of the child. In Nigerian customary law (as opposed to Federal statute – the Matrimonial Causes Act, Laws of the Federation of Nigeria (2004c)), for example, a father has exclusive custodial right over the children in a marriage and this right seems to extend to "ownership" of the children (Onokah, 2007). This legal perspective appears to have been informed by the patrilineal nature of some African societies and the dependence of paternity on the gift of the marriage symbol by the husband to the wife. It may also be informed by the cultural aversion to single-parent status. Consequently, the urgent need of the divorced woman would be to remarry and procreate within a new marriage rather than to busy herself with raising children "owned" by her ex-husband. That said, the attitude of Nigerian higher courts has been to uphold the "welfare" principle while paying close attention to cultural tendencies. In this way, adjudication has followed the pattern of granting the custody of older children to their fathers while the younger children (ostensibly in need of maternal care and succor) are typically left in the care of their mothers until they attain the age of three or four years, at which point they revert to the custody of their fathers who has the duty to economically maintain them (Onokah, 2007). Against this backdrop, forensic mental health experts who practice in African settings must be culturally informed while holding themselves up to the standard of considering the welfare of the child as paramount in child custody situations. Additionally, while they may be quite objective in their opinions on the mental health of parents involved in divorce proceedings and its implications for parenting capacity, their understanding of the legitimate interests of all parties in custody cases would aid them in their pursuit of fairness as well as humanizing the parties involved.

Tort cases

Forensic mental health experts may be involved in malpractice suits in which they could be invited to comment on standards of care in cases of negligent diagnosis, treatment or follow-up (Hicks, 2004), although this is not frequently observed yet in many African jurisdictions. Additionally, in employee compensation cases that recognize psychological injury, forensic psychiatrists may offer relevant expert testimony before the appropriate judicial body.

The expert witness role

The expert witness is defined by jurisdiction thus presupposing that socio-legal cultural factors arise in our understanding of such a role. From a socio-economic perspective, most countries in Africa suffer from significant mental health human resource constraints (Ogunlesi et al., 2012; United Nations, 2014; World Health Organization, 2018). There are few psychiatrists or psychologists who may serve as expert witnesses in the forensic mental health sense. Consequently, whenever they are able to provide expert services, they are likely to do so within a limited scope of cases – mainly in criminal cases involving murder or serious violence. The legal culture may also give priority to such cases because psychiatric testimony is likely to be more frequently requested in such situations compared with civil cases. Additionally, the aforementioned shortage in human resources may make a battle between experts a rarity in most African jurisdictions and this has been observed to be the pattern in many countries within the continent. Touari, Mesbah, Dellatolas and Bensmail (1993) suggest that even in situations where two experts are nominated by the courts for the purpose of psychiatric evaluation in criminal cases, they are expected to issue a joint report.

Furthermore, in the strong multi-ethnic and sometimes, multi-racial tensions that are found in African societies, the issue of truth telling constitutes not only an ethical burden but a rational and pragmatic consideration as well. Where the ends of justice are not served in systems fraught with ethnic stereotypes and prejudices, telling the truth in a bland and seemingly objective manner invariably leads the expert witness into participating in injustice. Griffith describes this attitude as the "dominant mode 'perspectivelessness,'" which refers to "a pretence by dominant group members to be objective and neutral while they embody an analytical stance that buttresses the specific cultural and political characteristics of the dominant group" (Griffith, 2003, p. 430). On the part of the expert witness in some patently unjust systems in which dominant cultural groups are seen to be prejudiced against the non-dominant class, Griffith (2003) contemplates a variant of truth-telling that is beneficent to the non-dominant offender while not sacrificing the legitimate interests of justice in a decent society. He calls this "good reasons to circumscribe the whole-truth-telling of forensic psychiatrists," thereby suggesting that in some cases, "partial truth" produced as a result of a permissible level of "excluded truth" may better serve the cause of justice. This perhaps modifies the dominant western view of "the whole truth and nothing but the truth." Certainly, this aim for beneficence does not excuse the African forensic mental health expert from the responsibility of honesty and striving for objectivity that represent the hallmark of impartiality (Niveau, Godet, & Völlm, 2019). Aiming for impartiality serves the interest of justice since it is expected to more readily achieve "fairness" in the trial process (Niveau & Welle, 2018; Niveau et al., 2019). The sound counsel of Hicks is instructive in this regard: "*Expert witnesses must be vigilant in monitoring their own potential biases. The ethnicity of the forensic psychiatrist, the ethnicity of the subject, and the interaction between dominant and non-dominant ethnic groups in the justice system may all affect an examiner's neutrality in complicated ways.*" (Hicks, 2004, p. 29).

Clinical and academic training

Given the colonial orientation of many countries in Africa, it is observed that most forensic mental health practitioners in East, West and southern Africa would be trained in essentially Western-based approaches – notably English and French orientations. The overwhelming impact of Islam in North Africa suggests that practitioners in those regions are more likely to be trained along a mixture of Islamic and European traditions with some French influences in countries like Algeria, Tunisia and Morocco while British customs would be expected to underpin Egyptian education. Be that as it may, it is important for Western-trained mental health professionals to adapt their training to the local cultures (currently existing as independent nations) within which they practice while still ensuring "global best practice." This cultural adaptation is more likely to be achievable if such professionals had been instructed in cross-cultural issues while in training. The clinician's ability to interpret psychopathological experiences within the context of religious and cultural norms is essential to establishing accurate diagnosis as well as providing reliable expert opinion on the accused's mental state at the time of an offense (Layde, 2004).

For clinicians working in foreign environments, an understanding of local norms is generally necessary depending on the extent to which the new environment differs from the individual's home culture. Preliminary information should be restricted to specific local customs, which if transgressed, could put the clinician or their patient in harm's way, or preclude the clinician from capably or safely administering care. Minor cultural differences will be negotiated as a clinician acclimates to their new surroundings. Moreover, communities and health care professionals indigenous to such communities need to be prepared for the foreign clinician who will be working in their jurisdiction as this can alleviate some initial resistance or discomfort from local patients and might allow the clinician to be vouched for and accepted to make the transition easier.

Parole decisions and rehabilitation

There have been major shifts in populations and levels of poverty in African settings with migration from rural poverty to urban scarcity in many cases. There is also the obvious absence of welfare provision of the kind that sustains forensic psychiatric after-care services in developed western countries. This understanding of the structure of rural and urban societies which are constantly changing is important in designing after-care and rehabilitation services.

In Nigeria as an African exemplar, a mentally ill individual who is found Not Guilty By Reason of Insanity (NGBRI) when granted amnesty/pardon under the governor's prerogative of mercy, is discharged to family members who must then undertake to guarantee that s/he would not harm others (Criminal Procedure Act, sections 230, 233 and 235, Laws of the Federation of Nigeria, 2004b). This reliance on family members perhaps taps into the African ideology of the extended family system which is regarded as a veritable support system when coping with mental disorders (Lasebikan, 2016). Contemporary experience, unfortunately, shows that this is gradually breaking down (Olaore & Drolet, 2017; Tanyi, André, & Mbah, 2018). Furthermore, it places an unreasonable amount of socio-legal responsibility on everyday citizens to regulate the conduct of adult individuals over whom they possess no legally enforceable restraining authority. A more realistic approach going forward would be a cultural shift towards the individualistic paradigm in which the paroled offender will have to be independently supported by the welfare structures of the state rather than by family members. In this regard, sections 37 and 40 of the Nigerian Correctional Service Act (2019) tersely address the role of government in ensuring the administration of a sustainable parole process.

Furthermore, what constitutes rehabilitation in prison settings and other custodial institutional settings appears to be different in Africa from the perception in Western settings. In an African setting, for example, good behavior, remorse, change in spiritual or religious beliefs or practice, acquisition of a skill or participation in further education might be given a lot of weight in terms of measuring the success of rehabilitative efforts. Those prisoners who fail in these areas for certain reasons (e.g., having a personality disorder or a mental disorder or disability) are likely to be seriously disadvantaged in terms of ease of achieving parole status. Clinicians in developing countries should be drawing attention to the plight of such vulnerable prisoners and ensure that they are processed through the criminal justice system equitably while paying attention to their unique mental health needs.

Offending or violence reduction programs are not well developed in African settings as in Europe and North America. These developments have been heavily influenced by cognitive sciences and social learning theory. In particular, the Risk-Need-Responsivity (RNR) model of offender rehabilitation (Bonta & Andrews, 2010) appears to be well-researched in Western cultures and could offer tangible benefits if culturally adapted to African settings. Principle 9 of the RNR model envisages a matching of treatment services with the bio-demographics of the individual offender including gender, ethnicity and age. Moreover, basic psycho-sociological research interrogating issues such as cognitions or distortions in thinking that support offending needs to take place using an ethnographic approach in order to better understand how these interventions may be deployed in a culturally appropriate manner.

Conclusions

Cultural sensitivity in African forensic mental health settings is crucial for effective service delivery given the multi-racial and multi-ethnic orientations in many countries within the continent. Central to its application is the concept of cultural competence which comprises scientific mindedness, dynamic sizing and cultural expertise. All of these are fundamental to valid forensic assessments, whether within the expert opinion-context or mental health service planning in secure forensic or criminal justice settings. The need for cultural sensitivity in psycho-legal issues such as mental capacity, dangerousness and involuntary hospitalization cannot be overemphasized. Additionally, the potent role of cultural factors in criminal matters and child-related issues must always command the attention of the culturally competent expert witness. This chapter provided several frameworks and specific recommendations for working effectively cross-culturally. Understanding some of the unique practices and idiosyncrasies of different cultural groups across the African continent, as described in this chapter, will allow for an improved ability to (i) effectively engage in cross-cultural clinical encounters, (ii) partake in self-reflexive clinical practices and (iii) provide meaningful culturally relevant services.

Note

1 While this definition contrasts with the recent DSM-5 definition (American Psychiatric Association, 2013) that notes that the belief is not shared by others in the individual's culture, it is more consistent with the original meaning proposed by Carl Wernicke (Rahman et al., 2019).

References

Adshead, G. (2003). Commentary on Szasz. *Journal of Medical Ethics, 29*(4), 230–232. https://doi.org/10.1136/jme.29.4.227.

African Charter on the Rights and Welfare of the Child (1990). https://www.unicef.org/esaro/African_Charter_articles_in_full.pdf.

Aggarwal, N. K. (2012). The psychiatric cultural formulation: applying medical anthropology in clinical practice. *Journal of Psychiatric Practice, 18*(2), 7310.1097/01.pra.0000413273.01682.05.

Alem, A., Jacobsson, L., Lynöe, N., Kohn, R., & Kullgren, G. (2002). Attitudes and practices among Ethiopian health care professionals in psychiatry regarding compulsory treatment. *International Journal of Law and Psychiatry, 25*(6), 599–610. https://doi.org/10.1016/S0160-2527(01)00112-1.

American Psychiatric Association (2013). *Diagnostic and statistical manual of mental disorders* (Fifth). Arlington, VA: American Psychiatric Association.

Andrews, D. A., & Bonta, J. (2010). *The psychology of criminal conduct* (5th ed.). New Providence, NJ: Matthew Bender & Company, Inc.

Ani v State. (2002). *10 N.S.C.Q.R 461.*

Aremu, L. (1980). Criminal responsibility for homicide in Nigeria and supernatural beliefs. *International and Comparative Law Quarterly, 29*(1), 112–131.

Arum v State. (1980). *1 N.C.R. 84.*

Barber Rioja, V., & Rosenfeld, B. (2018). Addressing linguistic and cultural differences in the forensic interview. *International Journal of Forensic Mental Health, 17*(4), 377–386.

Binder, R. L. (1999). Are the mentally ill dangerous? *Journal of American Academy of Psychiatry and the Law, 27*(2), 189–201.

Bonta, J., & Andrews, D. (2010). Viewing offender assessment and rehabilitation through the lens of the risk-need-responsivity model. In F. McNeill, P. Raynor, & C. Trotter (Eds.), *Offender supervision: New directions in theory, research and practice* (pp. 19–40). Abingdon: Routledge.

Coovadia, H., Jewkes, R., Barron, P., Sanders, D., & McIntyre, D. (2009). The health and health system of South Africa: Historical roots of current public health challenges. *The Lancet, 374*(9692), 817–834. https://doi.org/10.1016/S0140-6736(09)60951-X.

Das-Munshi, J., Lund, C., Mathews, C., Clark, C., Rothon, C., & Stansfeld, S. (2016). Mental health inequalities in adolescents growing up in post-apartheid South Africa: Cross-sectional Survey, SHaW study. *PLoS ONE, 11*(5), e0154478. https://doi.org/DOI:10.1371/journal.pone.0154478.

Denis, S., & Frances, N. (2014). Alternatives to instilling discipline in primary schools during the post-corporal punishment era in Uganda. *Journal of Human-Social Science, 14*(4), 21–26.

Deshpande, S. N., Kaur, J., Zaky, M., & Loza, N. (2013). Mental health legislation in Egypt and India: Ethical and practical aspects. *International Journal of Mental Health, 42*(1), 91–105. https://doi.org/10.2753/IMH0020-7411420106.

Dumin, J. (2006). Superstition-based injustice in Africa and the United States: The use of provocation as a defence for killing witches and homosexuals. *Wisconsin Women's Law Journal, 21*, 145.

Duncan, B. J. (1990). Cultural issues in forensic psychiatry. *Medicine and Law, 9*, 1220–1225.

Dupree, C. Y. (2000). The attitudes of black Americans toward advance directives. *Journal of Transcultural Nursing, 11*(1), 12–18. https://doi.org/10.1177/104365960001100104.

Eastman, N., Adshead, G., Fox, S., Latham, R., & Whyte, S. (2012). *Oxford specialist handbooks in psychiatry: Forensic psychiatry* (1st ed.). New York: Oxford University Press Inc.

Fabrega, H. (1991). Psychiatric stigma in non-Western societies. *Comprehensive Psychiatry, 32*(6), 534–551. https://doi.org/10.1016/0010-440X(91)90033-9.

Fernando, S., Ndegwa, D., & Wilson, M. (1998). *Forensic psychiatry, race and culture.* London: Routledge.

Fisher, R. J. (1993). Social desirability bias and the validity of indirect questioning. *Journal of Consumer Research, 20*(2), 303–315.

Gajwani, R., Parsons, H., Birchwood, M., & Singh, S. P. (2016). Ethnicity and detention: Are Black and minority ethnic (BME) groups disproportionately detained under the Mental Health Act 2007? *Social Psychiatry and Psychiatric Epidemiology, 51*(5), 703–711. https://doi.org/10.1007/s00127-016-1181-z.

Gose, M. (2002). *The African charter on the rights and welfare of the child.* Community Law Centre. https://web.archive.org/web/20110927035902/http://www.communitylawcentre.org.za/clc-projects/childrens-rights/other-publications/african_charter.pdf.

Grieger, L., & Hosser, D. (2014). Which risk factors are really predictive?: An analysis of Andrews and Bonta's "Central Eight" risk factors for recidivism in German youth correctional facility inmates. *Criminal Justice and Behavior, 41*(5), 613–634. https://doi.org/10.1177/0093854813511432.

Griffith, E. E. H. (2003). Truth in forensic psychiatry: A cultural response to gutheil and colleagues. *The Journal of the American Academy of Psychiatry and the Law, 31*(4), 4.

Gureje, O., Lasebikan, V. O., Ephraim-Oluwanuga, O., Olley, B. O., & Kola, L. (2005). Community study of knowledge of and attitude to mental illness in Nigeria. *The British Journal of Psychiatry, 186*(5), 436–441. https://doi.org/10.1192/bjp.186.5.436.

Gutierrez, L., Wilson, H. A., Rugge, T., & Bonta, J. (2013). The prediction of recidivism with aboriginal offenders: A theoretically informed meta-analysis. *Canadian Journal of Criminology and Criminal Justice, 55*(1), 55–99. https://doi.org/10.3138/cjccj.2011.E.51.

Halvorsrud, K., Nazroo, J., Otis, M., Hajdukova, E. B., & Bhui, K. (2019). Ethnic inequalities in the incidence of diagnosis of severe mental illness in England: a systematic review and new meta-analyses for non-affective and affective psychoses. *Social Psychiatry and Psychiatric Epidemiology, 54*(11), 1311–1323.

Hartwell, S. (2001). An examination of racial differences among mentally ill offenders in Massachusetts. *Psychiatric Services, 52*(2), 234–236. https://doi.org/10.1176/appi.ps.52.2.234.

Hempel, A. G., Levine, R. E., Reid Meloy, J., & Westermeyer, J. (2000). A cross-cultural review of sudden mass assault by a single individual in the oriental and occidental cultures. *Journal of Forensic Sciences, 45*(3), 582–588. https://doi.org/10.1520/JFS14732J.

Hicks, J. W. (2004). Ethnicity, race, and forensic psychiatry: Are we color-blind? *The Journal of the American Academy of Psychiatry and the Law, 32*(1), 13.

Hjelmeland, H., Akotia, C. S., Owens, V., Knizek, B. L., Nordvik, H., Schroeder, R., & Kinyanda, E. (2008). Self-reported suicidal behavior and attitudes toward suicide and suicide prevention among psychology students in Ghana, Uganda, and Norway. *Crisis, 29*(1), 20–31. https://doi.org/10.1027/0227-5910.29.1.20.

Igbinowanhia, N. G., & Akanni, O. (2019). Constraints, ethical dilemmas and precautions in psychiatric practice within non-contemporaneous mental health laws: A Nigerian experience with involuntary commitment. *Journal of Law, Policy and Globalization, 87*, 21–25. https://doi.org/10.7176/JLPG/87-03.

Iheanacho, T., Kapadia, D., Ezeanolue, C. O., Osuji, A. A., Ogidi, A. G., Ike, A., Patel, D., Stefanovics, E., Rosenheck, R., Obiefune, M., & Ezeanolue, E. E. (2016). Attitudes and beliefs about mental illness among church-based lay health workers: Experience from a prevention of mother-to-child HIV transmission trial in Nigeria. *International Journal of Culture and Mental Health*, *9*(1), 1–13. https://doi.org/10.1080/17542863.2015.1074260.

Jacob, K. S. (2019). Idioms of distress, mental symptoms, syndromes, disorders and transdiagnostic approaches. *Asian Journal of Psychiatry*, *46*, 7–8. https://doi.org/10.1016/j.ajp.2019.09.018.

Kerner, J., McCoy, B., Gilbo, N., Colavita, M., Kim, M., Zaval, L., & Rotter, M. (2020). Racial disparity in the clinical risk assessment. *Community Mental Health Journal*, *56*(4), 586–591. https://doi.org/10.1007/s10597-019-00516-3.

Keys, H. M., Kaiser, B. N., Kohrt, B. A., Khoury, N. M., & Brewster, A.-R. T. (2012). Idioms of distress, ethnopsychology, and the clinical encounter in Haiti's Central Plateau. *Social Science & Medicine*, *75*(3), 555–564. https://doi.org/10.1016/j.socscimed.2012.03.040.

Kidron, C. A., & Kirmayer, L. J. (2019). Global mental health and idioms of distress: The paradox of culture-sensitive pathologization of distress in Cambodia. *Culture, Medicine, and Psychiatry*, *43*(2), 211–235. https://doi.org/10.1007/s11013-018-9612-9.

Kirmayer, L. J., & Young, A. (1998). Culture and somatization: Clinical, epidemiological, and ethnographic perspectives. *Psychosomatic Medicine*, *60*(4), 420–430. https://doi.org/10.1097/00006842-199807000-00006.

Kisely, S., & Xiao, J. (2018). Cultural and linguistic diversity increases the likelihood of compulsory community treatment. *Schizophrenia Research*, *197*, 104–108. https://doi.org/10.1016/j.schres.2017.12.005.

Kleinman, A. (1996). How is culture important for DSM-IV? In J. E. Mezzich, A. Kleinman, H. Fabrega, & D.L. Parron (Eds.), *Culture and psychiatric diagnosis* (pp. 15–25). Washington DC: American Psychiatric Press Inc.

Kleinman, A., & Benson, P. (2006). Anthropology in the clinic: the problem of cultural competency and how to fix it. *PLoS Med*, *3*(10), e294.

Konkomba v Queen. (1952). *14 W.A.C.A 236.*

Lasebikan, V. O. (2016). Cultural aspects of mental health and mental health service delivery with a focus on Nigeria within a global community. *Mental Health, Religion & Culture*, *19*(4), 323–338. https://doi.org/10.1080/13674676.2016.1180672.

Latzman, R. D., Megreya, A. M., Hecht, L. K., Miller, J. D., Winiarski, D. A., & Lilienfeld, S. O. (2015). Self-reported psychopathy in the Middle East: a cross-national comparison across Egypt, Saudi Arabia, and the United States. *BMC Psychology*, *3*(1), 1–13.

Law and Development Associates. (2018). *Corporal punishment in Ghana: A position paper on the legal and policy issues.* Ghana: Department of Children, Ministry of Gender, Children and Social Protection and UNICEF. https://www.unicef.org/ghana/media/1956/file/Corporal%20Punishment%20in%20Ghana.pdf.

Law Commission (1995). *Mental Incapacity (Law Com No 231).*

Laws of the Federation of Nigeria (2004a). Criminal code act, CAP C38. Federal Ministry of Justice.

Laws of the Federation of Nigeria (2004b). Criminal procedure act CAP C41. Federal Ministry of Justice.

Laws of the Federation of Nigeria (2004c). Matrimonial Causes Act, CAP M7. Federal Ministry of Justice.

Layde, J. B. (2004). Cross-cultural issues in forensic psychiatry training. *Academic Psychiatry*, *28*, 34–39.

Lewis, G., Croft-Jeffreys, C., & David, A. (1990). Are British psychiatrists racist? *The British Journal of Psychiatry*, *157*(3), 410–415. https://doi.org/10.1192/bjp.157.3.410.

Lewis-Fernandez, R., Aggarwal, N. K., Baarnhielm, S., Rohlof, H., Kirmayer, L. J., Weiss, M. G., & Lu, F. (2014). Culture and psychiatric evaluation: operationalizing cultural formulation for DSM-5. *Psychiatry: Interpersonal and Biological Processes*, *77*(2), 130–154.

Marufu, G. (2019). *Characteristics of patients with recurrent involuntary admissions for 72 hour assessment at Kimberley hospital complex, Northern Cape province, Republic of South Africa* (Dissertation presented in fulfilment of the requirements for the degree of Master of Medicine in the Department of Family Medicine, School of Clinical Medicine, Faculty of Health Sciences). Free State.

Matshabane, O. P. (2019). *Exploring how a Genetic Attribution to disease relates to Internalised Stigma experiences of Xhosa people with Schizophrenia and Rheumatic Heart Disease in South Africa* (Dissertation presented in fulfilment of the requirements for the degree of Doctor of Philosophy in the Faculty of Health Science (Medicine), University of Cape Town). https://open.uct.ac.za/bitstream/handle/11427/31179/thesis_hsf_2019_matshabane_olivia_precious.pdf?sequence=4.

Menezes, S. B., Oyebode, F., & Haque, M. S. (2009). Victims of mentally disordered offenders in Zimbabwe, 1980–1990. *Journal of Forensic Psychiatry & Psychology*, *20*(3), 427–439. https://doi.org/10.1080/14789940802542907.

Mikton, C., & Grounds, A. (2007). Cross-cultural clinical judgment bias in personality disorder diagnosis by forensic psychiatrists in the UK: A case-vignette study. *Journal of Personality Disorders*, *21*(4), 400–417. https://doi.org/10.1521/pedi.2007.21.4.400.

Millet, P. E., Sullivan, B. F., Schwebel, A. I., & Myers, L. J. (1996). Black Americans' and White Americans' views of the etiology and treatment of mental health problems. *Community Mental Health Journal*, *32*(3), 235–242. https://doi.org/10.1007/BF02249425.

Moosa, M., & Jeenah, F. (2008). Involuntary treatment of psychiatric patients in South Africa. *African Journal of Psychiatry*, *11*(2), 109–112. https://doi.org/10.4314/ajpsy.v11i2.30261.

Moosa, M. Y. H., & Jeenah, F. Y. (2010). A review of the applications for involuntary admissions made to the Mental Health Review Boards by institutions in Gauteng in 2008. *South African Journal of Psychiatry*, *16*(4), 6. https://doi.org/10.4102/sajpsychiatry.v16i4.254.

Nathan, J. H., Wylie, A. M., & Marsella, A. J. (2001). Attribution and serious mental illness: Understanding multiple perspectives and ethnocultural factors. *American Journal of Orthopsychiatry*, *71*(3), 350–357. https://doi.org/10.1037/0002-9432.71.3.350.

Nichter, M. (2010). Idioms of distress revisited. *Culture, Medicine, and Psychiatry*, *34*(2), 401–416. https://doi.org/10.1007/s11013-010-9179-6.

Nigerian Correctional Service Act. (2019).

Niveau, G, & Welle, I. (2018). Forensic psychiatry, one subspecialty with two ethics? A systematic review. *BMC Medical Ethics*, *19*, 25.

Niveau, G., Godet, T., & Völlm, B. (2019). What does impartiality mean in medico-legal psychiatry? An international survey. *International Journal of Law and Psychiatry*, *66*, 101505. https://doi.org/10.1016/j.ijlp.2019.101505.

Nzimande, W. (2016). *Cultural defences in an open and democratic South Africa with specific reference to the custom of Ukuthwala and belief in witchcraft.* (Unpublished Dissertation submitted in partial fulfilment of the requirements for the degree Master of Law in Advanced Criminal Justice. Kwazulu-Natal).

Ogunlesi, A., Ogunwale, A., De Wet, P., Roos, L., & Kaliski, S. (2012). Forensic psychiatry in Africa: Prospects and challenges. *African Journal of Psychiatry*, *15*(1), 3–7. https://doi.org/10.4314/ajpsy.v15i1.1.

Ogunwale, A., Ogunlesi, A. O., & Majekodunmi, O. E. (2011). Psychiatric, psychological and witchcraft defences to murder in the Nigerian legal context. *Nigerian Journal of Psychiatry*, *9*(3), 17–24.

Ogunwale, A., & Oluwaranti, O. (2020). Pattern of utilization of the insanity plea in Nigeria: An empirical analysis of reported cases. *Forensic Science International: Mind and Law*, *1*, 100010. https://doi.org/10.1016/j.fsiml.2020.100010.

Olaore, A. Y., & Drolet, J. (2017). Indigenous knowledge, beliefs, and cultural practices for children and families in Nigeria. *Journal of Ethnic & Cultural Diversity in Social Work*, *26*(3), 254–270. https://doi.org/10.1080/15313204.2016.1241973.

Onokah, M. C. (2007). *Family law* (1st ed.). Ibadan: Spectrum Books Limited.

Pal, S. (1997). Mental disorders in abnormal offenders in Papua New Guinea. *Medicine and Law*, *16*, 87–95.

Perlin, M. L., & McClain, V. (2009). "Where souls are forgotten": Cultural competencies, forensic evaluations, and international human rights. *Psychology, Public Policy, and Law*, *15*(4), 257–277. https://doi.org/10.1037/a0017233.

Rahman, T., Meloy, J. R., & Bauer, R. (2019). Extreme overvalued belief and the legacy of Carl Wernicke. *The Journal of the American Academy of Psychiatry and the Law*, *47*(2), 8.

Rahman, T., Hartz, S. M., Xiong, W., Reid Meloy, J., Janofsky, J., Harry, B., & Resnick, P. J. (2020). Extreme overvalued beliefs. *J Am Acad Psychiatry Law*, *48*(3). https://doi.org/DOI:10.29158/JAAPL.200001-20.

Renteln, A. D. (2005). The use and abuse of the cultural defense. *Canadian Journal of Law and Society*, *20*(1), 47–74.

Sarkar, J. (2013). Mental health assessment of rape offenders. *Indian Journal of Psychiatry*, *55*(3), 235–243. https://doi.org/10.4103/0019-5545.117137-5545.117137.

Schwartz, R. C., & Blankenship, D. M. (2014). Racial disparities in psychotic disorder diagnosis: A review of empirical literature. *World Journal of Psychiatry*, *4*(4), 133–140. https://doi.org/10.5498/wjp.v4.i4.133.

Sheikh, T. L., Adekeye, O., Olisah, V. O., & Mohammed, A. (2015). Stigmatisation of mental illness among employees of a Northern Nigerian University. *Nigerian Medical Journal*, *56*(4), 244. https://doi.org/10.4103/0300-1652.169697.

Shepherd, S., & Willis-Esqueda, C. (2017). Indigenous perspectives on violence risk assessment: A thematic analysis. *Punishment & Society*, *20*(5), 599–627.

Shepherd, S. M. (2014). Finding color in conformity: A commentary on culturally specific risk factors for violence in Australia. *International Journal of Offender Therapy and Comparative Criminology*, *59*(12), 1297–1307. https://doi.org/10.1177/0306624X14540492.

Shepherd, S. M. (2016). Violence risk instruments may be culturally unsafe for use with Indigenous patients. *Australasian Psychiatry*, *24*(6), 565–567. https://doi.org/10.1177/1039856216665287.

Shepherd, S. M., & Lewis-Fernandez, R. (2016). Forensic risk assessment and cultural diversity: Contemporary challenges and future directions. *Psychology, Public Policy, and Law*, *22*(4), 427–438. https://doi.org/10.1037/law0000102.

Skeem, J. L., Edens, J. F., Camp, J., & Colwell, L. H. (2004). Are there ethnic differences in levels of psychopathy? A meta-analysis. *Law and Human Behavior, 28*(5), 505–527.

Stefan, S. (1996). Race, competence testing, and disability law: A review of the MacArthur competence research. *Psychology, Public Policy, and Law, 2*(1), 31–44. https://doi.org/10.1037/1076-8971.2.1.31.

Steffensmeier, D., Painter-Davis, N., & Ulmer, J. (2017). Intersectionality of race, ethnicity, gender, and age on criminal punishment. *Sociological Perspectives, 60*(4), 810–833. https://doi.org/10.1177/0731121416679371.

Sue, S. (1998). In search of cultural competence in psychotherapy and counseling. *American Psychologist, 58*(4), 440–448.

Sullivan, E. A., Abramowitz, C. S., Lopez, M., & Kosson, D. S. (2006). Reliability and construct validity of the psychopathy checklist-revised for Latino, European American, and African American male inmates. *Psychological Assessment, 18*(4), 382.

Szabo, C. P., Kohn, R., Gordon, A., & Hart, G. A. D. (2000). Ethics in the practice of psychiatry in South Africa. *South African Medical Journal, 90*(5), 498–503.

Szasz, T. (2003). Psychiatry and the control of dangerousness: On the apotropaic function of the term "mental illness." *Journal of Medical Ethics, 29*(4), 227–230. https://doi.org/10.1136/jme.29.4.227.

Tanyi, P. L., André, P., & Mbah, P. (2018). Care of the elderly in Nigeria: Implications for policy. *Cogent Social Sciences, 4*(1), 1–14. https://doi.org/10.1080/23311886.2018.1555201.

Touari, M., Mesbah, M., Dellatolas, G., & Bensmail, B. (1993). Association between criminality and psychosis: A retrospective study of 3984 expert psychiatric evaluations. *Revue d Epidemiologie et de Sante Publique, 41*, 218.

United Nations. (1966). *International covenant on civil and political rights. General Assemby resolution 2200A.* https://www.ohchr.org/Documents/ProfessionalInterest/ccpr.pdf.

United Nations. (2014). *2014wesp_country_classification.pdf.* https://www.un.org/en/development/desa/policy/wesp/wesp_current/2014wesp_country_classification.pdf.

van Horn, J. E., Eisenberg, M., Souverein, F. A., & Kraanen, F. (2018). The predictive value of the central eight criminogenic risk factors: A multi-group comparison of dually diagnosed violent offenders with other subgroups of violent offenders. *Journal of Addiction & Addictive Disorders, 5*(1), 1–11. https://doi.org/10.24966/AAD-7276/100014.

Weiss, R., & Rosenfeld, B. (2010). Cross-Cultural validity in malingering assessment: The dot counting test in a rural Indian sample. *International Journal of Forensic Mental Health, 9*(4), 300–307. https://doi.org/10.1080/14999013.2010.526680.

Weiss, R. A., & Rosenfeld, B. (2012). Navigating cross-cultural issues in forensic assessment: Recommendations for practice. *Professional Psychology: Research and Practice, 43*(3), 234–240. https://doi.org/10.1037/a0025850.

World Health Organization (1992). *The ICD-10 classification of mental and behavioural disorders.* Geneva: World Health Organization.

World Health Organization (Ed.) (2018). *Mental health atlas 2017.* Geneva: World Health Organization.

World Health Organization (2019). *Suicide.* https://www.who.int/news-room/fact-sheets/detail/suicide.

World Medical Association (1948). *Declaration of Geneva.* The World Medical Association Inc. https://www.wma.net/wp-content/uploads/2018/07/Decl-of-Geneva-v1948-1.pdf.

3 Forensic mental health care: Practice and policy in Africa

Jibril Abdulmalik, Olamiji Abiodun Badru, and Mary Ozioma Madu

Introduction

Forensic mental health is an area of specialization that involves the assessment and treatment of those who are both mentally ill and whose behavior has led, or could lead, to offending (Mullen, 2000). Because it deals with the interface of mental illness and the law, it is influenced by an interplay of a variety of factors specific to each region within which it is practiced. Such factors include historical developments, mental health systems and legal traditions (Eytan, Ngirababyeyi, Nkubili, & Mahoro, 2018), all of which play a role in legislations and the effect they have on the development of mental health policies and practices.

Forensic mental health services (FMHS) remain largely underdeveloped in Africa due to a number of factors such as lack of appropriate facilities, manpower deficiencies, lack of initiatives to involve relevant stake holders, as well as variations in legislative frameworks across various African countries (Ogunlesi, Ogunwale, & De Wet, 2012). Thus, FMHS across Africa are largely extensions of prisons, and are modeled on outdated mental health legislations (Eytan et al., 2018).

It is pertinent to recognize the strong nexus between mental health policy, practices and FMHS specifically. Thus, this chapter will describe the mental health policy and legislative situation across the continent; focus on forensic mental health practices and then close with recommendations for improving the situation. The overarching focus will be that of strengthening mental health systems across the continent.

Mental health policies and legislation

The World Health Organization's (WHO) Mental Health Atlas of 2017 indicated that 38% of countries globally lacked a mental health policy, 37% had no legislation on mental health, but 62% had revised their mental health policies and plans, while 42% had revised their mental health laws within the preceding five years (MH Atlas, 2017). Mental health legislation is lacking in most African countries. The few countries that have mental health laws operate outdated vestiges from colonial laws predating independence (Njenga, 2006; Esan et al., 2014).

Stigma, low prioritization by donors and low political priority are reasons why mental health remain low on the agenda for policy making across the continent.

Furthermore, inadequate mental health services and insufficient routine data collection on mental health ultimately leads to lack of data for planning and implementation (Abdulmalik, Kola, & Gureje, 2016).

West Africa

Mental health policies have been enacted in all English-speaking West African countries at different times. The newest policies are those of Gambia (2007), Sierra Leone (2009), Liberia (2009), Ghana (2012) and Nigeria (2013). These policies address service development and organization of mental health services – including FMHS, financing, medicines, advocacy, multi-sectoral collaboration, capacity building, human rights and decentralization of services. Poor implementation has limited the effect of existing mental health policies in the region (Omar, Green, & Bird, 2010).

Ghana's mental health laws, enacted in 2012, are the most refined in the region (Doku, Wusu-Takyi, & Awakame, 2012). Nigeria and Gambia still use obsolete laws enacted nearly a century ago. The legislation in Nigeria and Gambia failed to address access to care, protection of patients from involuntary admission and treatment, protection of rights of people with mental disorders, protection of rights of families and caregivers, quality assurance, protection of rights of vulnerable groups, substance use and issues related to legislative links with other sectors among others (Esan et al., 2014).

Strong and clear commitment from government, involvement of stakeholders and realistic goals such as issues in finance were lacking in the policies of Ghana. Furthermore, there was a failure to consult widely with important stakeholders during policy development, realism about what can be achieved and how were also not captured. Additionally, what was also lacking in Ghana was the need to radically reform services from an institutional model to one based on community care. Furthermore, deinstitutionalization was not addressed. Policies did not specifically promote the human rights of people with mental disabilities in the actions they prescribe.

Some of the other limitations include the absence of a strategic plan detailing what will be put in place to achieve the policy objectives and directions across the board.

Southern Africa

South Africa is the most visible and have developed the most comprehensive national mental health policy, following consultation with relevant stakeholders. Realistic goals such as issues in finance were lacking in the policies. However, there was promotion of policies for the integration of mental health care into general health services, as well as a community-oriented approach.

East Africa (Uganda)

A strong and clear commitment from government, involvement of stakeholders and realistic goals such as issues in finance were lacking in the mental health policies of Uganda. However, it promotes the integration of mental health care into general health services as well as a community-oriented approach.

South Central Africa (Zambia)

Strong and clear commitment from government, involvement of stakeholders and realistic goals such as issues in finance were lacking in the policies of Zambia. There was also a failure to consult widely with important stakeholders during policy development. There was no information on how to finance implementation of the policies.

Central West Africa

Equitorial Guinea, in Central West Africa, despite having the highest per capital investment in health, has a relatively poor organization for mental health, with only two research publications on mental health–related issues (Reuter, Mackail, Klim, & Reuter, 2016).

Forensic mental health policy, legislation and practice in Africa

It is critical to reiterate the strong interconnections between the governance structures of policy legislation on the practice of forensic mental health care services. Striking examples include the criminalization of suicidal attempts and homosexuality in several countries of Africa, where they are seen in most parts of Africa as criminal actions that are punishable by law. The situation is compounded by the dearth of information about forensic services on the continent (Njenga, 2006). In most countries there are few coordinated initiatives to involve all stakeholders, such as the police, departments of justice, prisons and hospitals, in the development of FMHS (Ogunlesi et al., 2012). An illustrative sub-regional overview is presented in Table 3.1.

Central/Eastern Africa (Rwanda)

In Rwanda, forensic psychiatry like other African countries is neglected. Part of the problems include the updating of pre-existing approvals, absence of forensic secured units and the need for international collaborations for supervision and training (Eytan et al., 2018).

North Africa

Forensic psychiatric practice in North Africa is not well organized, despite the fact that mental health legislation and human rights review bodies exist (El Hamaoui, Moussaoui, & Okasha, 2009). It is not a popular area of subspecialty interest in the region.

Table 3.1 Regional summary comparison of forensic mental health services across Africa (Ogunlesi et al., 2012)

Category	*East Africa*	*North Africa*	*Southern Africa*	*West Africa*
Origins	Colonial societies of the 1880s and the first half of the 1900s.	Colonial societies of the 1880s and the first half of the 1900s.	Colonial societies of the 1880s and the first half of the 1900s.	Colonial societies of the 1880s and the first half of the 1900s.
Mental Health Legislation	Kenya's (1989) legislation was revised in 2018 and passed in 2019.	Egypt was the first country in Africa, Asia and the World Health Organization Eastern Mediterranean Region (WHO-EMRO) to have a mental health act in 1944. The Egyptian 1944 Act was updated in April 2009. In addition, the Egyptian parliament had also passed a **law on substance abuse/addiction** in 1985, which provides for the involuntary admission of repeated drug offenders in hospitals rather than for their diversion into the criminal justice system. In Algeria, the Law 85-05 of December 1985 enacted for the promotion and protection of health, provides for procedures for admission of mentally ill patients and the protection of their rights. (El Hamaoui et al., 2009). Tunisia also enacted mental health legislation in 1992, which was reviewed in 2004.	Amendments to the South African Criminal Procedure Act and new mental health legislation, the Mental Health Care Act, No 17 of 2002 (shift from hospital care to community care, integration of general health care and protection of the mentally ill user's human rights)	Lunacy asylum order, Cap 79 of the former Gold Coast (Ghana) in 1888 and contained provisions for confining mentally ill patients to institutional care, and which virtually amounted to imprisonment. It was updated in line with global best practices in 2012. Sierra Leone still operates the Lunacy Act of 1902, but has recently evolved a new policy and strategic mental health plan. Nigeria: The Lunacy ordinance of 1916 and the Federal Law of 1958, provides for the establishment of the "asylums," which served as quasi-mental health hospitals/prisons in Calabar

(*Continued*)

Table 3.1 (Continued)

Category	*East Africa*	*North Africa*	*Southern Africa*	*West Africa*
				(established in 1903), Yaba (established in 1907) and Lantoro (established in 1944). Although these asylums initially only provided custodial care (while waiting for the requisite legislation to define their functions), they have since developed into proper psychiatric hospitals. Nigeria is in the process of reviewing a draft mental health Bill.
				Liberia passed a new Mental Health Legislation in 2017, while Gambia still operates a "Suspected Lunacy" Act of 1964 (Kretzschmar, Nyan, Mendy, & Janneh, 2012).
Human Resources	Psychiatric evaluations of mentally ill offenders are conducted by general psychiatrists, many of whom are in government service.	Psychiatric evaluations of mentally ill offenders are conducted by general psychiatrists, many of whom are in government service.	Few are actively involved in forensic psychiatry (Mars, Ramlall, & Kaliski, 2012).	Psychiatric evaluations of mentally ill offenders are conducted by general psychiatrists, many of whom are in government service.

Training	There is no formal training in forensic psychiatry.	No certified training programs in forensic psychiatry within North Africa. However, according special courses held for trainee-psychiatrists in forensic psychiatry in Egypt which would be synthesized into a certified training program (El Hamaoui et al., 2009).	Postgraduate programs, introduced into some academic departments and publishing of texts to standardize the overall practice of forensic mental health (Kaliski, 2006; Zabow, 1998). There is a Diploma in Forensic Psychiatry, and subsequently the Health Professions Council of SA has accepted, by proclamation in the Government Gazette, the recognition of forensic psychiatry formally as a subspecialty in South Africa.	There is a critical shortage of trained personnel that may hinder the implementation of a new training curriculum developed by the West African College of Physicians.
Facilities	There is no designated forensic psychiatric facility. Some services are provided within existing prison services.	Presence of institutions dedicated for the rehabilitation of mentally ill offenders, for example, in Egypt, the Abassia Hospital in Cairo and the El-Khanka Hospital in Kalyobia. Hitherto, only the Berrechid Hospital and the Tit Mellil were selected for a similar purpose in Morocco but, at present, all psychiatric institutions in the country may admit convicted persons with mental illness. Similarly, in Tunisia, the Manouba and in Algeria the Frantz Fanon Hospitals are designated forensic hospitals.	There are no dedicated forensic psychiatric hospitals but some facilities have dedicated units and beds for forensic psychiatric assessments and treatments. In the Eastern Cape, these would be Komani Hospital and Fort England Hospital (FEH), Grahamstown.	Generally, the prisons have also had to provide alternative rudimentary forensic psychiatric services in some countries in West Africa. There is no designated forensic psychiatric hospital, but some facilities have dedicated beds for forensic observations and treatment such as the Aro Neuropsychiatric Hospital, Abeokuta, Nigeria.

Southern Africa (South Africa)

There is paucity of information around forensic psychiatry in South Africa. For instance, there is no research data on forensic psychiatric service provision in the Eastern Cape, Republic of South Africa (Sukeri, Betancourt, Emsley, Nagdee, & Erlacher, 2016). Their recommendation was for the Provincial Department of Health to develop and implement strategies for the effective roll-out of forensic psychiatric services. The establishment of an inter-departmental task team, which includes Health, Justice and Constitutional Development and Correctional Services would also be useful in this regard (Sukeri et al., 2016).

West Africa (Nigeria)

Forensic psychiatric services are poorly organized and not readily available across the country, with just a handful of facilities offering any semblance of forensic psychiatric services. While the West African College of Physicians has developed curriculum for subspecialty training in forensic psychiatry, a dearth of competent trainers may be a stumbling block to effective implementation across the region. A summary table depicting the regional comparison of policy, legislation and forensic psychiatry services across the region, as extracted from Ogunlesi et al. (2012) and augmented by currently available literature, is presented in Table 3.1.

Discussion

The current parlous state of forensic mental health policy and practice across the continent should be of grave concern to stakeholders and policy makers. This is especially pertinent given some of the peculiarities of the criminal justice system as well as pattern of incarceration across the continent. For instance, while it is established that the prevalence of mental health problems is much higher among incarcerated persons in low- and middle-income countries including Africa, as compared to the general population (Baranyi et al., 2019); there is no commensurate availability of FMHS to respond to this need. Furthermore, a unique feature across the continent is the large proportion of awaiting trial inmates, with a recent systematic review and meta-analysis indicating that in 36% of the included studies, the majority of the participants were incarcerated while still awaiting trial; and had not yet been convicted of any crime (Lovett, Kwon, & Kidia, 2019). Yet some of them had been in prison for as high as ten years (Abdulmalik et al., 2014). In other studies, an average of 40% of incarcerated persons on the African continent were awaiting trial inmates (Gureje & Abdulmalik, 2019).

The common challenges across all subregions of the African continent include the low priority accorded to mental health generally, and forensic psychiatry, specifically. Secondly, a weak mental health system governance structure is in place across all the regions. Governance structures such as mental health policies, legislation, programs and plans, as well as funding, are necessary to provide an enabling framework for services to be developed and implemented in a co-ordinated and sustainable manner. The obsolete mental health legislation in most countries and the absence of a mental health policy (that should mention forensic services) makes it an uphill task to advocate for the development of services. Thirdly, there is a severe shortage of competent personnel to provide FMHS as well as to provide training for others. This is worsened by the waves of periodic brain drain that occurs intermittently, based on the needs and policy restrictions (or ease) of Western countries.

Yet it must be borne in mind that the thrust of the sustainable development goals (SDGs) is to ensure equitable access to health care services (including mental health care) for all citizens – including those who are incarcerated or in contact with the criminal justice system. Specifically, the SDG 3 aspires for equitable access to quality health care for all citizens (Patel et al., 2018). Thus, it would be a major failing to ignore the huge unmet needs of the large proportion of citizens incarcerated in prisons, and who are at greater risk of mental health problems. Baranyi et al. (2019) reported that about two-thirds of the world's prison population is in low- and middle-income countries, including Africa. Thus, it is a specific problem that is deserving of concerted attention for the African continent.

Recommendations

Deriving from the identified challenges hindering the development of FMHS across the continent, a raft of feasible and pragmatic strategies will be recommended for improving the practice and policy interface for accessible and qualitative FMHS.

1. Mental health system strengthening: An effective governance structure including mental health policies. Legislation that is in tandem with global best practices and conforms with the UN Convention on the Rights of Persons with Disabilities (CRPD), as well as funding streams, needs to be put in place. Provide an enabling environment, without which it will be exceedingly difficult to develop FMHS. Stakeholders should be engaged in the formulation process of policies and legislation to ensure future buy-in and increase the chances of successful implementation.
2. Task shifting: The grossly insufficient numbers of mental health professionals available and interested in providing FHMS makes it imperative to consider pragmatic but equally effective intervention strategies. The task shifting approach that will involve training non-specialist correctional officers and other health workers to provide mental health interventions, with appropriate referrals as may be indicated, appears to be the low-hanging fruit approach to solving the problem of acute manpower shortage. The WHO's mental health gap action program intervention guide (mhGAP-IG) can be deployed in this regard, with supportive supervision provided by mental health professionals (Gureje, Abdulmalik, & Kola, 2015). Innovative use of mobile technology and telepsychiatry can also be used to augment service provision with expert

support from remote locations. There is sufficient evidence of the efficacy of psychosocial interventions in low and middle income countries (LMICs), that is delivered by non-specialists (Barbui et al., 2020).

3. Community rehabilitation: Individuals who are incarcerated and also have mental health challenges are doubly at risk of having poor rehabilitation outcomes into the society. Community integration approaches that promote smooth transition from prisons and into the community, as well as provisions of mental health services within the community that complements their rehabilitation needs to be developed.
4. Funding: Once the governance structure is in place and there are policies as well as legislation backing the development and provision of FMHS, budget lines and funding streams should naturally follow that process. It is impossible to improve services without funding to back the process.
5. Brain drain reversal: The African continent can benefit from reverse brain drain by engaging with African forensic psychiatrists in the diaspora, many of whom are looking for ways to give back to their countries of origin. They can be engaged to provide short-term trainings, remote consultations via telepsychiatry, as well as provisions of materials and resources. Some may even be willing to plan physical visits and oversee the development and implementation of programs and services, in active partnership with locally trained experts who are more conversant of the context and potential pitfalls to avoid.
6. Implementation science research: It is important to conceive of research that is driven by local realities and needs, which seeks to provide pragmatic and evidence-based solutions. Such topics may be longitudinal studies from risk factors, to reception, incarceration process, as well as transition and rehabilitation into the community.
7. Ethical issues: Issues regarding individual freedoms and civil liberties, the right to treatment (or the right to refuse treatment), involuntary hospitalization, patient's needs vs social needs and human rights, legality vs morality and many more are areas that need to be resolved in line with global best practices in a way that also carries along all stakeholders (Ogunlesi & Ogunwale, 2018).
8. Mental health advocacy: Sustained mental health advocacy that highlights the relevance of updated mental health legislation as well as improved mental health services for all citizens can also push the policymakers to take action. Specific attention should be directed at the vulnerable persons who are incarcerated (Jack et al., 2018). Other areas of focus should include reducing stigma and discrimination.

Conclusion

The landscape of forensic mental health practice and policy in Africa is underdeveloped and further hampered by numerous challenges, but there are glimmers of hope and several pragmatic strategies that can be leveraged upon to improve the situation moving forward. With consistent and systematic advocacy for reforms, progress should be assured in the not-too-distant future.

References

Abdulmalik, J. O., Adedokun, B. O., & Baiyewu, O. O. (2014). Prevalence and correlates of mental health problems among awaiting trial inmates in a prison facility in Ibadan. *African Journal of Medical and Health Sciences, 43*(Suppl. 1), 193–199.

Abdulmalik, J., Kola, L., & Gureje, O. (2016). Mental health system governance in Nigeria: Challenges, opportunities and strategies for improvement. *Global Mental Health,* 3, e9. doi: 10.1017/gmh.2016.2

Baranyi, G., Scholl, C., Fazel, S., Patel, V., Priebe, S., & Mundt, A. P. (2019). Severe mental illness and substance use disorders in prisoners in low-income and middle-income countries: A systematic review and meta-analysis of prevalence studies. *Lancet Global Health, 7*(4), e461–e471. doi: 10.1016/S2214-109X(18)30539-4

Barbui, C., Purgato, M., Abdulmalik, J., Acarturk, C., Eaton, J., Gastaldon, C., Gureje, O., Hanlon, C., Jordans, M., Lund, C., Nosè, M., Ostuzzi, G., Papola, D., Tedeschi, F., Tol, W., Turrini, G., Patel, V., & Thornicroft, G. (2020). Efficacy of psychosocial interventions for mental health outcomes in low-income and middle-income countries: An umbrella review. *The Lancet Psychiatry, 7*(2), 162–172. https://doi.org/10.1016/S2215-0366(19)30511-5

Doku, V. C. K., Wusu-Takyi, A., & Awakame, J. (2012). Implementing the mental health act in Ghana: Any challenges ahead? *Ghana Medical Journal, 46*(4), 241–250.

El Hamaoui, Y., Moussaoui, D., & Okasha, T. (2009). Forensic psychiatry in North Africa. *Current Opinion in Psychiatry, 22*(5), 507–510.

Esan, O., Abdulmalik, J., Eaton, J., Kola, L., Fadahunsi, W., & Gureje, O. (2014). Mental health care in anglophone West Africa. *Psychiatric Services, 65,* 1084–1087.

Eytan, A., Ngirababyeyi, A., Nkubili, C., & Mahoro, P. N. (2018). Forensic psychiatry in Rwanda. Global Health Action, *11*(1), 1509933.

Gureje, O., & Abdulmalik, J. (2019). Severe mental disorders among prisoners in low-income and middle-income countries: Reaching the difficult to reach. *Lancet Global Health, 7*(4), e392–e393. doi: 10.1016/S2214-109X(19)30057-9

Gureje, O., Abdulmalik, J., & Kola, L., et al. (2015). Integrating mental health into primary care in Nigeria: Report of a demonstration project using the mental health gap action programme intervention guide. *BMC Health Services Research, 15,* 242.

Jack, H. E., Fricchione, G., Chibanda, D., Thornicroft, G., Machando, D., & Kidia, K. (2018). Mental health of incarcerated people: A global call to action. *Lancet Psychiatry, 5*(5), 391–392.

Kaliski, S. Z. (2006). Introduction. In Kaliski S. Z., (Ed.). *Psycholegal Assessment in South Africa* (pp. 1–7).Cape Town: Oxford University Press.

Kretzschmar, I., Nyan. O., Mendy. A., & Janneh, B. (2012). Mental health in the Republic of The Gambia. *International Psychology, 9*(2), 38–40.

Lovett, A., Kwon, H. R., Kidia, K., et al. (2019). Mental health of people detained within the justice system in Africa: Systematic review and meta-analysis. *International Journal of Mental Health Systems, 13,* 31. https://doi.org/10.1186/s13033-019-0273-z

Mars, M., Ramlall, S., & Kaliski, S. (2012). Forensic telepsychiatry: A possible solution for South Africa? *African Journal of Psychiatry, 15,* 244–247.

Mullen, P. E. (2000). Forensic mental health. *The British Journal of Psychiatry, 176*(4), 307–311.

Njenga, F. G. (2006). Forensic psychiatry: The African experience. *World Psychiatry, 5* (2), 97.

Ogunlesi, A. O., & Ogunwale, A. (2018). Correctional psychiatry in Nigeria: Dynamics of mental healthcare in the most restrictive alternative. *BJPsych International, 15*(2), 35–38. https://doi.org/10.1192/bji.2017.13

Ogunlesi, A. O., Ogunwale, A., De Wet, P., et al. (2012). Forensic psychiatry in Africa: Prospects and challenges. *African Journal of Psychiatry, 15*, 3–7.

Omar, M. A., Green, A. T., Bird, P. K., et al. (2010). Mental health policy process: A comparative study of Ghana, South Africa, Uganda and Zambia. *International Journal of Mental Health System, 4*, 24.

Patel, V., Saxena, S., Lund, C., Thornicroft, G., Baingana, F., Bolton, P., Chisholm, D., Collins, P. Y., Cooper, J. L., Eaton. J., et al. (2018). The Lancet commission on global mental health and sustainable development. *Lancet, 392*(10157), 1553–1598.

Reuter, P. R., Mackail, S., Klim, M., & Reuter, E. (2016). Public health professionals perceptions of mental health services in Equitorial Guinea, Central-West Africa. *Pan African Medical Journal, 25*, Article 236. doi: 10.11604/pamj.2016.25.236.10220.

Sukeri, K., Betancourt, O. A., Emsley, R., Nagdee, M., & Erlacher, H. (2016). Forensic mental health services: Current service provision and planning for a prison mental health service in the Eastern Cape. *The South African Journal of Psychiatry: SAJP: The Journal of the Society of Psychiatrists of South Africa, 22*(1), 787. https://doi.org/10.4102/sajpsychiatry.v22i1.787

WHO. (2018). Mental health atlas 2017. Geneva: WHO.

Zabow, T. (1998). Forensic psychiatric evaluation: Clinical, ethical and procedural issues in South Africa. *Medical Law, 17*, 69–75.

4 Best practices in service planning for prisoners in Africa

Aishatu Yusha'u Armiya'u and Abdulkareem Jika Yusuf

Introduction

Correctional facilities all over the world are established to serve as reformational and rehabilitation centers for individuals who violate the rules and regulations of their society. However, prisons also serve as homes for several mentally challenged individuals who actually require treatment. Research shows consistently higher rates of mental illness in prisoners, with more people with mental disorders in prisons than in psychiatric hospitals in some countries (Fazel, Hayes, Bartellas, Clerici, & Trestman, 2016). While correctional facilities were absolutely not meant to cater to those with mental illnesses, today they have become one of their principal responsibilities. This problem is more glaring in Africa despite the paucity of mental health resources on the continent. In Africa, the criminal justice system has treated the mentally challenged with the same detachment conferred on criminal offenders generally, resulting in impacts that have been catastrophic. In Africa, penal systems inherited from colonial rule have largely remained unchanged, particularly in terms of the legislative and infrastructural frameworks. Even though attempts have been made by some countries to improve the conditions of correctional facilities, the institutions still remain archaic and inadequate to cater to the needs of inmates with or without mental health challenges. As such, the conditions of prisons across Africa are perilous for the mental health of offenders, due to overcrowding, poor sanitary facilities, violence, lack of privacy, absence of meaningful activities, isolation from family and friends, provision of poor-quality nutrition, uncertainty about life after prison and lack of or inadequate health services. The inadequate knowledge of mental health issues by warders, poor funding, etc. also negatively impact prisoners in many parts of the continent. The consequences of these problems will therefore be worsened for prisoners whose thinking and emotional responses are already impaired by major depression, schizophrenia, bipolar disorder and other mental illnesses. The societal rejection and the prevalent myths about mental illness, coupled with the judicial inadequacies, result in prisoners with mental health challenges going without treatment in the prison.

Despite population explosion on the continent and an increase in crime as a result of urbanization, the capacity in many prisons has remained the same or is even reduced in several countries, with negative impact on offenders (UNOWA, 2007). Rapid urbanization results in the chaotic expansion of urban spaces. This disables the national and local government's capacity to provide security and adequate basic social infrastructure such as affordable housing, health, education, sewage and water supply (UNOWA, 2007). It is within this context that urban crime in Africa is on the rise, largely due to weak governance systems, limited infrastructure and servicing (Owusu, Wrigley-Asante, Oteng-Ababio, & Owusu, 2015, 2016a, 2016b). Consequent to that, many of the continent's prison systems are in a state of crisis, burdened with overcrowding. The prison cells are poorly lit, have inadequate ventilation, prisoners sleep on damp and dirty floors and use overflowing buckets that serve as toilet facilities within the cells. Washing facilities lack adequate water supply, which results in poor sanitary hygiene and possible outbreaks of communicable diseases (Owusu et al., 2015, 2016a, 2016b). There is also the inability or unwillingness of the government to protect the human rights of prisoners – a constituency marginalized and widely despised by politicians and the public alike (Schonteich, 2015).

In North African countries, due to scarce human and financial resources, there are no formally trained forensic psychiatrists or forensic psychiatry institutions. Therefore, forensic psychiatry is disorganized in these countries (Hamaoui, Moussaoui, & Okasha, 2009). In Morocco, several mentally ill individuals are in prison and remain there due to lack of forensic psychiatry facilities and the slow judicial procedure. As such, they spend a long time in the prison without taking their mental state into account. This is found in almost all the North African countries (Ministry of Health Morocco and WHO, 2006; Administration Centrale Pénitentiaire Morocco, 2006; Ministry of Health Tunisia and WHO, 2008). However, Egypt has dedicated institutions for the rehabilitation of mentally ill offenders but currently has no certified training programs for forensic psychiatry like many other African countries (Ogunlesi, Ogunwale, Wet, Roos, & Kaliski, 2012).

Statistics on female prisoners across Africa are scanty, apart from a few countries such as South Africa, Nigeria, Zambia, Kenya, Uganda, Egypt, Tunisia, Rwanda and Cameroon, respectively. As outlined in Figure 4.1, South Africa has a total prison population of 163,015 with a female population of 2.6%. It is the largest prison population on the continent and the ninth in the world. Nigeria's prison population stands at 72,627 with a female population of 1.9% (Institute for Crime and Justice Policy Research, 2020). Female inmates in Zambia are approximately 3.0% of the total prison population of 22,823 (Institute for Crime and Justice Policy Research, 2020). Zambia has one exclusive female prison out of 86 prisons in the country. Kenya and Uganda have a total prison population of 51,130 and 55,229, respectively, with female populations of 6.3% and 4.5%, respectively. In Egypt, the total prison population is 106,000 with 3.7% female population, while Tunisia has a female prison population of 2.8% with a total population of 222,663 (Institute for Crime and Justice Policy Research, 2020). Cameroon's prison population stands at 30,701 in the year 2017, according to the Ministry of Justice, with a female population of 2.7% (Institute for Crime and Justice Policy Research, 2020).

S/N	Countries	Total Prison Population	Female
1	South Africa	163,015	2.6%
2	Nigeria	72,627	1.9%
3	Kenya	51,130	6.3%
4	Uganda	55,229	4.5%
5	Egypt	106,000	3.7%
6	Tunisia	222,663	2.8%
7	Cameroon	30,701	2.7%

Figure 4.1 Summary of countries total prison population and percentage of female inmates (Institute for Crime and Justice Policy Research, 2020).

Prisons around the world are separated by gender, with research showing demographic and criminal characteristics of female prisoners differing from that of their male counterparts (Fazel et al., 2016). However, in some countries both genders share the same prison environment (Samakaya-Makarati, 2003). Cameroon has no exclusive female prison, with women sharing the same compound with men, even toilet facilities in some case in Cameroon (Fontebo, 2013). A prison in Cameroon wakes female prisoners at 5 a.m. to have access to the bathroom before the men. By implication, the female prisoners in this prison have no access to the bathroom during the daytime (Fontebo, 2013).

The rate of conviction is higher among young girls than adult women (Van Hout & Mhlanga-Gunda, 2019). According to a report in 2015, the vulnerability of girls in the criminal justice system is unique due to issues relating to abuse and violence, unstable environment, presence of mental and physical health conditions and discrimination (Penal Reform International, 2017). Being incarcerated worsens their mental health challenges and exposes them to more traumatic experiences, including sexual abuse. A girl's remand home in Ghana was reported to be located on the same compound with that of the boys (Commonwealth Human Rights Initiative CHRI, Africa Office, 2011). The mixing of girls, boys and adult prisoners results in continuous threats of sexual abuse and violence to the young girls and boys that are vulnerable. Additionally, the lack of basic necessities in the prison, such as food, makes them more prone to manipulation by the older, powerful and wealthier adult prisoners, making them easy targets for sexual abuse (Topp et al., 2016). Apart from sexual abuse, these young offenders are subjected to humiliation and degrading treatment like stripping young female prisoners during searches in Swaziland as reported by the Department of States Bureau of Democracy, Human Rights and Labor (DRL) (DRL, 2017). This hinders their development and transition into adulthood, with subsequent unsuccessful reintegration into the community at the time of discharge (Lambie & Randell, 2013).

In Zambia and Sudan, basic health care services are not provided for female detainees (Todrys & Amon, 2011a; IRIN Africa, 2003). Therefore, mental health services were not discussed since basic health needs are unmet. This amounts to human rights violations of women who are already isolated and are separated from their children and spouses. All of the above could lead to mental health challenges. Studies from Africa reported physical abuse (Cape, 2009), rape and sexual violence (Kron, 2009) against female inmates. The Federal Bureau of Justice (BJS) in the United States of America reported an alleged increase in the incident of sexual victimization among prisoners. It increased by 180% from 2011 to 2015 (Bliss, 2018).

In many prisons in Africa, there are no measures put in place by policy makers to tackle specific gender issues relating to pregnant women, mothers with children, menstruation and privacy. Moreover, they do not consider that imprisonment poses a strain on mothers and their children. In prisons across Africa, infants are separated from their imprisoned mothers after birth. Early separation from mothers is traumatic and worse for the children, with negative implications for the cognitive development of the children.

Global data available showed that about one million young children were in incarceration in 2010, with an intended upcoming report in 2019 by the UN Global Study on Children Deprived of Liberty (Van Hout & Mhlanga-Gunda, 2019). Demographic data of young people incarcerated in Sub-Saharan Africa (SSA) showed an age range between 12 and below 18 years. This evidence was found in 37 of 49 SSA countries, with 11 referring to juvenile detention centers (Van Hout & Mhlanga-Gunda, 2019). Incarceration should be a last resort for young people who come into conflict with the law and for the shortest possible time (United Nations, 1989). Young people in detention have specific and unmet health needs and may be disproportionately affected by risky health behaviors, self-harm, suicide, learning disabilities and poorer mental health (Barnert, Perry, & Morris, 2016; Lennox, 2014; Lambie & Randell, 2013). Potentially life-threatening harsh penal conditions were reported from 2012 to 2017 from 16 SSA countries that include Central African Republic, Mali, Rwanda, Senegal and Gabon, among others (Van Hout & Mhlanga-Gunda, 2019). Overcrowding was also reported in the young people's detention center. This was reported in a Togolese study in 2014 where young inmates were kept in tiny cellblocks measuring 6 m × 5 m (Y Care International, 2014). Other studies in Zambia and Nigeria found similar reports of overcrowding in a detention center for youth (Atilola, 2013; Topp et al., 2016).

Housing young people while on detention vary across the SSA countries. Although some countries have separate places for young people, others mix young people with adults in the same facility. This mixing is attributed to lack of resources in such countries to house the minors separately (Sarkin, 2008). A Zambian prison official reported that *"As a father it pains me that children do not have their own facilities ...—we need to build a separate area for juvenile offenders"* (Human Rights Watch HRW, 2010). Another young boy in detention in a mixed facility said *"... We sleep with the adults, but they told us to say we sleep in a juvenile cell. If we don't say we sleep in a separate cell, they will beat us. We are given punishment when we start talking. But we are scared we might die here ..."* (Todrys & Amon, 2011b). This situation results in the young people being victims of sexual and physical assault. The traumatic experiences ultimately result in mental health challenges for such young, incarcerated persons. The prevalence of male rape in the juvenile section of a South African correctional facility was found with a frequency of about two to three a week (African Commission on Human and Peoples' Rights ACHPR, 2004). In Zambia, adult prisoners establish relationships with young people due to the failure of protection by the prison officials *"... Mainly the juveniles are very vulnerable. As young people coming into prison, we are full of fear. The convicts take advantage of us by providing us with food and security. We enter their dragnet, but by the time we discover this it is too late ... ."* (Human Rights Watch HRW, 2010). In other SSA countries, the prison officials traffic the young people to adult inmates in exchange for money to be abused. A young boy commented that *"... Forced sexual activity is very common. The way we sleep, we are in one another's lap"* (Todrys & Amon, 2011b).

The elderly population has received little attention in the criminal justice system, despite a rapid increase in their population in prisons globally (Ojo & Okunola, 2014). This also contributes to the overcrowding in the prison system. Elderly inmates have unique problems that pose challenges to the correctional services. They have been presented in categories: those who are recidivists (repeat offenders), those who grow old in prison and those who committed their first offense in old age (Kakoullis, Le Mesurier, & Kingston, 2010; Nowotny, Cepeda, James-Hawkins, & Boardman, 2016). A major challenge with the elderly prisoners is health care service delivery in correctional facilities. They face more serious problems than younger offenders. Due to their age, they are faced with multiple health problems (Davies, 2011) and comorbidities (Armiya'u, Obembe, et al., 2013).

The elderly are fragile and some have been in prison since a young age. Prison in itself can lead to psychological damage, particularly for those with a life sentence (Davies, 2011). About eight in ten studied elderly inmates had depression, while a few had epilepsy. With no concrete means to help this vulnerable group of offenders due to the absence of mental health services, their mental health deteriorates (Ojo & Okunola, 2014). Another area of concern is the lack of proper bedding, clothing and nutrition for the elderly inmates. Clothing and bedding are prerequisites for the elderly. This will protect them from harsh weather. Coupled with poor and inadequate feeding, their health rapidly deteriorates (Ojo & Okunola, 2014).

Profile of mentally ill offenders

Worldwide, there are over 10.74 million people detained in penal institutions (Walmsley, 2018) with an increased risk for negative outcomes that include self-harm, suicide, victimization, violence and death (Fazel et al., 2016). Sexual abuse is on the increase in prisons both between the prisoners and between the correctional officers and prisoners (Van Hout & Mhlanga-Gunda, 2019). The prevalence of mental health disorder in Africa is alarming and a major concern. This is because of the difficult and poor access to mental health services across Africa (Lovett et al., 2019). Resource constraints for mental health services and shifts toward community-based care from institutions for individuals with chronic mental health have resulted in the rise in the number of forensic patients (Yusuf & Nuhu, 2009).

The prevalence of mental illness differs between the prison population and general population, with higher rates among prisoners (Fatoye, Fatoye, Oyebanji, & Ogunro, 2006; Armiya'u et al., 2013). Among adult prisoners across Africa, the prevalence of mental illness was found to be 59%, 61% among youths and 44% among inpatients in forensic wards (Lovett et al., 2019). The disproportionately higher rate of mental disorders in prison relates to several factors including the general belief that people with mental disorders are dangerous, intolerance towards mentally disordered people due to disturbing behaviors, failed promotion of treatment, care and rehabilitation and poor access to mental health services in several African countries. These disorders are likely to be present before imprisonment and worsen during imprisonment or contacted while in prison. The prison condition itself could precipitate a mental health disorder. Factors such as isolation from social networks, lack or inadequate health care, lack of medication, overcrowding and uncertainty about the outcome of their cases as well as their future can raise the risk for suicide and other mental health problems among prisoners.

In the adult prison population across Africa, mood disorder was found in 22%, psychotic disorder in 33% and substance use disorder in 38%; among youths, mood disorder was found in 24% and 22% had substance use disorder (Lovett et al., 2019). Female prisoners have higher levels of mental disorders (i.e., depression) than male prisoners (Weissman, DeLamater, & Lovejoy, 2013). Other disorders include sleep disorder, stress, generalized anxiety disorder (Boxer, Middlemass, & Delorenzo, 2009) as well as post-traumatic stress disorder (PTSD) (Baranyi et al., 2018). Female prisoners are vulnerable, with complex needs. Higher suicide and self-harm rates have also been reported among this group of offenders (Fazel et al., 2016). The prison environment in itself can predispose them to new mental illness or exacerbate an already existing mental illness (United Nations Office on Drugs and Crime UNODC, 2010). Adaptation to prison environment is poor, especially by female prisoners who had a prior history of mental illness, sexual and or physical abuse, abusive relationships or abuse of alcohol and drugs (Van Voorhis, Wright, Salisbury, & Bauman, 2010). The following quotes were two responses from different prison officials about female inmates from a study conducted in Nigeria about coping with the prison environment. It was stated that:

> *... they are mostly withdrawn from their colleagues, they keep to themselves, some of them are even difficult to deal with by the staff, they find rules and regulations guiding their stay very difficult to keep to ... some don't eat, some don't clean up properly or do their laundries ... a lot of them talk to themselves and easily break down in tears at slighest provocation while some engage in fights ...*
>
> (Prison Official)

> *... sometimes, their adjustment is dependent on their experience with the Police before they are brought to the Prison ... some of them may have been brutalized, dehumanized and treated so badly by the police that they will still remain in shock and trauma for a long time after getting here ....*
>
> (Prison Official) (Van Voorhis et al., 2010)

The overrepresentation of the mentally ill in prisons worldwide, including Africa, is not without consequences. This is because there are about ten times more individuals with serious mental illness (SMI) in prisons than in psychiatric hospitals (Torrey et al., 2010). Serious mental illness includes schizophrenia, bipolar affective disorder and major depression. A systematic review in Africa found psychotic disorder in 33% of the adult prison population (Lovett et al., 2019). Imprisonment of individuals with mental illness is a major public health challenge, which comes with clinical, economic and social implications (Al-Rousan et al., 2017). The balance between providing safety for the public and human rights has become a challenge in the provision of adequate and appropriate treatment for these individuals by the correctional services (Al-Rousan et al., 2017).

The link between mental illness and violence has been established by several researchers. Some specific factors have been identified such as psychotic and/or delusional symptoms as well as substance use disorders that are known to be associated with violent behaviors in individuals with mental illness (Coid et al., 2013; Kuhns & Clodfelter, 2009). Researches have shown high rates of psychiatric morbidity among homicide and other violent offenders in the prison (Fatoye et al., 2006; Armiya'u & Adole, 2015).

Schizophrenia is a major mental disorder that has been associated with violent crimes and reported among prisoners worldwide, Africa inclusive. Studies have found schizophrenia to be 20 times more common in individuals who committed homicide than the general population (Fazel & Grann, 2006). An estimated 6.5% of homicide cases were committed by individuals with schizophrenia, from a meta-analysis (Large, Smith, & Nielssen, 2009). Positive symptoms of schizophrenia have been implicated in crime commission, specifically delusions of persecution (Coid et al., 2013). A recent comparative study in Nigeria among homicide and non-homicide offenders showed that psychosis was found only among homicide offenders, with none of the non-homicide offenders meeting the diagnostic criteria for psychosis (Armiya'u, 2019). The neurocognitive dysfunction, which is a core feature of psychosis, is likely to contribute to the violent aggression manifesting in these persons (Stratton, Brook, & Hanlon, 2017). It is important and necessary to institute initial mental health assessment for all offenders admitted into the prison. This is because an early and accurate diagnosis is key to the treatment and rehabilitation of the mentally ill offender to avoid further violence inside the prison due to lack of medication.

Studies have shown that among the incarcerated population, elderly prisoners with mental health illness are the fastest-growing subgroup and with a worse health outcome (Chodos, Ahalt, Cenzer, & Goldenson, 2013; Pro & Marzell, 2017). They have the highest somatic (Moschetti et al., 2015) and mental health disorders rate (Nowotny et al., 2016). Mental health problems found in older inmates include substance use disorder, depression, anxiety disorder, psychotic disorder and age-related neuropsychiatric disorders like dementia (Haesen et al., 2019). A Nigerian study reported depression among older male prisoners, which was associated with current medical care, prison location and condition (Majekodunmi, Obadeji, Oluwole, & Oyelami, 2017). Major predictors of depression in these inmates were the presence of physical comorbidity and inmates' perception of the prison environment.

Epilepsy accounts for 0.5% of the 13.1% global burden of disease for neuropsychiatric disorders. Its prevalence is highest in low- and middle-income countries (LAMIC), which includes 80% of countries found in SSA where treatment is unavailable to the majority (Chin, 2012). These countries represent the poorest in the world and depend heavily on assistance from developed countries for health, with most targeted to treating communicable diseases. By 2050, the UN population division estimates the population of SSA to double to over 1.75 billion (Chin, 2012). The risk of mental health disorders is increased in epilepsy compared to the general population. Those with epilepsy have higher rates for depression, generalized anxiety disorder and suicide (Rai et al., 2012). They also have an increased frequency for psychosis, which increases violence (Clancy, Clarke, Connor, Cannon, & Cotter, 2014). In the prison, the prevalence of epilepsy tends to be higher than the general population. It is therefore important for those working in the correctional services to understand this neurological disorder so as to handle the inmates with epilepsy appropriately. Certain factors in the prison increase triggers for convulsions. These include high stress level, low sugar level and possible drug abuse (Mersey Region Epilepsy Association, 2019). Epilepsy was reported to be prevalent among inmates aged 40–49 years and those 50 years and above. It was also found to be common in recidivists when compared to first-time offenders, and alcohol dependence was four times more likely to be found in inmates with epilepsy (Stawinska-Witoszynka, Czechowska, & Wieckwska, 2019). Long-term alcohol use alone can increase the risk of an epileptic seizure by two to ten times, depending on daily consumption (Restel & Rola, 2014). Violence and/or aggression in epilepsy occurs during different phases of the seizure. Ictal violence is rare and is linked to frontal lobe epilepsy. Violence in epilepsy occurs more commonly in the post-ictal phase and can be hours to days after the initial periods of confusion. It is usually undirected and may relate to post-ictal psychosis. Inter-ictal violence is the most aggressive behavior in people with epilepsy (Brower & Price, 2000). The biological behaviors seen in patients with epilepsy are a result of a brain injury and not the seizure discharge (Marsh & Krauss, 2000). Therefore, the violence and aggression are because of the location of the brain injury and not the seizure discharge.

Substance use, abuse and dependence are more prevalent in the criminal justice population than the general population (Gray & Littlefield, 2002; United States Department of State Bureau of Democracy, Human Rights and Labor, 2014). Studies conducted in prisons in Africa found a high prevalence of substance use disorders in inmates (Uganda Prisons Service, 2009; Armiya'u et al., 2013; Kinyanjui & Atwoli, 2013). Most studies on alcohol abuse/dependence link such behavior with violent behaviors, especially homicide offenses, while cannabis and other drugs were more linked to the offense of robbery. Alcohol has a direct effect on violence due to disruption of the normal brain function. Consumption of alcohol weakens the mechanism of the brain that normally restrains impulsive behaviors and inappropriate aggression (Gustafson, 1994). After the ingestion of alcohol, the information-processing capacity of an individual is likely going to be impaired and could result in misjudging social cues, with an overreaction to any perceived threat (Miczek, 1997). These are some reasons why such inmates in prison need to be managed appropriately before reintegration into the community.

Intellectual disability impacts the functional abilities of an individual and could result in frustration, shame and deficits in social skills. These could prompt the individual to engage in antisocial behavior and ultimately unlawful acts, such as criminal behavior. A study conducted in Nigeria among convicted inmates found intellectual disability in 18% of the participants; however, the specific intellectual disability could not be determined (Adewunmi, 2018). In Zambia, prisoners with intellectual disability are discriminated against and routinely disadvantaged (Jacobson et al., 2017). Like all other inmates, they experience harsh and brutal conditions in the prison, and because of their disability, such experiences are felt more severely. The disability can be aggravated by the detention or the non-availability of health care within the prison environment (Jacobson et al., 2017). A South African study reported that offenders with suspected intellectual disability (ID) are commonly referred for forensic evaluation by courts of law. Of the 120 study participants, 70.8% had a mild intellectual disability. The majority of them were found neither competent to stand trial nor criminally responsible for their offenses because of their ID (Mosotho et al., 2020). Another study in Ghana assessed the life of persons with disabilities in prison. The majority of the disabilities were acquired, with drug-related mental disabilities being the third most common among inmates with disabilities (Dogbe et al., 2016). The study identified 1.6% of prison inmates as suffering from some form of disability, which includes mental disabilities.

Mental health services

A recent systematic review across Africa revealed a shortage of personnel in prison mental health services, insufficient human resources for health, lack of psychosocial services, absence of timely psychiatric assessment, limitation in rehabilitation, vocational and recreational space and also community re-integration services (Lovett et al., 2019). There is insufficient food, psychiatric medications, physical resources and dearth of knowledge of mental health principles among the workers in the correctional system. In South Africa, the Eastern Cape has 45 correctional centers with a population of 19,265 (449 females; 18,816 males). With the second-highest occupancy rate in the country, it does not have any policy for long-term management of mentally ill prisoners or a reintegration plan for these patients either to the hospital or back to community-based services (Sukeri et al., 2016). Correctional services have no permanent psychological services and psychiatric services are non-existent. Twenty-two psychologists are found in all the correctional centers in South Africa, but no on-site psychiatrist exists (NICRO submission, 2011). The implication of this is that mentally ill individuals are detained due to the absence of preliminary assessments to ascertain their mental health status (Sukeri et al., 2016).

In West Africa, Nigeria specifically, the current prison statistics stand at 48,807 prisoners (pre-trial/remand), which is 72.6% of the total prison population across 240 holding facilities (Institute for Crime & Justice Policy Research, 2020). While the Prisons Service Act confers on the prison authorities the responsibility to arrange for the treatment of mentally ill offenders in prison, (Laws of the Federation of Nigeria, 2004), the elevated rates of mental disorders among the prisoners, coupled with the absence of mental health workers and poor funding, are constraints that overstretch the prison system (Ogunlesi & Ogunwale, 2018). Three prototypes of mental health care services exist in Nigerian prisons and their health systems are characterized by inadequate workforce, poor funding, security and safety issues as well as numerous ethical challenges (Ogunlesi & Ogunwale, 2018). The three prototypes are described in Table 4.1.

Model II, described by Ogunlesi and Ogunwale (2018), is used at a maximum-security prison in Plateau state Nigeria. Volunteers from two non-governmental organizations are part of the mental health team and the members of the mental health team provide and ensure adequate supply of medication for the mentally challenged inmates receiving treatment at the prison clinic. So far it has yielded positive outcomes, with inmates holding leadership positions within the prison environment and has resulted in a calm prison environment. With the team fully on the ground, running weekly clinics, stigma and the discrimination of inmates with mental illness reduced remarkably. In addition, fellow inmates and prison staff are able to identify and refer new cases of inmates with mental illness to the mental health team. The clinical psychologist in the prison is the first point of contact who assesses the inmates and refers the inmate to the psychiatrist when the need arises. On discharge from the prison, about 40% of the inmates undergo follow-up at the tertiary hospital to continue medication. This has led to a

Table 4.1 Prototypes of mental health service provision in correctional facilities in Nigeria

Prototype	*Description*
I	The most common prototype is the provision of mental health care by non-psychiatric doctors, nurses and support staff in the correctional service facility clinic. The correctional service and/or inmate's relatives provide funds for the medications.
II	Less common than prototype I but more frequently practiced than prototype III. A visiting psychiatrist from a tertiary health care facility within the state the correctional facility is located provides mental health care services to the inmates. The correctional service clinic provides support services and nursing care. Medication is funded by the correctional service or occasionally by relatives of the inmates.
III	A visiting psychiatrist (and a multidisciplinary team where available) and a stationed mental health nurse who runs daily morning shifts only (excluding weekend) from a tertiary health facility in which the prison is located provide mental health services. The correctional service clinic staff provides support services. The correctional service also provides funds for the medication or the inmate's relatives. This is the least practiced model in the country.

Source: Ogunlesi and Ogunwale (2018).

reduction in the rate of recidivism at the prison facility between 2017 and 2019 (Armiya'u et al., in press).

Young people face the same or worse challenges with getting standard health care services while in detention. Prison-based health care services were described to be virtually non-existent in the Republic of Benin and Guinea-Bissau (cited in Van Hout & Mhlanga-Gunda, 2019). The majority of the SSA countries do not have mental health and psychiatric services available or accessible to young people while in detention (Van Hout & Mhlanga-Gunda, 2019). The absence or lack of adequate health facilities resulted in the presence of anxiety and suicidal and depressive symptoms among some participants studied in a Nigerian remand home (Bella, Atilola, & Omigbodun, 2010).

In Egypt, under their prison act, when an offender with mental illness is brought into the prison, the offender is sent to the hospital for assessment

> *If the prison physician believes any sentenced prisoner has a mental defect; his case shall be reviewed by the director of the Prisons Medical Department. Should it be deemed necessary to send him to the mental hospital for verification, the director shall do so promptly. If it is proven that the prisoner has a mental defect, the prisoner shall remain in the hospital and the public prosecutor shall be notified to issue a committal order until the prisoner is cured. Upon cure, the hospital administration shall inform the public prosecutor, who shall order the prisoner's return to prison. The time served in the hospital shall be deducted from his sentence.*
>
> Article 35, Prisons Law (Egyptian Initiative for Personal Rights, 2014)

Convicted mentally disordered offenders are kept in two facilities where they receive treatment. Following recovery, they are referred back to the judicial system. Although the law exists and clearly stipulates what should be done, these inmates are held with other inmates and subjected to inhumane treatment and continual abuse (Egyptian Initiative for Personal Rights, 2014). This makes them vulnerable to harm by fellow inmates or the prison authorities. However, in Morocco, convicted offenders with mental disorders are kept in psychiatric hospitals, occupying regular psychiatric beds for a long period of time (Hamaoui et al., 2009).

Research findings from North Africa showed the importance of mental health care, but this is lacking in the prison despite its importance. Prisons lack social workers or psychological specialists, and they do not have programs for psychological or vocational rehabilitation, which are important to support and aid prisoners before they are released into society (Egyptian Initiative for Personal Rights, 2014).

Human rights abuse as it relates to mental health

According to the World Health Organization, every human being deserves to enjoy the highest attainable standard of physical and mental health as a fundamental human right without discrimination. However, this is not so for prisoners as they suffer a disproportionate weight of health problems due to the neglect of their health care needs. The United Nations (1990) Basic Principles for the Treatment of Prisoners set out that "prisoners shall have access to the health services available in the country without discrimination on the grounds of their legal situation" (Principle 9, A/RES/45/111). Regardless of the environment the mentally ill individual finds him/herself, the human rights principle should be adhered to. The intent is to provide the required mental health treatment to accommodate the special needs of the prison population. However, challenges arise in unskilled manpower, individuals with various degrees, severity of mental illness (Naudts et al., 2005), emphasis on punishment rather than psychiatric support, physical and verbal abuse, neglect by staff and worsening of mental illness due to isolation and confinement (Fellner, 2006).

In 2016, the Commission on Crime Prevention and Criminal Justice (CCPCJ), a governing board of the United Nations Office on Drugs and Crime (UNODC), reported that prisons in 114 countries were filled beyond capacity. This was in respect of 198 countries with available data. In developing countries, overcrowding affects the prison system disproportionately. The highest rates were found in five regions, including Central, East and West Africa. Prisoners in overcrowded facilities are vulnerable to human rights violations, which qualified in 2013 as an inhumane treatment and torture according to the European Court of Human Rights. High rates of mental illness are experienced by prisoners, which could lead to violence and abuse, the by-products of overcrowding with marked consequences (Bantjes, Swartz, & Niewoudt, 2017).

Human rights violations occur often among the prison population, especially the mentally ill prisoners. An example of this was reported in a study on human rights and mental health in post-apartheid South Africa, where participants explained that the prison is primarily meant to focus on control, security and confinement, and not a therapeutic environment. They further reported that it is difficult or impossible to institute any form of psychological intervention or provide any care to prisoners with mental health challenges (Bantjes et al., 2017). A participant reported that *"The correctional services are little more geared to treating people with more normal physical, not mental health symptoms, and once they then become severe they would say, transfer the person to hospital … ."* This is because health care facilities within the prison are more equipped to manage medical or physical conditions, rather than psychiatric or psychosocial care (Bantjes et al., 2017).

In an Egyptian prison, reports showed that mentally ill inmates are brutally beaten for unacceptable behaviors, even though they are not responsible for such behaviors due to their mental incapacity. They are left on their own until they deteriorate. Inmates also reported maltreatment in their first contact with the prison. These include insults, body searches described as degrading and aimed at breaking the prisoner upon arrival (Egyptian Initiative for Personal Rights, 2014). A documentary from Kenya showed human rights abuses at Mathari Psychiatric Hospital, where a dead person was found lying next to another live person with a psychosocial disability in a seclusion cell (McKenzie, 2011). Additionally, in Kenya, a report from the Special Rapporteur on torture says solitary confinement cannot be justified as a form of treatment or therapy for mentally disordered offenders – "prolonged solitary confinement and seclusion of persons may constitute torture or ill-treatment" says the report (McKenzie, 2011).

Mental health legislation as it relates to the treatment of prisoners across Africa

In Africa, 64% of the countries have either non-existent or obsolete mental health laws. Most of the mental health laws have remained as they were inherited from the colonial era. For instance, in Nigeria there is no new national mental health legislation that provides for the proper treatment of prisoners with mental illness (Ogunlesi & Ogunwale, 2018). However, the Lagos state of Nigeria succeeded in passing a state law in 2019. The Lunacy Law in current use within the country has no sufficient provision for the treatment of offenders with mental health challenges while incarcerated (Laws of Nigeria, 1948). The Nigerian Lunacy Law of 1959 (originally enacted as an "ordinance" in 1916) is still the legislation in place, despite ongoing attempts to pass a proposed mental health and substance abuse law, which was last deliberated upon in the Nigeria senate in 2019. Egypt was the first country in Africa to have a Mental Health Act in 1944. This was revised in 2009 by the Egyptian parliament and termed "Care of Psychiatric Patients Act" (Hamaoui et al., 2009). It included changes in the penal code and introduced for the first time the concept that there is no criminal responsibility for individuals who have lost their perception and diminished responsibility for individuals who lack perception (Hamaoui et al., 2009). Tunisia enacted its law in 1992 and reviewed it in 2004. It focuses on conditions of hospitalization for individuals with mental disorders and mechanisms to oversee involuntary treatment practices (Ministry of Health Tunisia and WHO, 2008). Algeria, on the other hand, created its law in 1985 that highlights mechanisms for the protection of the mentally ill, the promotion of mental health and the processes for the admission of mentally ill patients, as well as how to protect their rights (Touari & Bensmail, 1990).

Kenya passed a new law in 1989 but is yet to implement the law due to lack of funds to train the multidisciplinary staff (Bartlett et al., 2011). However, the law was revised in 2012 as Mental Health Act chapter 248 (Ndetei et al., 2017). Mental Health Care Act 2002 in South Africa has transformed mental health services and particularly improved the quality of care of persons with mental disorders. It successfully resulted in the shifting of care from psychiatric institutions to general hospitals (Ramlall, 2012). However, infrastructural constraints and shortage of mental health professionals hampered the integration of services into primary health care. Little attention was given to health promotion, prevention and rehabilitation (Ramlall, 2012). Resource constraint for the mental health review boards, weak political will and administrative challenges all impeded the comprehensive implementation of the Act. Greater resource investment is needed to ensure its success (Ramlall, 2012). Uganda has a new Mental Health Law with the latest international human rights standards that highlighted the protection and promotion of human rights, deinstitutionalization, social inclusion, community integration of mental health care, safety and quality and intersectoral collaboration (Mental Health and Poverty project, 2010). Ghana passed the Mental Health Act into law successfully in 2012, which was a major milestone (Doku, Wusu-Takyi, & Awakame, 2012). It addressed the issues of mental health and human rights protection of persons with mental health disorders in Ghana. However, there are numerous challenges for the implementation of the Ghana Mental Health Act (Doku et al., 2012). A recent study in Zimbabwe identified five themes as key to mental health services delivery in the country, which included Mental Health Law and Policy (Kidia, Machando, Mangezi, Hendler, & Crooks, 2017). The priorities were to explore forensic care and mental health integration. The authors highlighted forensic services as central components of the mental health system which has been a neglected concept (Kidia et al., 2017).

Many of the obsolete laws placed emphasis on incapacity and involuntary treatment and failed to adequately promote voluntary treatment on the basis of informed consent. This goes contrary to the International standards on human rights. Older laws presumed people with mental health challenges lacked the capacity to consent for treatment and to make decisions or exercise their fundamental human rights. Institutional care was promoted in the old laws especially in psychiatric institutions where the violation of human rights of mentally ill persons is often prevalent. The laws also failed to promote respect, autonomy and dignity of persons with mental health challenges. The aim of the new mental health legislation in many countries is the promotion, protection and improvement of the lives and mental well-being of those with mental disorders.

Services planning and evidence-based approach: A model for African prison settings

The primary purpose of legislation relating to mental health is to promote high standards of care and best practices in mental health services delivery. Persons with mental health challenges have an array of needs that could be biological, psychological and/or social. They may therefore need to have access to several professionals, not only doctors and nurses but also psychologists, social workers, occupational therapists and other professionals. For a comprehensive and holistic mental health service to persons with mental health challenges, research has provided evidence for a multidisciplinary team approach (McKenna et al., 2015). This was found to be the most effective means of service delivery. The strength of this approach is the coming together of various professionals to deliver seamless services through combined expertise. The multidisciplinary team working in the prison system focuses on ensuring continuity of care across a range of needs for prisoners even as they transit the gate (Jarrett et al., 2012). This model of care impacts positively as it detects those in need of assistance (Pillai et al., 2016) and improves their engagement with mental health services post-release. It increasingly focuses on reducing re-offending post-release.

The US Department of Justice made a program statement for the treatment and care of inmates with mental health challenges. This follows a change in service provision for this category of inmates. The modifications incorporated the establishment of detailed and prioritized evidence-based practices for the treatment and care of mentally challenged offenders in prison. Operationalization of mental health care at systematic levels, which include diagnostic, impairment and intervention-based criteria with additional care-level-based treatment as well as documentation when required is important. Team-based approach to mental health care provision, as well as enhanced procedures for screening; evaluation and intervention with inmates' restrictive housing setting were emphasized. Mental health training for staff was outlined and specialty training for interested staff. The establishment of a mental health companion program for inmates with mental health challenges so as to provide peer support and assistance for one another during incarceration was stressed. For inmates who participate in the mental health programming, achievement awards were given. Finally, the procedures for mentally challenged inmates were updated and refined with respect to designation, transfer and release, with emphasis on continuity of care both across institutions and to the community (US Department of Justice, 2014).

Policies and legislations are increasingly focusing on interagency collaboration for mental health services in the prisons (Department of Health and Concordat signatories, 2014). These involve the police, criminal justice system, mental health providers and also the social services. This collaboration involves a range of functions including joint decision making with limited shared resources to fully integrate services. The three core principles involved are information sharing, joint decision making and coordinated intervention (Home Office, 2013, 2014). Even though the police often serve as the first contact for persons with mental health challenges, mental illness is poorly recognized and poorly handled by the police. Therefore, several people end up detained rather than receiving treatment at the right place (Sainsbury Centre for Mental Health, 2009).

Therapeutic jurisprudence involves collaborating with the legal system to view cases from the therapeutic lens (Kenna, Skipworth, & Pillai, 2017). For instance, psychosocial challenges could result in criminal behavior and without understanding this, offenders may revolve in and out of the prison doors. Mental illness, substance dependence and social care needs are all linked to crime and therefore understanding this through the legal lens will go a long way in dealing with reoffending (Kenna et al., 2017). Through this solution-focused approach, courts took advantage of using the legal process to encourage people to address the causes of offending and involve the social agencies that can assist the individuals (Wiener, Winick, Georges, & Castro, 2010). This is better than the old-fashioned punishment for a crime approach, without understanding the cause.

A paradigm shift in youth justice custodial services showed trauma-informed model of care involves collaboration with families and wider social networks to facilitate and support the recovery and resilience of young people (Ford, Kerig, Desai, & Feierman, 2016). Evidence from research showed that youths who are involved in the justice system are usually exposed to high rates of trauma. Traumatic exposure could result in offending behaviors due to the negative impact of the trauma. This increases the likelihood for mental illness and involvement with the criminal justice system (Ford et al., 2016). Trauma-informed model of treatment can be used for the treatment of traumatized inmates, both males and females. Studies have found post-traumatic stress disorder and exposure to violence to be higher among prisoners than the general population (Miller & Najavits, 2012). Other trauma triggers such as environmental, sensory and perceived presence of authority can all become threats to incarcerated individuals. Evidence shows that trauma-informed care and using evidence-based cognitive behavioral therapy (CBT) has promise in reducing criminal risk factors. It supports the integrated program for substance-abusing offenders with co-occurring disorders (Miller & Najavits, 2012).

Psychologically Informed Planned Environments (PIPEs) are designed specifically for staff members so as to have additional training to enable them to have psychological understanding in the context of their work (Castledine, 2015). In correctional settings, it serves to develop a supportive environment to facilitate the development of inmates, especially those with mental health challenges. The environment is built on an already-existing structure, to enhance the promotion of a healthy environment for inmates, thus reducing risk behaviors, improving psychological well-being and encouraging prosocial life (Castledine, 2015). It is for inmates with personality disorders or complex needs.

Evidence-based practices in African prisons for the treatment of mentally disordered offenders is almost non-existent. The forensic psychiatry field is shrouded in confusion as many of those working in the field are self-taught individuals or forced by time to be in the field (Njenga, 2006). Many African countries do not have current Mental Health Legislation (MHL). In Nigeria, the Correctional Service Act which was signed into law on 8th of August 2019, repealed the Prison Service Act and changed the "Nigeria Prisons Service" to "Nigeria Correctional Service." This new Act provides changes and modifications to the repealed Act. The current Act (section 25) empowers authorities to transfer inmates who are of unsound mind or are seriously ill to the hospital. The Correctional Service Act sections 24–25 discussed the management of mentally disordered offenders. In the area of training for forensic mental health personnel, a publication by Ogunlesi et al. (2012) reported that international collaboration for forensic psychiatry training is difficult in Africa due to the variation in legislative frameworks of several countries. This may, to an extent, limit the continent's ability to provide a consensual evidence-based practice on the subject. Teamwork involving intersectoral collaboration with criminal justice system, police and social welfare among others in Africa as a whole is difficult. This is due to religious, cultural and linguistic challenges. Mentally challenged persons in the prison have more total needs on average and significantly more unmet needs than their general adult patient counterparts (Harty, Tighe, Leese, Parrott, & Thornicroft, 2003). The unmet needs include psychological distress, psychotic symptoms, daytime activities, money, welfare benefits, food and company (Harty et al., 2003). These needs cannot be handled by a single professional. Due to their vulnerability in the correctional setting, mentally ill inmates may have several challenges in the areas of accommodation, work, education, discipline and transfer. By using the team approach model, this is feasible because the needs of inmates with mental illness are identified and addressed. With teamwork, mental health symptoms are recorded, conflicts in cells with cell mates are prevented, leisure/work deficits are known, bullying and abuse by other inmates are reported and escalation of dangerous behavior is prevented.

The provision of basic care benefits prisoners with mental health challenges. When such needs are unmet, their mental well-being deteriorates. Some of the expected changes in Africa should include the domains of accommodation, physical and mental health needs of mentally ill inmates and safety consideration. For example, Section 14 (8b) of the Correctional Services Act of Nigeria says that "The correctional service shall take adequate step to ensure the prevention of inhumane and degrading treatment against inmates." Furthermore, Section 14 (1) of the 2019 Correctional Services Act of Nigeria states that the "correctional service shall provide opportunities for education, training. Vocational training, as well as training in modern farming techniques and animal husbandry for inmates" (Nigerian Correctional Service Act, 2019).

With a recovery-oriented program model, a lot can be achieved for inmates with mental illness. In said model of treatment, recovery should be the guiding principle. This is the ability to live, work, learn and participate fully in the community. According to the National Consensus Statement on Mental Health Recovery, ten fundamental components of recovery were listed. These include self-direction, individualized and person-centered care, empowerment, holistic treatment, nonlinear progression, strengths-based focus, peer support, respect, responsibility and hope (Harty et al., 2003). A study by Durcan (2008) of men, women, young men, and juvenile prisoners' views of their needs reported that "having someone to talk to" was the best way to improve their mental health. This could be a psychiatrist, therapist or peer mentor. Doing something meaningful was reported as a need for inmates. Prisoners need to be active and those with mental health problems are not different. There is strong evidence that work helps mentally challenged inmates to recover (cited in World Health Organization, 2014). In the prison for young adults and children, education should be part of a purposeful activity to keep them engaged. They also saw therapy and medication as a need. This entails getting the right medication and support to use it. Advocacy was recognized as a need by the studied inmates due to the harsh nature of the prison environment, especially for mentally disordered inmates. Even when the right help is available, seeking it might be difficult. Therefore, the need to have someone who can talk for them and represent their needs, such as health professionals, is significant for them.

Challenges associated with the increasing prevalence of severe and persistent mentally ill offenders in prisons have come to stay and may not disappear in a long time, especially in Africa. Homegrown methods for providing better mental health care for such populations need to be explored. In pursuance of this objective, developing an acute care psychiatric unit within the prison can be an option. The advantage of creating an acute psychiatric unit within the prison is that it will provide a therapeutic milieu compatible with the correctional service mission. It also ensures a safe and proper implementation of specialized treatment, which includes involuntary administration of medication for offenders with serious mental illness who are not compliant and proper implementation of therapeutic restraints as well as seclusion (Daniel, 2007). This model will incur additional expenditure on the part of the correctional services. It will, however, reduce the expenditure that will be incurred with the transfer of offenders back and forth between the prisons and mental health hospitals, mitigate the ensuing security challenges, as well as conflicts within departments and the problems with communication in the handling of offenders. The conflicts will include admission criteria, type and level of care, and also access to medical records. Lastly, when the offender returns to the prison, conflicts in handling conduct violation may arise (Daniel, 2007).

On the other hand, the expansion of psychiatric hospitals to include the provision of secure units for offenders with mental health challenges that require admission into the hospital outside the correctional service facility is an alternative. Such resources will provide inpatient and outpatient treatment in a secure mental health system (Lamb & Weinberger, 2005). It will serve severe mentally ill persons and divert those individuals who are most difficult to treat and manage away from the correctional services setting. Establishing these secure units within psychiatric hospitals will not just be appropriate for the treatment of this population, it will also prevent their labeling as criminals. It will likely not cost much and might even be less expensive than providing such care in the correctional service facility (Lamberg, 2004). A hybrid model of a separate mental health service facility in the prison and the provision of secure units in psychiatric hospitals to cater for the severely mentally ill may be the better direction to go.

In the context of Nigeria and most other parts of Africa, correctional services have not been privatized. Therefore, an exploration of a partnership between the psychiatric hospitals and correctional services, where the hospitals provide manpower and structure while the correctional service pays the bill for treatment as well as provides security while the mentally ill inmate is on admission at the hospital may be considered. There could also be partnerships between the correctional services, the psychiatric hospitals and security organizations with defined roles each partner will provide. In addition, with the privatization of correctional services in some developed countries and South Africa on the African continent, is there a potential for the private sector to provide both correctional-related facilities and treatment services outside the government-established correctional facilities? This is an issue that deserves consideration in an era where the private sector is increasingly becoming dominant actors in health and security provision.

Finally, in times of epidemics and pandemics, it is important to have guiding principles in correctional facilities. This is because correctional facilities typically house large numbers of persons in closed and overcrowded conditions for long periods of time. The recent COVID-19 pandemic highlights the importance of outbreak prevention and containment preparedness, particularly in congregate settings like correctional services. This group of people may be more vulnerable than others to the psychosocial effects of pandemics. Those at heightened risk include individuals living in congregate settings (prisoners generally), prisoners with pre-existing physical, mental, substance-use disorders and aged prisoners. These individuals are at an increased risk for adverse psychosocial outcomes (Pfefferbaum & North, 2020). Outbreaks in correctional facilities can easily spread to the surrounding community. As such, correctional facilities must remain vigilant for infectious/communicable disease outbreaks and should have prevention and control plans in place (Ogunwale, Majekodunmi, Ajayi, & Abdulmalik, 2020).

All correctional facilities should designate a frontline staff or first responder to oversee disease control efforts, psychosocial needs of prisoners and to work with partners in the facility (e.g., administrative and medical staff) as well as in the community (e.g., health departments). Education and training regarding psychosocial issues should be provided to health system leaders, first responders and health care professionals. With the consent of the facility's chief medical officer, first responders should follow explicit protocols that are adapted for the specific condition. These conditions vary depending on the severity of the disease as well as the mode and rapidity of transmission such as COVID-19 infections. The first responder must establish clear definitions for possible and confirmed cases, categorize cases appropriately and update this information as needed (Parvez, Lobato, & Greifinger, 2010).

Multidisciplinary planning among the medical leadership, correctional facility administration and the staff unions is essential. Ongoing communication, education and transparency with staff and inmates will allay fears. Likewise, an ongoing partnership with local or state health departments is critical for preparedness. Correctional staff should develop policies and protocols that complement local emergency preparedness plans for mental health and psychosocial needs, and they should work with local public health authorities to ensure that correctional facilities are included in local emergency plans for the allocation of resources (e.g., isolation rooms, masks, medications, among others) (Parvez et al., 2010). Recent research suggests that policy makers should implement criminal justice policies that will protect the health of inmates and correctional staff without endangering public safety (Yang, 2020). Some of the responses in pandemics should include releasing medically vulnerable inmates, including those with severe mental health challenges (Ogunwale et al., 2020), and limiting pre-trial detention for persons charged with non-violent offenses.

References

Adewunmi, A. T. (2018). Learning disabilities evidences among convicts with criminal behaviour in Ibadan prison. *AJPSSI*, *21*(3), 1–14.

Administration Centrale Pénitentiaire (Morocco). (2006). Bulletin Statistique.

African Commission on Human and Peoples' Rights (ACHPR). (2004). South Africa: Prisons and Detention Conditions – 2004/South Africa/States/ACHPR. Gambia. http://www.achpr.org/states/south-africa/missions/prisons-2004/. Accessed 26 December 2019.

Al-Rousan, T., Rubenstein, L., Sieleni, B., Deol, H., et al. (2017). Inside the nation's largest mental health institution: A prevalence study in a state prison system. *BMC Public Health*, *17*, 342. doi: 10.1186/s12889-017-4257-0

Armiya'u, A. Y. (2019). Psychiatric morbidity and factors among homicide offenders in a Nigerian prison: A comparative analysis. Unpublished thesis submitted to Universidad Central De Nicaragua.

Armiya'u, A. Y., & Adole, O. (2015). Relationship between sociodemographic characteristics, psychiatric burden and violent offence in a maximum-security prison in north-central Nigeria. *Journal of Forensic Science & Criminology*, *3*(2), 1–6. doi: 10.15744/2348-9804.2.502

Armiya'u, A. Y., Audu, M. D., Obembe, A., Umar, U. M., & Adole, O. (2013). A study of psychiatric morbidity and co-morbid physical illness among convicted and awaiting trial inmates in Jos prison. *Journal of Forensic and Legal Medicine*, *20*, 1048–1051.

Armiya'u, A. Y., Obembe, A., Audu, M. D., & Afolaranmi, T. O. (2013). Prevalence of psychiatric morbidity among inmates in Jos maximum security prison. *Open Journal of Psychiatry*, *3*, 12–17.

Atilola, O. (2013). Juvenile/youth justice management in Nigeria: Making a case for diversion programmes. *Youth Justice*, *13*, 3–16.

Bantjes, J., Swartz, L., & Niewoudt, P. (2017). Human rights and mental health in post-apartheid South Africa: Lessons from health care professionals working with suicidal inmates in the prison system. *BMC International Health and Human Rights*, *17*, 29. doi: 10.1186/s12914-017-0136-0

Baranyi, G., Cassidy, M., Fazel, S., Priebe, S., et al. (2018). Prevalence of posttraumatic stress disorder in prisoners. *Epidemiologic Reviews*, *40*(1), 166.

Barnert, E. S., Perry, R., & Morris, R. E. (2016). Juvenile incarceration and health. *Academic Pediatrics*, *16*, 99–109.

Bartlett, P., Jenkins, R., & Kiima, D. (2011). Mental health law in the community: thinking about Africa. *International Journal of Mental Health Systems*, *5*(1), 1.

Bella, T. T., Atilola, O., & Omigbodun, O. O. (2010). Children within the juvenile justice system in Nigeria: Psychopathology and psychosocial needs. *Annals Ibadan Postgraduate Medicine*, *8*, 34–39.

Bliss, K. W. (2018). BJS Report find prisoner sexual abuse allegations continue to rise. Available on http://www.prisonlegalnews.org/news/2018/dec/7/bjs-report-finds-prisoner-sexual-abuse-allegations-continue-rise. Accessed 27 January 2020.

Boxer, P., Middlemass, K., & Delorenzo, T. (2009). Exposure to violent crime during incarceration: Effects on psychological adjustment following release. *Criminal Justice and Behaviour*, *38*(8), 793–807.

Brower, M. C., & Price, B. H. (2000). Epilepsy and violence: When is the brain to blame? *Epilepsy Behaviour*, *1*, 145–149.

Cape Argus. (2009). South Africa: Local woman in hospital after prison beating. Retrieved from http://allafrica.com/stories/200902160947.html. Accessed 18 January 2020.

Castledine, S. (2015). Psychologically informed and planned environments: A community perspective. *Probation Journal*, *62*(3), 273–280.

Chin, J. (2012). Epilepsy treatment in sub-Saharan Africa: Closing the gap. *African Health Sciences*, *12*, 186–192.

Chodos, A. H., Ahalt, C., Cenzer, I. S., & Goldenson, J. (2013). Characteristics of older adults who use the emergency room prior to jail detainment. *Journal of General Internal Medicine. Conference: 36th Annual Meeting of the Society of General Internal Medicine, SGIM 2013. Denver, CO United States. Conference Start: 20130424.Conference End: 20130427. Conference Publication: (var.pagings)* (p. 28).

Clancy, M. J., Clarke, M. C., Connor, D. J., Cannon, M., & Cotter, D. R. (2014). The prevalence of psychosis in epilepsy: A systematic review and meta-analysis. *BMC Psychiatry*, *14*, 75.

Coid, J. W., Ullrich, S., Kallis, C., Keers, R., et al. (2013). The relationship between delusions and violence: Findings from East London first episode psychosis study. *JAMA Psychiatry*, *70*, 465–471.

Commonwealth Human Rights Initiative (CHRI), Africa Office. (2011). Juvenile Justice in Ghana. A study to assess the status of juvenile justice in Ghana. Commonwealth Human Rights Initiative (CHRI), Africa Office, Accra, 2011. www.humanrightsinitiative.org/publications/ghana/JuvenileJusticeinGhana.pdf. Accessed 20 December 2019.

Daniel, A. (2007). Care of the mentally ill in prisons: Challenges and solutions. *Journal of American Academy of Psychiatry Law*, *35*, 406–410.

Davies, Mathew. (2011). The reintegration of elderly prisoners: An exploration of services provided in England and Wales. *Internet Journal of Criminology* www.internetjournalofcriminology.com Retrieved on 13 January 2020.

Department of Health and Concordat signatories. (2014). *Improving outcomes for people experiencing mental health crisis*. London: HM Government.

Dogbe, J., Owusu-Dabo, E., Edusei, A., et al. (2016). Assessment of prison life of persons with disability in Ghana. *BMC International Health and Human Rights*, *16*, 20. http://doi.org/10.1186/s12914-016-0094-y

Doku, V. C. K., Wusu-Takyi, A., & Awakame, J. (2012). Implementing Mental Health Act in Ghana: Any challenges ahead? *Ghana Medical Journal*, *46*(4), 241–250.

Durcan, G. (2008). *From the inside: Experiences of prison mental health care*. London, Sainsbury Centre for Mental Health, 2008. http://www.centreformentalhealth.org.uk/pdfs/From_the_Inside.pdf. Accessed 10 April 2020

Egyptian Initiative for Personal Rights. (2014). Health in Egyptian Prisons: A field study on the determinants of health behind bars. Retrieved from https://eipr.org>reports>pdf. Accessed 14 May 2020.

Fatoye, F. O., Fatoye, G. K., Oyebanji, A. O., & Ogunro, A. S. (2006). Psychological characteristics as correlates of emotional burden in incarcerated offenders in Nigeria. *East Africa Medical Journal*, *83*(10), 545–552.

Fazel, S., & Grann, M. (2006). The population impact of severe mental illness on violent crime. The American Journal of Psychiatry, *163*(8), 1397–1403.

Fazel, S., Hayes, A. J., Bartellas, K., Clerici, M., & Trestman, R. (2016). The mental health of prisoners: A review of prevalence, adverse outcome and intervention. *Lancet Psychiatry*, *3*(9), 871–881. doi: 10.1016/S2215-0366(16)30142-0

Fellner, J. (2006). A corrections quandary: Mental illness and prison rules. *Harvard Civil Rights – Civil Liberties Law Review*, *41*, 391–412.

Fontebo, H. N. (2013). Prison conditions in Cameroon: The narrative of female inmates. Retrieved from https://www.semanticscholar.org/paper/Prison-conditions-in-Cameroon%3A-the-narratives-of-Fontebo/2e72e8c915475d23a570beebaeb467e407d842fe. Accessed 24 January 2020.

Ford, J. D., Kerig, P. K., Desai, N., & Feierman, J. (2016). Psychosocial interventions for traumatized youth in the juvenile justice system: Research, evidence base, and clinical/legal challenges. *OJJDP Journal of Juvenile Justice*, *5*, 31–49.

Gray, M., & Littlefield, M. B. (2002). Black women and addiction. In: S. L. A. Straussner, & S. Brown (Eds.). The Handbook of Addiction Treatment for Women: Theory and Practice (pp. 301–322). San Francisco: Jossey-Bass.

Gustafson, R. (1994). Alcohol and aggression. *Journal of Offender Rehabiltation*, *21*(3-4), 41–48.

Haesen, S., Merkt, H., Imber, A., & Elger, B. et al. (2019). Substance use disorder and other mental health disorders among older prisoners. *International Journal of Law and Psychiatry*, *62*, 20–31.

Hamaoui, Y. El., Moussaoui, D., & Okasha, T. (2009). Forensic psychiatry in North Africa. *Current Opinion in Psychiatry*, *22*, 507–510.

Harty, M. A., Tighe, J., Leese, M., Parrott, J., & Thornicroft, G. (2003). Inverse care for mentally ill prisoners: Unmet needs in forensic mental health services. *The Journal of Forensic Psychiatry and Psychology*, *14*(3), 600–614.

Home Office. (2013). *Multi-agency working and information sharing project early findings*. London: Home Office.

Home Office. (2014). *Multi-agency working and information sharing project: Final report*. London, UK: Home Office.

Human Rights Watch (HRW). (2010). Unjust and unhealthy HIV, TB, and abuse in Zambian prisons 2010. New York. https://www.hrw.org/report/2010/04/27/unjust-and-unhealthy/hiv-tb-and-abuse-zambian-prisons. Accessed 24 January 2020.

Institute for Crime and Justice Policy Research. (2020). World Prison Brief Data. https://prisonstudies.org/map/africa. Accessed 12 February 2020.

IRIN Africa. (2003). Sudan: Women and children in prison. Retrieved from http://www.irinnews.org.Report.aspx?ReportId=45598. Accessed 20 January 2020.

Jacobson, J., Sabuni, P., & Talbot, J. (2017). Disability and the criminal justice system in Zambia. *Journal of Intellectual Disabilities and Offending Behaviour*, *8*(2), 59–69. http://doi.org/10.1108/JIDOB-12-2016-0023

Jarrett, M., Thornicroft, G., Forrester, A., et al. (2012). Continuity of care for recently released prisoners with mental illness: A pilot randomised controlled trial testing the feasibility of a Critical Time Intervention. *Epidemiology and Psychiatric Sciences*, *21*, 187–193.

Kakoullis, A., Le Mesurier, N., & Kingston, P. (2010). The mental health of older prisoners. *International Psychogeriatrics*, *22*(5), 693–701. https://doi.org/10.1017/S1041610210000359

Kenna, B. M. C., Skipworth, J., & Pillai, K. (2017). Mental health care and treatment in prisons: A new paradigm to support best practice. *World Psychiatry*, *6*(1), 3–4.

Kidia, K., Machando, D., Mangezi, W., Hendler, R., & Crooks, M. (2017). Mental health in Zimbabwe: A health systems analysis. *The Lancet Psychiatry*, *4*(11), 876–886.

Kinyanjui, D. M. C., & Atwoli, L. (2013). Substance use among inmates at the Eldoret prison in Western Kenya. *BMC Psychiatry*, *13*, 53. doi: 10.1186/1471-244X-13-53

Kron J. (2009). 20 women raped in DR Congo Prison Riot. Daily Nation. Available on http://www.nation.co.ke/News/africa/-/1066/614476/-/139e937z/-/index.html. Accessed 18 January 2020.

Kuhns, J. B., & Clodfelter, T. A. (2009). Illicit drug-related psychopharmacological violence: The current understanding within a causal context. *Aggression and Violent Behavior*, *14*(1), 69–78.

Lamb, H. R., & Weinberger, L. E. (2005). The shift of psychiatric inpatient care from hospitals to jails and prisons. *Journal of the American Academy of Psychiatry and the Law*, *33*, 529–534.

Lamberg, L. (2004). Efforts grow to keep mentally ill out of jails. *JAMA*, *292*, 555–556.

Lambie, I., & Randell, I. (2013). The impact of incarceration on juvenile offenders. *Clinical Psychology Review*, *33*, 448–459.

Large, M., Smith, G., & Nielssen, G. (2009). The relationship between the rate of homicide by those with schizophrenia and the overall homicide rate: A systematic review and meta-analysis. *Schizophenia Research*, *112*(1–3), 123–129.

Laws of the Federation of Nigeria. (2004). *Criminal Procedure Act CAP.* C41 Vol. 4, Federal Ministry of Justice.

Laws of Nigeria. (1948). *Lunacy Ordinance*, Vol. IV, CAP. 121, Government Printer.

Lennox, C. (2014). The health needs of young people in prison. *British Medical Bulletin*, *112*, 17–25.

Lovett, A., Kwon, H., Kidia, K., Machando, D., et al. (2019). Mental health of people detained within the criminal justice system in Africa: Systematic review and meta-analysis. *International Journal of Mental Health Systems*, *13*, 31. https://doi.org/10.1186/s13033-019-0273-z

Majekodunmi, O. E., Obadeji, A., Oluwole, L. O., & Oyelami, O. (2017). Depression and associated physical comorbidities in elderly prison inmates. *International Journal of Mental Health*, *46*(4), 269–283. doi: 10.1080/00207411.2017.1345040

Marsh, L., & Krauss, G. C. (2000). Aggression and violence in patients with epilepsy. *Epilepsy & Behavior*, *1*, 160–168.

McKenna, B., Skipworth, J., Tapsell, R., et al. (2015). A prison mental health in-reach model informed by assertive community treatment principles: Evaluation of its impact on planning during the pre-release period, community mental health service engagement and reoffending. *Criminal Behaviour and Mental Health, 25*, 429–439.

McKenzie, D. (2011). Rights groups accuse Kenya of patient abuse. Part of complete coverage on World's Untold Stories, CNN World. Retrieved from www.cnn.com>africa>kenya.health. Accessed 27 June 2020.

Mental Health and Poverty project. (2010). Mental Health Law reform in Uganda. Retrieved from https://assets.publishing.service.gov.uk/media/57a08b0aed915d622c000a71/MHPB_Uganda3.pdf. Accessed 28 January 2020.

Mersey Region Epilepsy Association. (2019). Epilepsy in prison – A guide for prison staff. Retrieved from www.epilepsymersey.org.uk/docs/prison.pdf. Accessed 25 January 2020.

Miczek, K. A. (1997). Alcohol, GABA-Benzodiazepine receptor complex and aggression. In M., Galanter (Ed.), *Recent development in alcoholism* (Vol. 13, pp. 139–171). New York: Plenum Press.

Miller, N. A., & Najavits, L. M. (2012). Creating trauma-informed correctional care: A balance of goals and environment. *European Journal of Psychotraumatology, 3*, 17246. doi: 10.3402/ejpt.v3i0.17246.

Ministry of Health Morocco and WHO. (2006). A report of the assessment of the mental health system in Morocco using the World Health Organization: Assessment Instrument for Mental Health Systems (WHO-AIMS). Rabat, Morocco.

Ministry of Health Tunisia and WHO. (2008). A report of the assessment of the mental health system in Tunisia using the World Health Organization - Assessment Instrument for Mental Health Systems (WHO-AIMS). Tunis, Tunisia.

Moschetti, K., Stadelmann, P., Wangmo, T., Holly, A., Bodenmann, P., Wasserfallen, J. B., & Gravier, B. (2015). Disease profiles of detainees in the Canton of Vaud in Switzerland: Gender and age differences in substance abuse, mental health and chrocic health conditions. *BMC Public Health, 15*, 872. https://doi.org/10.1186/s12889-015-2211-6

Mosotho, N. L., Bambo, D., Mkhombo, T., Mgidlana, C., Motsumi, N. Matlhabe, T., Joubert, G., & Roux, H. E. L. (2020). Demographic, clinical, and forensic profiling of alleged offenders diagnosed with an intellectual disability. *Journal of Forensic Psychology Research and Practice, 4*, 362–376. doi: 10.1080/24732850.2020.1742004. http://doi.org/10.1080/24732850.2020.1742004

Naudts, K. H., Cosyns, P., Mcinnery, T., Audenaert, K., et al. (2005). Belgium and its internees: A problem for human rights and a stimulus for service change. *Criminal Behaviour and Mental Health, 15*, 148–153.

Ndetei, D. M., Muthike, J., & Nandoya, E. S. (2017). Kenya's mental health law, *The British Journal of Psychiatry, 14*(4), 96–97.

NICRO submission. (2011). Department of correctional Services Budget Vote 21. http://www.issafrica.org/crimehub/uploads/110316nicro_0.pdf

Nigerian Correctional Service Act. (2019). Nigerian Service Act, 2019 – Policy and Legal Advocacy Center. Retrieved from https://placng.org/Nigerian-Correctional-Service-Act-2019.pdf. Accessed 13 July 2020.

Njenga, F. G. (2006). Forensic psychiatry: The African experience. World Psychiatry, *5*(2), 97.

Nowotny, K. M., Cepeda, A., James-Hawkins, L., & Boardman, J. D. (2016). Growing old behind bars: Health profiles of the older male inmate population in the United States. *Journal of Aging and Health*, *28*(6), 935–956. https://doi.org/10.1177/0898264315614007

Ogunlesi, A. O., & Ogunwale, A. (2018). Correctional psychiatry in Nigeria: Dynamics of mental healthcare in the most restrictive alternative. *BJPSYCH International*, *15*(2), 35–38. doi: 10.1192/bji.2017.13

Ogunlesi, A. O., Ogunwale, A., Wet, P. De., Roos, L., & Kaliski, S. (2012). Forensic psychiatry in Africa: Prospects and challenges. *African Journal of Psychiatry*, *15*, 3–7.

Ogunwale, A., Majekodunmi, O. E., Ajayi, S. O., & Abdulmalik, J. (2020). Forensic mental health service implications of COVID-19 in Nigeria. *Forensic Science International: Mind and Law*, *1*, 100026. http://doi.org/10.1016/j.fsiml.2020.100026

Ojo, M. O. D., & Okunola, R. A. (2014). The plights of aged inmates in Nigerian prison system: A survey of two prisons in Ogun state, Nigeria. *Bangladesh e-Journal of Sociology*, *11*(1), 54–73.

Owusu, G., Wrigley-Asante, C., Oteng-Ababio, M., & Owusu, A. Y. (2015). Crime prevention through environmental design (CPTED) and built-environmental manifestations in Accra and Kumasi, Ghana. *Crime Prevention & Community Safety*, *17*(4), 270–290.

Owusu, G., Oteng-Ababio, M., Owusu, A. Y., & Wrigley-Asante, C. (2016a). Can poor neighbourhoods be correlated with crime? Evidence from urban Ghana. *Ghana Geographical Jou*, *8*(1), 11–31. Special Issue.

Owusu, G., Owusu, A. Y., Oteng-Ababio, M., Wrigley-Asante, C., & Agyapong, I. (2016b). An assessment of households' perceptions of private security companies and crime in urban Ghana. *Crime Science*, *5*(5), 1–11. doi: 10.1186/s40163-016-0053-x

Parvez, F. M., Lobato, M. N., & Greifinger, R. B. (2010). Tuberculosis control: Lessons from outbreak preparedness in Correctional facilities. *Journal of Correctional Health Care*, *16*(3), 239–242. doi: 10.1177/1078345810367593.

Penal Reform International. (2017). Global prison trends 2017. Penal Reform International. London. https://www.penalreform.org/resource/globalprison-trends-2017/. Accessed 22 January 2020.

Pfefferbaum, B., & North, C. S. (2020). Mental health and COVID-19 pandemic. *The New England Journal of Medicine*, *383*(510–512), 1–3. doi: 10.1056/NEJMp2008017

Pillai, K., Rouse, P., McKenna, B., & Skipworth, J., Cavney, J., Tapsell, R., & Madell, D. (2016). From positive screen to engagement in treatment: A preliminary study of the impact of a new model of care for prisoners with serious mental illness. *BMC Psychiatry*, *16*(1), 9.

Pro, G., & Marzell, M. (2017). Medical parole and aging prisoners: A qualitative study. *J Correct Health Care*, *23*(2), 162–172. https://doi.org/10.1177/1078345817699608

Rai, D., Kerr, M. P., McManus, S., Jordanova, V., Lewis, G., & Brugha, T. S. (2012). Epilepsy and psychiatric comorbidity: A nationally representative population-based study. *Epilepsia*, *53*(6), 1095–1103.

Ramlall, S. (2012). The Mental Health Care Act no 17 South Africa. Trials and triumphs: 2002–2012. *African Journal of Psychiatry*, *15*(6), 407–410.

Restel, M., & Rola, R. (2014). Epileptic seizures and epilepsy in case of people with alcohol dependency syndrome. *Neurologia Po Dyplomie*, *9*(5), 41–49.

Sainsbury Centre for Mental Health. (2009). *Diversion: A better way for criminal justice and mental health*. London: Nuffield Press.

Samakaya-Makarati, J. (2003). Female prisoners in "male" prisons. In C. Musengezi, & I. Staunton (Eds.), *A tragedy of lives: Women in prison in Zimbabwe*. Harare: Weaver Press.

Sarkin J. (2008). Prisons in Africa: An evaluation from a human rights perspective. *Sur Rev Int Direitos Hum, 5*, 22–51.

Schonteich, M. (2015). Hidden cruelties: Prison conditions in Sub-Saharan Africa. Retrieved from https://www.wporldpoliticsreview.com/articles/15366/hidden-cruelties-prison-conditions-in-sub-saharan-africa. Accessed 25 January 2020.

Stawinska-Witoszynka, B., Czechowska, K., & Wieckwska, B. (2019). The prevalence of epilepsy and its co-occurrence with alcohol dependence among Polish prisoners. *International Journal for Equity in Health, 18*, 102. https://doi.org/10.1186/s12939-019-1009-z

Stratton, J., Brook, M., & Hanlon, R. (2017). Murder and psychosis: Neuropsychological profiles of homicide offenders with schizophrenia. *Criminal Behaviour and Mental Health, 27*(2), 146–161. http://doi.org/10.1002/cbm.1990

Sukeri, K., Betancourt, O. A., Emsley, R., Nagdee, M., & Erlacher, H. (2016). Forensic mental health services: Current services provision and planning for a prison mental health service if the Eastern Cape. *South African Journal of Psychiatry, 22*(1), a787. http://dx.doi.org/10.4102/ sajpsychiatry. v22i1.787

Todrys, K. W., & Amon, J. J. (2011a). Health and human rights of women imprisoned in Zambia. *BMC International Health and Human Rights, 11*, 8. https://doi.org/10.1186/1472-698X-11-8

Todrys, K. W., & Amon, J. J. (2011b). Human rights and health among juvenile prisoners in Zambia. *Int J Prison Health, 7*(1), 10 – 17.

Topp, S., Moonga, C., Luo, N., Kaingu, M., Chileshe, C., et al. (2016). Exploring the drivers of health and healthcare access in Zambian prisons: A health systems approach. *HPP, 31*, 1250–1261.

Torrey, E. F., Kennard, A. D., Eslinger, D., et al. (2010). *More mentally ill persons are in jails and prisons than hospitals: A survey of the states*. Treatment Advocacy Center Arlington, VA.

Touari, M., & Bensmail, B. (1990). Epidemiology in legal psychiatry in the Constantinois: Results of a survey from 1963 to 1986. *Actualite's Psychiatriques, 20*, 28–31.

Uganda Prisons Service. (2009). *A Rapid Situation Assessment of Hiv/Sti/Tb and Drug Abuse Among Prisoners in Uganda*. Uganda Prisons Service and United Nations Office on Drugs and Crime, Prisons Service, Kampala, Uganda.

United Nations. (1989). United Nations (UN) general assembly. Convention on the rights of the child general comment no 24. CRC/C/GC/24. New York. Retrieved from http://www.ohchr.org/en/professionalinteresrt/pages/crc.aspx. Accessed 28 December 2019.

United Nations. (1990). Basic principles for the treatment of prisoners. Retrieved from: http://www.un.org/ruleoflaw/blog/document/basic-principles-for-the-treatment-of--prisoners.

United Nations. (2008). *Handbook for prison managers and policy makers on women and imprisonment: Criminal justice handbook series*. New York: United Nations.

United Nations Office on Drugs and Crime (UNODC). (2010). *International statistics on crime and justice*. Helsinki: European Institute for Crime Prevention and Control.

US Department of Justice. (2014). Review of the Federal Bureau of prison's. Use of restrictive housing for inmates with mental illness. Retrieved from: http://oig.justice.gov/report/2017/e1705.pdf.

United States Department of State Bureau of Democracy, Human Rights and Labor. (2014). Mali 2014 human rights report. Washington, DC. https://www.state.gov/documents/organization/236592.pdf. Accessed 20 January 2020.

United States Department of State Bureau of Democracy, Human Rights and Labor. (2017). Senegal 2017 human rights report. Washington, DC. https://www.state.gov/documents/organization/277283.pdf. Accessed 11 January 2020.

United States Department of State Bureau of Democracy, Human Rights and Labor. (2017). Gabon 2017 Human Rights Report. Washington, DC. https://www.state.gov/documents/organization/277245.pdf. Accessed 11 January 2020.

United States Department of State Bureau of Democracy, Human Rights and Labor. (2017). Swaziland 2017 Human Rights Report. Washington, DC. https://www.state.gov/documents/organization/277297.pdf. Accessed 24 December 2019.

UNOWA. (2007). Urbanization and insecurity in West Africa: Population movements, mega cities and regional stability, Dakar: UNOWA.

Van Hout, M-R, & Mhlanga-Gunda, R. (2019). Prison health situation and health rights of young people incarcerated in Sub-Saharan Africa prisons and detention centers: A scoping review of extant literature. *BMC International Health and Human Rights*, *19*, 17. https://doi.org/10.1186/s12914-019-0200-z

Van Voorhis, P., Wright, E. M., Salisbury, E. J., & Bauman, A. (2010). Women's risk factors and their contributions to existing risk/needs assessment: The current status of a gender-responsive supplement. *Criminal Justice and Behaviour*, *37*, 261–288.

Walmsley, R. (2018). World Prison Population List (12th ed.). Institute for Criminal Policy Research. Retrieved from http://www.prisonstudies.org. Accessed 13 April 2020.

Weissman, M., DeLamater, L., & Lovejoy, A. (2013). Women's choices: Case management for women leaving jails and prisons. *The Source*, *12*(1), 9–12.

Wiener, R. L., Winick, B. J., Georges, L. S., & Castro, A. (2010). A testable theory of problem-solving courts: Avoiding past empirical and legal failures. *International Journal of Law and Psychiatry*, *33*(5–6), 417–427. PMID: 20980056

Y Care International. (2014). Young people in conflict with the law in Togo, West Africa 2014. Y care international. London. http://www.ycareinternational.org/wp-content/uploads/2015/06/YCI_Young-people-inconflict-with-the-law-in-Togo_3.pdf. Accessed 11 January 2020.

Yang, C. (2020). Assessing the effect of the COVID-19 pandemic on correctional institutions. The Harvard Gazette. Retrieved from https://news.harvard.edu/gazette/story/2020/04. Accessed 15 June 2020.

Yusuf, A. J., & Nuhu, F. T. (2009). The profile of mentally ill offenders in Katsina, Northern Nigeria. *African Journal of Psychiatry*, *12*, 231–232.

World Health Organization. (2014). *Prison and health.* In S. Enggist, L. Moller, G. Galea, & C. Udesen (Eds.). Regional Office for Europe. Retrieved from www.euro.who.int. Accessed 10 April 2020.

5 Ethics and the forensic mental health system in Africa

Oladipo Adeolu Sowunmi, Omokehinde Olubunmi Fakorede, and Adegboyega Ogunwale

Introduction

The word "forensic" is derived from the root word "forum" in Latin (which is also translated as "court" in English). Forensic psychiatry deals with both the living and the dead (Shokry, 2014) and it is the interaction of the scientific and clinical aspects of psychiatry on one hand and the law (comprising criminal, correctional and legislative matters) on the other hand (Arboleda-Florez, 2006). (AAPL, 2005; Bloch & Green, 2013; Griffith, 1998; Griffith, Darby, Weinstock, Glancy, & Simpson, 2018; Norko, 2005; Taborda, Abdalla-Filho, & Garrafa, 2007; Weinstock, 1998). It is worth noting that initially, the legal aspects covered in forensic psychiatry were essentially criminal matters, but the discipline has evolved to include civil matters (Arboleda-Florez, 2006). While this may be considered a significant development, the practice of forensic psychiatry by mental health experts who have minimal or no training in law and jurisprudence remains a daunting challenge (Schouten, 2001). The greater challenge is the ability to dive successfully and not drown amidst the three disciplines of medicine, law and ethics which form the critical building blocks of forensic mental health practice. In Africa, particularly West Africa, the training of doctors in forensic psychiatry and ethics is usually at the postgraduate (residency) level (Ewuoso, 2016; Pobee, 1982). Despite this, there is hardly any structured training in forensic psychiatry in many parts of the continent. Thus, in many African jurisdictions, the only available expert is a non-forensically qualified one. This relative scarcity of adequately trained mental health expert witnesses had been noted by some authors in Western climes as well (Appelbaum, 1997, 2008; Bloch & Green, 2013; Gaughwin, 2004; Rosner & Scott, 2003; Shaboltas, Gorbatov, Arbuzova, & Khaleeva, 2020; Stone, 2008; Weinstock, Leong & Silva, 1990).

That said, the concept of ethics to a practicing physician is fundamentally grounded in the principles of autonomy, justice, beneficence and non-maleficence (Varkey, 2020), with most scholars convinced that the fourth is most paramount as the Latin axiom "*primum non nocere*" (above all, do no harm) seems to confer primacy upon it (Varkey, 2020). However, this principle-based ethical posture may not hold true for the forensic mental health expert witness. Unlike the general adult psychiatrist, the expert's loyalty is not to the patient but to the cause of justice (Hatta, 2018). In a situation where the expert witness also doubles as the treating psychiatrist, he is not only bound to the court but also to the patient. This dilemma may explain why some authors have suggested a different ethical code for forensic psychiatric expert witnesses working in different jurisdictions. They propose that this guideline should entertain considerations of culture and ethnicity alongside compassion (Sanders, 2009). Such a code would necessarily address the ethical premise of therapeutic engagements as well as that of expert witness roles.

Unfortunately, the African forensic mental health expert witness does not readily have an explicit ethics code to work with; rather, he/she is left to extrapolate from general medical codes of ethics or rely on outdated mental health laws whenever medico-legal issues arise in practice (Calcedo-Barba, 2010; Griffith, 1998; Grisso & Appelbaum, 1992; Hudgins, 1996; Kohn & Levav, 2000; Konrad, 2010; Konrad & Opitz-Welke, 2014; Niveau, Godet, & Völlm, 2019; Niveau & Welle, 2018; Ugochukwu et al., 2020). Furthermore, local or regional ethical codes are not available for taking into account cultural differences in the application of ethical codes. Even where general ethical codes exist, social and economic factors are usually considered during the implementation of such codes. This may be sometimes unfavorable for patients, especially when social values predominate or when economical values dominate in high profile cases. In a practical sense, whether a code exists or not, an expert witness should inform an evaluee that his obligations are primarily to the court and that information obtained during the interview may be used by the court for or against him (Strasburger, Gutheil, & Brodsky, 1997; AAPL, 2005; Franke, Speiser, Dudeck, & Streb, 2020; Goethals, Gunn, & Calcedo-Barba, 2012; Kapoor, Young, Coleman, Norko, & Griffith, 2011; Lish, 2018; Norko, 2005; Szasz, 2003; Taborda et al., 2007; Totsuka, 1989; Weinstock, 1998).

On the other hand, the treating psychiatrist managing prisoners on probation and awaiting trial inmates and convicted offenders should also inform their patients that although the treatment at that point is therapeutic and the principles of beneficence and non-maleficence apply in strictly clinical terms, the relationship in the future can be changed to that of examiner–examinee, in which case, ethical principles shift slightly in focus from pursuing the good of the patient to the pursuit of the ends of justice (AAPL, 2005; Appelbaum, 1997; Gaughwin, 2004; Griffith et al., 2018; Gutheil & Hilliard, 2001; Verdun-Jones, 2000).

In order to address these bottlenecks, authors had proposed that before therapeutic alliance is reached or at the point of first contact, the onus is on the expert witness to intimate the client that the interview is not geared toward therapy, and that contents/results of assessment are not confidential. The evaluee may refuse to answer any question (though it will be noted) and he/she has the free will to take reasonable breaks from the interview (Bloch & Green, 2013; Goethals et al., 2012; Rosner & Scott, 2003; Weinstock et al., 1990). While this approach may prevent the expert witness from potentially hurting the client inadvertently, the former should also understand the merits of practicing within the ambience of confidentiality, informed consent, honesty and objectivity (Strasburger et al., 1997). He must also be able negotiate complex situations that place a great demand on his/her knowledge and practice of both psychiatry and ethics. Such situations include forensic opinions in the absence of examination, performance/expectations in a dual role, the hired gun problems, query about his/her qualification and the extent of his/her opinion in court (Gaughwin, 2004; Griffith et al., 2018; Shaboltas et al., 2020; Stone, 2008).

Forensic psychiatry is a road less traveled in the African context. Potential clients who may benefit from the services of expert witnesses (e.g., having committed a crime under the influence of gross psychotic disturbance such as commanding hallucinations) are not sufficiently positioned to secure such opportunity. This is because in some parts of Africa, there appears to be a penchant for jungle justice and some of these offenders would have been lynched or even murdered before getting the attention of the social worker or law enforcement agents (The Nation Nigeria, 2020).

Standards relating to confidentiality

A psychiatrist, in an expert witness role, requires some level of confidentiality to conduct an objective examination, report of which will be useful for court proceedings. It is also his/her duty to ensure that the relationship remains "evaluator–evaluee" throughout the course of the interview. This is because the client may revert to a doctor–patient relationship unconsciously (AAPL, 2005; Appelbaum, 1997, 2008; Calcedo-Barba, 2010; Taylor, Graf, Schanda, & Völlm, 2012). The age-long tradition of total openness to one's priest, attorney and physician is a popular belief in the African setting, but this belief cannot hold sway in this examiner–examinee contract.

Confidentiality is also highly prioritized in the African setting but delineation between therapeutic confidentiality and confidentiality associated with forensic interview is not usually done. This may reflect the deficit in the training obtained by the expert witness, one that is much worse with the forensic subspecialty. The extent to which the expert can reveal the information received from his/her interview is not cast in stone. As such, personal experience and the advice of more senior practitioners may be of help.

Standards and issues of consent

Before the commencement of a forensic interview, it is important that informed consent be obtained, following an explanation of the nature and purpose of the interview as well as limitations on confidentiality (Shapiro, 1991). The client should also understand that there is a difference between consent for evaluation and consent for treatment. Also, it should be understood that while the courts send patients to the hospital for evaluation by forensic experts in situations like competence to stand trial or criminal responsibility, the final decision is entirely that of the court (judge) irrespective of its alignment or non-alignment with the opinion of the expert witness (Canela et al., 2019; Casey, 2003; Konrad, 2010; Konrad & Opitz-Welke, 2014; Lish, 2018; Totsuka, 1989). For instance, if the forensic interview reveals incompetence to stand trial, the expert should understand his limitation of being restricted to opinion only while awaiting the court's verdict (Hudgins, 1996; Kapoor et al., 2011; Kohn & Levav, 2000; Taborda et al., 2007). The content and context of the forensic interview may not be elaborately presented in the process of consent seeking in some African settings. This is not because of any malevolent intentions but rather because of the likely familiarity that could be bred by the dual agency of being treating physician and expert witness. Consent-related malpractice suits are not common in Africa (Chima, 2018). Furthermore, consent in the African setting could be obtained from a significant other, usually the funder of the treatment (Igbinomwanhia & Akanni, 2019), which is not the normative practice in the West.

Honesty and striving for objectivity

The ethical code of an attorney requires frenzied representation of their client whether as the prosecuting or the defense team. This is however not so for the evaluating forensic psychiatrist whose code of ethics should hinge on honesty, objectivity and logical opinion in spite of pressure of unintended bias (AAPL, 2005; Calcedo-Barba, 2010; Cantor, 1966). Furthermore, another closely related concept is that of "a hired gun," which implies that an expert witness should resist the temptation of financial motivation to manipulate his professional opinion (Griffith, 1998; Konrad, 2010; Konrad & Opitz-Welke, 2014; Szasz, 2003).

In the main, it may be more reasonable to interpret the codes of honesty and objectivity together. According to the American Academy of Psychiatry and the Law (AAPL) guideline, it states that "*when psychiatrists function as an expert within the legal process, they should adhere to the principle of honesty and should strive for objectivity. Although they may be retained by one party to a civil or criminal matter, psychiatrists should adhere to these principles when conducting evaluations, applying clinical data to legal criteria, and expressing opinions.*" The emphasis is on striving for objectivity and not just objectivity such that self-reflection, transparent reasoning and an effort to explore all aspects is incorporated into the interview process (AAPL, 2005; Griffith, 1998). Thus, exploration of the inconsistencies and goals of forensic report by either or both counsels should be perceived as a norm, and not attack, by the forensic expert. Therefore, the expert should conduct a thorough and extensive review of relevant information within the limits of the rule of admissibility and subsequently communicate to the court. Nevertheless, it is important to note also that some have queried the usefulness of a professional opinion in legal issues (Dodier et al., 2019). Similarly, another situation which places demand on the honesty and objectivity of the expert is also in the area of child custody litigation where all parties (beyond the nuclear family) cannot be said to be comprehensively investigated (Deed, 1991; Franke et al., 2020; Lish, 2018; Niveau et al., 2019; Niveau & Welle, 2018; Shaboltas et al., 2020).

Forensic opinions in the absence of examination

As much as the direct interview of the client by the expert witness seems sacrosanct, it may not be possible in all cases. Psychological autopsy of the dead, malpractice litigation on behalf of the dead, post-mortem will contest and client's refusal to be interviewed are some of these instances (Goethals et al., 2012; Miller, Maier & Kaye, 1986; Rosner & Scott, 2003; Shulman et al., 2020; Totsuka, 1989; Young, 1992). In these situations, the forensic expert should endeavor to indicate that his/her professional opinion has this limitation. In addition, the use of the expert's subjective yardstick for standard of care in his/her evaluation, in malpractice suits, should be avoided as it violates the standard of striving for objectivity (Shaboltas et al., 2020; Szasz, 2003). To surmount this obstacle, the mental health ethical expert should ensure that his/her standards are defined and are compatible with the demographic and sociocultural practice of the setting in question. Despite the fulfillment of the above, the expert must be ready to subject himself/herself to cross-examination and be willing to objectively agree that there might be contradictions, unknown areas and limitations with respect to available data on current practice (Shaboltas et al., 2020; Szasz, 2003).

Dual role complexity

According to the AAPL code, "*psychiatrists who take on a forensic role for a patient they are treating may adversely affect the therapeutic relationship with them. Forensic evaluation usually requires interviewing corroborative sources, exposing information to public scrutiny, or subjecting clients and treatment itself to potential damaging cross-examination. The forensic evaluation and the credibility of the practitioner may also be undermined by conflicts inherent in differing clinical and forensic roles. Treating psychiatrists should, therefore, generally avoid acting as the expert witness for their own patients or performing evaluations of their patients for legal purposes. (I, Section IV).*" Unfortunately, this situation arises because attorneys may want to avoid expert fees, may be ignorant of any conflict between the roles or may want to take advantage of the passion of the treating psychiatrist to help his case (AAPL, 2005; Franke et al., 2020; Niveau & Welle, 2018). In African settings, dual agency scenarios are likely to be driven by human resource constraints. Notwithstanding this, dual roles may not only be detrimental to patient's treatment but will also imperil the expert's duty of striving for objectivity. Table 5.1 best summarizes the peculiarities of each role.

Financial benefit and quest for objectivity

From the time of the M'Naghten case, high-profile cases have attracted both public sympathy and condemnation. A major issue arises when the opinion of the psychiatry is at variance with that of the public (Chin, Lutsky, & Dror, et al., 2019). If the expert presents an opinion suggesting that the defendant was suffering from mental disorder at the time of the offense which could potentially lessen culpability or exculpate entirely in cases such as murder, she/he could be

Table 5.1 Comparing the ethical duties of treating psychiatrist with those of the expert witness

Ethical concept/issues	*Treating psychiatrist*	*Expert witness*
Summary of role	*Health care provision* (Schouten, 1993)	*Educator of court* (Andrew, 2006) *Evaluation of examinee* (Gutheil, 2008)
Obligation to whom?	*Obligation to protect the patient (client)*	*Obligation to assist the court* (Weissberger, 2007)
Confidentiality of records and communication	*Patients are encouraged to make full disclosure of experiences, interpretations and planned actions. The Hippocratic oath binds the clinician to maintain utmost confidentiality except in cases of imminent danger to the client or public where extra measures are necessary*	*The client needs to know* ab initio *that the information he/she volunteers in the course of being examined by the treating psychiatrist is not confidential and can be made available to the court of law on request*
Beneficence and non-maleficence	*Doing good and not harming the patient are core ethical principles that must be maintained in this relationship* (Cambra-Badii et al., 2020)	*Whether the outcome harms the subject or not is not relevant. What is sacrosanct is that any resultant harm from the outcome must not stem from the expert's self-interest (e.g., to obtain financial remuneration)* (Kass & Rose, 2016)

seen as working toward the defendant's acquittal. This is more likely to be the case if the expert is retained by the defense. On another hand, there may also be forensic experts who are willing to provide a preferred testimony for economic gain rather than sticking to honesty and the need for the objective examination (Calcedo-Barba, 2010; Griffith, 1998; Robert Weinstock et al., 1990). The AAPL code therefore advices that fee for service should not be tied to the result of the case – so-called "contingency fee." However, professional charges legitimately due to the expert whether or not the outcome of the case is favorable to the commissioning party are regarded as appropriate.

The issues raised in the foregoing may constitute things that could be somewhat theoretical in a sense. Given a number of uncertainties regarding forensic examinations (e.g., attempting to ascertain the mental state at the time of a crime which occurred several months before the evaluation), the validity and reliability of forensic evaluations, on their own, may not be without question. Furthermore, conflict may also arise when personal factors such as morals or religious upbringing of the forensic expert are brought to bear during the forensic interview (MacLean, Smith, & Dror, 2020). An expert witness should be guided by the fact that every client, irrespective of the complaint/crime, is entitled to a defense and she/he (expert) is not bound to take cases that are in clear opposition to his/her personal beliefs and values (Kapoor et al., 2011; Shaboltas et al., 2020; Taborda et al., 2007), which may clearly constitute conflicts of interest.

Evidence of academic qualification and presentation of clinical findings in legal settings

The practice of forensic psychiatry requires that one's knowledge, skill, training and experience should be disclosed from the onset to the retaining lawyer and one should not attempt to hide these facts during the court proceedings (Appelbaum, 2008; Niveau & Welle, 2018). This is to prevent misrepresentation of the actual level of his/her expertise and undermining of the value of the professional opinion given. Another twist to this issue is the clarity of the expert on the limitations of his/her opinion such as the guarantee of recurrence/non-recurrence of a clinical condition (Appelbaum, 2008; Niveau & Welle, 2018).

Secondly, whether an expert witness should state the conclusion of his/her professional opinions in the frame of the "ultimate question" remains controversial and jurisdiction-bound. Some authors are of the opinion that there should be no conclusion but rather a statement on his/her findings while others believe that the ultimate question should be answered (Frierson & Joshi, 2020). However, the onus is on the expert witness to be conversant with the local customs, retaining lawyer's advice and the implications of judicial instructions during a court proceeding (Appelbaum, 2008; Franke et al., 2020; Niveau & Welle, 2018; Rosner & Scott, 2003; Taborda et al., 2007).

Ethical controversy in forensic and general psychiatry

The timing of clinical evaluation after the offense

The timing for the clinical evaluation of a suspect remains controversial – whether immediately after an arrest or after assignment to a counsel. According to the AAPL guideline (1, Sect III, Commentary) "*Absent a court order, psychiatrists should not perform forensic evaluation for the prosecution or the government on persons who have not consulted with legal counsel when such persons are known to be charged with criminal acts; under investigation for criminal or quasi-criminal conduct; held in government custody or detention; or being interrogated for criminal or quasi-criminal conduct, hostile acts against a government or immigration violations*" (AAPL, 2005). This guideline is protective of the client because his counsel would have informed him of the importance of guarding his statements as well as refraining from answering potentially incriminating questions during the forensic interview. However, opposing scholars maintain that in the spirit of honesty and objectivity, the best time to obtain a "true confession" about a crime is in the immediate post-crime period (Franke et al., 2020; Kapoor et al., 2011; Szasz, 2003).

Ethical issues in expert evaluation of cases involving the insanity defense

Perhaps one of the most complex and fundamental assessments in forensic psychiatry is the evaluation of a subject for the insanity defense. It is a duty that requires a forensic expert to be meticulous and precise in an effort to bridge the gap between the clinical and legal domains (Calcedo-Barba, 2010; Franke et al., 2020; Griffith et al., 2018; Kapoor et al., 2011; Niveau et al., 2019; Niveau & Welle, 2018; Shaboltas et al., 2020; Weinstock et al., 1990). There are two major issues that a forensic expert will need to answer. First is the issue of determining criminal responsibility retrospectively. Secondly, there is the issue of disposition. Despite the rigor required, this evaluation is fraught with ethical pitfalls because the expert witness may be perceived as identifying with the suspect or perpetrator, when in fact, this is not so. The main reason that has been projected by the public is that the verdict "not guilty by reason of insanity" does not confer any clear disposition to the suspect/perpetrator. It appears as if they are given a free pass to continue the perceived crime with the physician using his power to protect/promote the premature release of a purported mentally disordered individual (Calcedo-Barba, 2010; Franke et al., 2020; Griffith et al., 2018; Kapoor et al., 2011; Niveau et al., 2019; Niveau & Welle, 2018; Shaboltas et al., 2020; Robert Weinstock et al., 1990).

Psychiatric testimony in psychological injury cases

Another interesting area is the management of clients with psychological injury. This evaluation is more subjective than objective and as such exaggeration of symptoms and malingering are common. In a bid to be objective, the treating psychiatrist is torn between guarding the truth and avoiding confronting a potentially hurting client. This he must navigate to hope for a successful evaluation (Calcedo-Barba, 2010; Franke et al., 2020; Griffith et al., 2018; Kapoor et al., 2011; Niveau et al., 2019; Niveau & Welle, 2018; Shaboltas et al., 2020; Robert Weinstock et al., 1990).

The dual agent in forensic treatment settings

The forensic hospital and prison services both involve incarceration with different ethical issues. More often than not, both services provide treatment and evaluation because of resource constraint. As a result, forensic psychiatrists in prison, for example, may encounter ethical stalemates in the course of their duties (Calcedo-Barba, 2010; Franke et al., 2020; Griffith et al., 2018; Kapoor et al., 2011; Niveau et al., 2019; Niveau & Welle, 2018; Shaboltas et al., 2020; Robert Weinstock et al., 1990). A patient committed into the forensic facility based on insanity may be evaluated and observed not to have the underlying illness by the treating psychiatrist in charge. What is to be done by the psychiatrist in such cases is not immediately clear because it may constitute the forensic expert trying to reverse the decision of a court of competent jurisdiction. On the other hand, it is hardly ethical to hospitalize or treat an individual for a mental disorder when one does not objectively exist. Other issues that may arise may include spontaneous confessions of crime or criminal activities in the correctional facility or disclosure of setting-related rape, murder, escape or riot plans. The solution to these knotty issues is to have clear guidelines or protocols that experts can work with.

The forensic expert and the death penalty in African settings

The death penalty has remained a sensitive issue worldwide and despite decline in its support in the West, Nigeria and Egypt have been reported to be responsible for an increase in implementing the death penalty. This has been opined to be related to their cultural tilt toward it. It is believed to serve as a form of deterrence or retribution and that it supports public opinion.

Unfortunately, the involvement of the psychiatrist in death penalty cases constitutes an ethical dilemma. For instance, one problem is the psychiatrist's participation in certifying a prisoner for execution and the other is the need to treat prisoners who are sick only for them to be eventually executed, the so-called grotesque situation.

The stand of most medical bodies has been to conduct evaluations of those handed the death penalty when judgment has already been passed (Calcedo-Barba, 2010; Franke et al., 2020; Griffith et al., 2018; Kapoor et al., 2011; Niveau et al., 2019; Niveau & Welle, 2018; Shaboltas et al., 2020; Robert Weinstock et al., 1990). Moreover, personal, clinical and official attitudes toward the death penalty play a vital role in the subjective attitude of the expert.

Leading authors have divergent opinions about the role of a treating psychiatrist, with some arguing that they should not withhold their services to a convict on death penalty while others clamor that experts should not be involved in proceedings that lead to harm, in this case, death (Calcedo-Barba, 2010; Franke et al., 2020; Griffith et al., 2018; Kapoor et al., 2011; Niveau et al., 2019; Niveau & Welle, 2018; Shaboltas et al., 2020; Robert Weinstock et al., 1990). Currently there is no consensus and there is no hope for one in the nearest future. What is important is that a balance must be struck between saving a suspect from or supporting execution (Calcedo-Barba, 2010; Franke et al., 2020; Griffith et al., 2018; Kapoor et al., 2011; Niveau et al., 2019; Niveau & Welle, 2018; Shaboltas et al., 2020; Weinstock et al., 1990). Furthermore, because an expert witness is an elective and voluntary role and his/her main duty is to protect the truth of the opinion from both lawyers and to preserve independence and objectivity, he/she may occasionally, as a last resort, choose to withdraw at any point during the proceeding.

Conclusion

Ethical issues in African forensic mental health contexts are not different from those observable from more developed climes. However, these issues are complicated by factors such as human resource constraints and cultural nuances as well as the glaring absence of ethical codes of practice that are critical to decision making, whether in the therapeutic sense or within the expert witness role. By far the most daunting challenge for African forensic mental health practitioners is the dual agency position in which the treating physician doubles as the expert witness. While this may represent a pragmatic response to the human resource shortages, it carries with it the potential risk of harm to the patient and damage to the reputation of the expert. The presence of the death penalty in some African countries also raises significant ethical questions regarding the role of psychiatrists in the assessment and treatment of persons who have been sentenced to death. It is crucial for African forensic mental health experts to engage with these issues by emphasizing the need for continuing professional development as well as the establishment of ethical codes of practice. A highly measured approach to dual agency is, without question, a most significant resolution mechanism to some of the ethical quandaries that must arise.

References

American Academy of Psychiatry and the Law. (2005). *Ethics guidelines for the practice of forensic psychiatry*. https://aapl.org/guidelines-and-practice-resources.

Andrew, L. B. (2006). Expert witness testimony: The ethics of being a medical expert witness. *Emergency Medicine Clinics, 24*(3), 715–731. https://doi.org/10.1016/j.emc.2006.05.001.

Appelbaum, P. S. (1997). A theory of ethics for forensic psychiatry. *Journal of the American Academy of Psychiatry and the Law, 25*(3), 233–247.

Appelbaum, P. S. (2008). Ethics and forensic psychiatry: Translating principles into practice. *Journal of the American Academy of Psychiatry and the Law, 36*(2), 195–200.

Arboleda-Florez, J. (2006). Forensic psychiatry: Contemporary scope, challenges and controversies. *World Psychiatry, 5*(2), 87–91. https://www.ncbi.nlm.nih.gov/pmc/articles/PMC1525122/.

Bloch, S., & Green, S. A. (2013). The scope of psychiatric ethics. *Psychiatric Ethics*, 3–8. https://doi.org/10.1093/med/9780199234318.003.0001.

Calcedo-Barba, A. (2010). Objectivity and ethics in forensic psychiatry. *Current Opinion in Psychiatry, 23*(5), 447–452. https://doi.org/10.1097/YCO.0b013e32833cd1e6.

Cambra-Badii, I., Pinar, A., & Baños, J.-E. (2020). The Good Doctor and bioethical principles: A content analysis. *Educación Médica.* https://doi.org/10.1016/j.edumed.2019.12.006'Q.

Canela, C., Buadze, A., Dube, A., Jackowski, C., Pude, I., Nellen, R., Signorini, P., & Liebrenz, M. (2019). How do legal experts cope with medical reports and forensic evidence? The experiences, perceptions, and narratives of Swiss judges and other legal experts. *Frontiers in Psychiatry, 10*, 18.

Cantor, B. J. (1966). The expert witness. *American Bar Association Journal, 52*(12), 946–948.

Casey, P. (2003). Expert testimony in court. 1: General principles. *Advances in Psychiatric Treatment, 9*(3), 177–182.

Chima, S. C. (2018). An investigation of informed consent in clinical practice in South Africa. *LLD Thesis, University of South Africa (UNISA), Viewed, 1.*

Chin, J. M., Lutsky, M., & Dror, I. E. (2019). The biases of experts: An empirical analysis of expert witness challenges. *Man. LJ, 42*, 21.

Deed, M. L. (1991). Court-ordered child custody evaluations: Helping or victimizing vulnerable families. *Psychotherapy: Theory, Research, Practice, Training, 28*(1), 76.

Dodier, O., Melinder, A., Otgaar, H., Payoux, M., & Magnussen, S. (2019). Psychologists and psychiatrists in court: What do they know about eyewitness memory? A comparison of experts in inquisitorial and adversarial legal systems. *Journal of Police and Criminal Psychology, 34*(3), 254–262.

Ewuoso, O. C. (2016). Bioethics education in Nigeria and West Africa: Historical beginnings and impacts. *Global Bioethics, 27*(2–4), 50–60.

Franke, I., Speiser, O., Dudeck, M., & Streb, J. (2020). Clinical ethics support services are not as well-established in forensic psychiatry as in general psychiatry. *Frontiers in Psychiatry, 11*(March), 1–8. https://doi.org/10.3389/fpsyt.2020.00186.

Frierson, R. L., & Joshi, K. G. (2020). Called to court? Tips for testifying. *Current Psychiatry, 19*(1), 50–52.

Gaughwin, P. C. (2004). A consideration of the relationship between the Rules of Court and the Code of Ethics forensic psychiatry. *Australian and New Zealand Journal of Psychiatry, 38*(1–2), 20–25. https://doi.org/10.1111/j.1440-1614.2004.01293.x.

Goethals, K., Gunn, J., & Calcedo-Barba, A. (2012). Selling forensic psychiatry: Recruiting for the future, establishing services. *Criminal Behaviour and Mental Health, 1*(22), 261–270. https://doi.org/10.1002/cbm.

Griffith, E. E. H. (1998). Ethics in forensic psychiatry: A cultural response to Stone and Appelbaum. *Journal of the American Academy of Psychiatry and the Law, 26*(2), 171–184.

Griffith, E. E. H., Darby, C., Weinstock, R., Glancy, G. D., & Simpson, A. (2018). *Ethics Challenges in Forensic Psychiatry and Psychology Practice, 206*(9), 2018.

Grisso, T., & Appelbaum, P. S. (1992). Is it unethical to offer predictions of future violence? *Law and Human Behavior, 16*(6), 621–633. https://doi.org/10.1007/BF01884019.

Gutheil, T. G., & Hilliard, J. T. (2001). The treating psychiatrist thrust into the role of expert witness. *Psychiatric Services (Washington, DC), 52*(11), 1526–1527. https://doi.org/10.1176/appi.ps.52.11.1526.

Gutheil, T. G. (2008). Forensic psychiatry. In S. Bloch & S. A. Green (Eds.), *Psychiatric Ethics*. Oxford: Oxford University Press.

Hatta, M. (2018). The position of expert witnesses in medical malpractice cases in Indonesia. *Al-Ahkam, 28*(1), 47–72.

Hudgins, A. (1996). An autobiographer's lies. *American Scholar, 65*(4), 541.

Igbinomwanhia, N., & Akanni, O. (2019). Constraints, ethical dilemmas and precautions in psychiatric practice within non-contemporaneous mental health laws: A Nigerian experience with involuntary commitment. *JL Pol'y & Globalization, 87*, 21.

Kapoor, R., Young, J. L., Coleman, J. T., Norko, M. A., & Griffith, E. E. H. (2011). Ethics in forensic psychiatry publishing. *Journal of the American Academy of Psychiatry and the Law, 39*(3), 332–341.

Kass, J. S., & Rose, R. V. (2016). Ethical challenges for the medical expert witness. *AMA Journal of Ethics, 18*(3), 201–208. https://doi.org/10.1001/journalofethics.2016.18.3.ecas1-1603.

Kohn, R., & Levav, I. (2000). Ethics in the practice of psychiatry in South Africa. *South African Medical Journal = Suid-Afrikaanse tydskrif vir geneeskunde, 90*(5), 498–503.

Konrad, N. (2010). Ethical issues in forensic psychiatry in penal and other correctional facilities. *Current Opinion in Psychiatry, 23*(5), 467–471. https://doi.org/10.1097/YCO.0b013e32833bb2f2.

Konrad, N., & Opitz-Welke, A. (2014). The challenges of treating the mentally ill in a prison setting: The European perspective. *Clinical Practice, 11*(5), 517–523. https://doi.org/10.2217/cpr.14.44.

Lish, D. L. (2018). Ethics challenges in forensic psychiatry and psychology practice. *American Journal of Psychiatry, 175*(10), 1024–1025. https://doi.org/10.1176/appi.ajp.2018.18060663.

MacLean, C. L., Smith, L., & Dror, I. E. (2020). Experts on trial: Unearthing bias in scientific evidence. *UBCL Rev.*, *53*, 101.

Mentally-ill man lynched for killing five siblings—The Nation Nigeria. (2020, May 24). *Latest Nigeria News, Nigerian Newspapers, Politics.* https://thenationonlineng.net/mentally-ill-man-lynched-for-killing-five-siblings/.

Miller, R. D., Maier, G. J., & Kaye, M. (1986). The right to remain silent during psychiatric examination in civil and criminal cases—A national survey and an analysis. *International Journal of Law and Psychiatry*, *9*(1), 77–94.

Niveau, G., Godet, T., & Völlm, B. (2019). What does impartiality mean in medico-legal psychiatry? An international survey. *International Journal of Law and Psychiatry*, *66*(June), 101505. https://doi.org/10.1016/j.ijlp.2019.101505.

Niveau, G., & Welle, I. (2018). Forensic psychiatry, one subspecialty with two ethics? A systematic review. *BMC Medical Ethics*, *19*(1), 1–10. https://doi.org/10.1186/s12910-018-0266-5.

Norko, M. A. (2005). Commentary: Compassion at the core of forensic ethics. *Journal of the American Academy of Psychiatry and the Law*, *33*(3), 386–389.

Pobee, J. O. M. (1982). Postgraduate medical education for physicians in West Africa. *Journal of the Royal College of Physicians of London*, *16*(4), 242–244. https://www.ncbi.nlm.nih.gov/pmc/articles/PMC5377594/.

Rosner, R., & Scott, C. L. (Eds.). (2003). Principles and practice of forensic psychiatry, In: *Principles and practice of forensic psychiatry* (3rd ed., p. 1096). CRC Press. ISBN 9781482262285. Published January 18, 2017. https://doi.org/10.1201/b13499.

Sanders, J. (2009). Science, law, and the expert witness. *Law and Contemporary Problems*, *72*(1), 63–90. JSTOR. https://www.jstor.org/stable/40647166.

Schouten, R. (1993). Pitfalls of clinical practice: The treating clinician as expert witness. *Harvard Review of Psychiatry*, *1*(1), 64–65.

Schouten, R. (2001). Law and psychiatry: What should our residents learn? *Harvard Review of Psychiatry*, *9*(3), 136–138.

Shaboltas, A. V., Gorbatov, S. V., Arbuzova, E. N., & Khaleeva, M. V. (2020). The ethical problems in forensic psychological expert evaluation: A view from modern Russia. *Psychology in Russia: State of the Art*, *13*(1), 11–21. https://doi.org/10.11621/pir.2020.0102.

Shapiro, D. L. (1991). Informed consent in forensic evaluations. *Psychotherapy in Private Practice*, *9*(1), 145–154.

Shokry, D. A. (Ed.). (2014). The practice of forensic science in Egypt: A story of pioneering. In *The Global Practice of Forensic Science* (pp. 73–81). Wiley Online Library.

Shulman, K., Herrmann, N., Peglar, H., Dochylo, D., Burns, C., & Peisah, C. (2020). The role of the medical expert in the retrospective assessment of testamentary capacity. *The Canadian Journal of Psychiatry*, 0706743720915007. doi: 10.1177/0706743720915007.

Stone, A. A. (2008). The ethical boundaries of forensic psychiatry: A view from the Ivory Tower. *Journal of the American Academy of Psychiatry and the Law*, *36*(2), 167–174.

Strasburger, L. H., Gutheil, T. G., & Brodsky, A. (1997). On wearing two hats: Role conflict in serving as both psychotherapist and expert witness. *American Journal of Psychiatry*, *154*(4), 448–456.

Szasz, T. (2003). Psychiatry and the control of dangerousness: On the apotropaic function of the term "mental illness." *Journal of Social Work Education*, *39*(3), 375–381. https://doi.org/10.1080/10437797.2003.10779144.

Taborda, J. G. V., Abdalla-Filho, E., & Garrafa, V. (2007). Ethics in forensic psychiatry. *Current Opinion in Psychiatry*, *20*(5), 507–510. https://doi.org/10.1097/YCO.0b013e32827851eb.

Taylor, P. J., Graf, M., Schanda, H., & Völlm, B. (2012). The treating psychiatrist as expert in the courts: Is it necessary or possible to separate the roles of physician and expert? *Criminal Behaviour and Mental Health*, *22*(4), 271–292.

Totsuka, E. (1989). Ethics and forensic psychiatry: Developments in the international community*Current Opinion in Psychiatry*, *2*(6), 723–728. https://doi.org/10.1097/00001504-198912000-00002.

Ugochukwu, O., Mbaezue, N., Lawal, S. A., Azubogu, C., Sheikh, T. L., & Vallières, F. (2020). The time is now: Reforming Nigeria's outdated mental health laws. *The Lancet Global Health*, *8*(8), e989–e990.

Varkey, B. (2020). Principles of clinical ethics and their application to practice. *Medical Principles and Practice*, *30*(1), 17–28. doi: 10.1159/000509119.

Verdun-Jones, S. N. (2000). Forensic psychiatry, ethics and protective sentencing: What are the limits of psychiatric participation in the criminal justice process? *Acta Psychiatrica Scandinavica, Supplement*, *101*(399), 77–82. https://doi.org/10.1111/j.0902-4441.2000.007s020[dash]18.x.

Weinstock, R. (1998). A theory of ethics for forensic psychiatry. *The Journal of the American Academy of Psychiatry and the Law*, *26*(1), 151–155.

Weinstock, R., Leong, G. B., & Silva, J. A. (1990). The role of traditional medical ethics in forensic psychiatry. In: R. Rosner, & R. Weinstock (Eds.), *Ethical Practice in Psychiatry and the Law* (vol. 7, pp. 31–51). Boston, MA: Springer. https://doi.org/10.1007/978-1-4899-1663-1_3.

Weissberger, E. (2007). The ethics forum: The ethics of being an expert witness. *Limnology and Oceanography Bulletin*, *16*(4), 86–87. https://doi.org/10.1002/lob.200716486.

Young, T. J. (1992). Procedures and problems in conducting a psychological autopsy. *International Journal of Offender Therapy and Comparative Criminology*, *36*(1), 43–52.

Part II

Forensic mental health assessment

6 The state-of-the-art of violence risk assessment in Africa

Adegboyega Ogunwale and Katrina I. Serpa

Introduction

Estimating an individual's risk of violence has occupied the minds of researchers for several decades (Grisso & Appelbaum, 1992; Monahan, 1981, 1996; Mossman, 1994; Torrey, Stanley, Monahan, & Steadman, 2008). This has been largely driven by society's interest in public safety (Dahlberg & Mercy, 2009). Research has shown a disturbing link between violence and specific types of severe mental disorder (Arseneault, Moffitt, Caspi, Taylor, & Silva, 2000; Fazel et al., 2006; Fazel, Gulati, Linsell, Geddes, & Grann 2009; Fazel, Buxrud, Ruchkin, & Grann, 2010; Hodgins, Alderton, Cree, Aboud, & Mak, 2007; Lindqvist & Allebeck, 1990; Swanson, Holzer, Ganju, & Jono, 1990; Wallace et al., 1998; Wallace, Mullen, & Burgess, 2004; Witt, van Dorn, & Fazel, 2013) and this has contributed to renewed interest in accurately estimating violence risk among individuals with mental disorders with a view to achieving harm prevention. Importantly, this interest in harm prevention also has relevance to violent offenders without mental illness. To date, assessing the risk of violence is rife with challenges and retains a level of controversy within the field of risk assessment. Attempts to provide reliable and valid assessments of risk have resulted in an evolution from unstructured clinical assessments to structured approaches (Douglas, Cox, & Webster, 1999; Douglas et al., 2014; Douglas, Pugh, Singh, Savulescu & Fazel, 2017; Webster, Douglas, Eaves, & Hart, 1997). This chapter reviews the key sociocultural and legal issues that underpin the widespread use of unstructured clinical judgment in Africa and the inherent risks of employing this method of assessment. We will also focus on how these existing frameworks in different African countries impact on the use of actuarial and Structured Professional Judgment (SPJ) tools in risk assessment. Finally, research designs which will afford the validation of internationally developed risk instruments within African settings will be discussed. The potential for the development of locally derived and culturally sensitive risk assessment instruments will be explored as a pragmatic prospect as well.

A conceptual view of violence risk assessment

Definition

Violence has been observed to have several definitions (Webster et al., 1997). In strictly legal terms, violence may be defined as: "Unjust or unwarranted use of force, usually accompanied by fury, vehemence, or outrage; physical force unlawfully exercised with the intent to harm" (Garner, 2001, p. 1564). In the 2002 World Report on Health, Krug, Mercy, Dahlberg, and Zwi (2002) provided a more inclusive definition as follows: "The intentional use of physical force or power, threatened or actual, against oneself, another person or against a group or community that either results in or has a high likelihood of resulting in injury, death, psychological harm…" (p. 1084). Webster et al. (1997) suggested a descriptive and operational approach to the definition in stating that: "violence is actual, attempted, or threatened harm to a person or persons. Threats of harm must be clear and unambiguous (e.g., 'I am going to kill you!'), rather than vague statements of hostility." Adopting a practical and more importantly, operational definition, of violence is crucial to criterion definition for the intended outcome in the particular population of individuals being assessed. This is a critical factor in view of the sometimes-complex statistical procedures that are utilized to develop structured risk assessment procedures. Specifically, Heilbrun, Brooks Holliday, and King (2013) suggest that the specification of the "target behavior" (i.e., the type violence) is relevant to the base rate of violence. Hart (2003) also submits that the potential for bias in violence risk estimation may occur because of varying definitions of criterion behavior. Thus, tensions can arise between the validity and reliability of risk estimates as well as comparability of findings from different studies adopting varied definitions of violence.

Risk factors

A long literature has identified a concert of risk factors associated with violence (Andrews, Bonta, & Wormith, 2006; Douglas et al., 1999, 2017). In defining violence risk, it is important both from a clinical and statistical point of view, to define reliable risk factors for violence. Research aimed at developing violence risk assessment instruments (Harris, Rice, & Quinsey, 1993; Webster et al., 1997) have identified key factors in this regard. For example, 12 predictors of violent recidivism were identified by Harris et al. (1993). They included eight positive predictors, namely: psychopathy, separation from parents under age 16, "never married" marital status, elementary school maladjustment, failure on prior conditional release, property offense history, alcohol abuse history and presence of personality disorder. The remaining four predictors (presence of schizophrenia, victim injury in index offense, female victim at index offense and age at index offense) demonstrate negative correlations with violent recidivism. Factors similar to these have been highlighted by Webster et al. (1997); these include, among others: previous violence, young age at first violent incident, relationship instability, employment problems, substance-use problems, major mental illness, psychopathy, early maladjustment, personality disorder, prior supervision failure, impulsivity, lack of insight, stress, lack of personal support and non-compliance with remediation attempts. A meta-analysis by Bonta, Law, and Hanson (1998) revealed similar risk factors for violent recidivism: adult criminal history, juvenile delinquency, antisocial personality disorder, non-violent criminal history, institutional adjustment, hospital admissions, substance abuse, family problems, violent history and single marital status. Partly consistent with the findings of Harris et al. (1993), negative predictors included: mentally disordered offender status, not guilty by reason of insanity, psychosis and age. In addition to these factors predictive of violent recidivism and general violence, there are others that are predictive of more specific forms of violent behavior.

Protective factors

Despite the overwhelming emphasis on risk factors for violence, emerging research and clinical observations have increasingly centered their focus on "strengths," "protective factors" or "buffer" factors that serve to reduce or mitigate the likelihood of violent outcomes (Webster, Martin, Brink, Nicholls, & Desmarais, 2009). It is being advocated that these protective factors or strengths should have their place in violence risk assessment and management plans. While some tools essentially encompass protective factors in the formulation of risk (Webster et al., 2009), others are entirely made up of protective factors (de Vries Robbé, de Vogel, & de Spa, 2011; de Vries Robbé, Geers, Stapel, Hilterman, & de Vogel, 2015).

Approaches to violence risk assessment

Unstructured professional judgment

Historically, violence risk assessments were conducted using "clinical judgment" (this was largely demonstrated in the 1966 *Baxstrom case* in the United States and validated in Barefoot v Estelle (1983)) which rested on unstandardized clinical discretion (i.e., "gut feeling"). Such assessments had little scientific reliability and produced predictive validity estimates no better than chance (Monahan, 2000). Despite the obvious limitations of unstructured clinical judgments regarding violence risk, they portray important merits that include flexibility based on individualized contexts, accommodation of dynamic factors and the ability to inform treatment and harm prevention.

Actuarial approach

An actuarial approach to violence risk assessment is a formal method of assessment that utilizes "an equation, a formula, a graph, or an actuarial table to arrive at a probability, or expected value, of some outcome" (Grove & Meehl,

1996, p. 293). It entails the inclusion of predictors often determined through a process of statistical modeling, focusing on an outcome of interest (Heilbrun, Holliday, & King, 2013). The predictor variables included in the model are not assumed to possess any "causal" relationship with the violence being investigated (Jackson & Guyton, 2008).

One of the earliest and most widely used actuarial violence assessment instrument is the Violence Risk Appraisal Guide (VRAG) (Harris et al., 1993) that is intended to predict long-term violence risk among individuals with prior violent episodes. It has 12 items, and each item is scored according to a weighting procedure. Total scores range from –26 to +38. The total scores are then used to categorize individuals into "bins" that are associated with levels of risk for violent recidivism (Harris et al., 1993). In the initial validation, Harris et al. (1993) reported a correlation of 0.44 between total VRAG scores and violent recidivism ($p < 0.01$). The AUC was observed to be equally high (0.76) indicating acceptable predictive accuracy.

Criticisms of actuarial approaches have been highlighted (Hart, 2003; Hart, Michie, & Cooke, 2007; Jackson & Guyton, 2008). First, while high scores on actuarial instruments suggest an increased probability of violence, like other risk instruments, they neither indicate certainty nor establish the level of violence potential. Second, the designation of risk level by actuarial instruments is on a group basis, although this is not unique to them. However, it may be misleading to directly apply that risk level to every individual who falls into the group. For example, such methods do not allow distinction in the violence risk levels of two individuals in the same "bin." Statistically speaking, it is not clear to which extent one may apply the error rates and confidence intervals reported for the aggregate data to the individual patient. Third, it appears that actuarial instruments tend to focus on risk prediction alone without significant emphasis on treatment and/or management. Many of them with a few exceptions largely focus on "static" risk factors for violence rather than including dynamic (changeable) items to risk prediction and management. Fourth, actuarial instruments are utilized within a rigid framework in which the input of clinical discretion is limited or disallowed. Finally, they are constructed on specific samples that can impact their ability to generalizable beyond the construction sample.

Structured professional judgment

Structured Professional Judgment (SPJ) utilizes specified risk factors for violence that are commonly identified through a review of literature or through clinical consensus. Upon selection, the risk factors are carefully "operationalized" to ensure their reliable coding. Evaluators conducting the assessment consider the presence and context of risk factors and determine a risk rating that relates to the client's level of risk and the expected level of management, supervision or treatment needs. Typically, the items are not summed into a total score except for research purposes (Webster et al., 1997).

Here, the SPJ tools differ somewhat from actuarial tools. Moreover, the recourse to clinical discretion in making a final risk judgment also significantly differentiates them.

A leading SPJ tool is the Historical/Clinical/Risk Management – 20 (HCR – 20). It is a 20-item checklist of risk factors for violent behavior and organized as follows: ten historical factors, five clinical items and five risk management issues (Webster et al., 1997). The items are coded on a three-point scale (0 – risk factor is absent, 1 – risk factor is partially or possibly present, 2 – risk factor is definitely present). Where there is absence of information regarding an item, it may be omitted, although the omission option is to be used sparingly. It has been noted that the HCR-20 may be used in an actuarial fashion for research purposes (Webster et al., 1997) with items scores summed up into a total score ranging from 0 to 40 and total scores used to estimate risk levels. A recent meta-analysis has shown that SPJ tools are frequently used in an additive manner (Singh, Grann, & Fazel, 2011). However, the HCR-20 has no cut-off point to determine risk and arbitrary points are not advisable for clinical settings (Webster et al., 1997). Extensive research into the HCR-20 in different contexts has demonstrated its reliability and predictive accuracy (McNiel, Gregory, Binder, & Sullivan, 2003; Singh et al., 2011). Adjorlolo and Chan (2019) have equally demonstrated fairly satisfactory predictive accuracy for the HCR-20v3 among offenders in Ghana with AUC values ranging from 0.69 to 0.88. Notwithstanding the foregoing, existing literature suggests that the HCR-20 may reflect culturally determined variations in its predictive accuracy (Fujii, Tokioka, Lichton, & Hishinuma, 2005) and this appears to be common among violence risk assessment instruments (Singh et al., 2011).

Another commonly used SPJ tool is the Short-Term Assessment of Risk and Treatability (START), largely because of its dual emphasis on both strengths and vulnerabilities (Webster et al., 2009). It is a brief, clinical guide for the historical and dynamic assessment of seven defined risk domains. It is designed for interdisciplinary use, although it may be rated by an individual clinician. It contains 20 dynamic items and each is coded for both strength and vulnerability according to the descriptions in the manual. The aim of the START is not to compute an actuarial score but to obtain a comprehensive assessment of risks and to identify strengths that are relevant to the client's functioning (Webster et al., 2009). For clinical uses, the scores on the items are not summed into a total but for research purposes, the item scores may be summed up separately. That said, SPJ tools are not without criticisms. In creating room for flexibility based on professional opinion, risk judgments using the SPJ framework may be prone to biases fueled by cultural presuppositions and negative (or positive) stereotypes on the part of the assessor that may have significant impact on the accuracy of risk measurement (Shepherd & Spivak, 2020). Additionally, the typical absence of cut-off scores, while further allowing clinician flexibility, represents a practical limitation of SPJ approaches because the clinician has no empirically supported benchmark upon which an ultimate determination regarding violence risk can be made (Jackson & Guyton, 2008).

What are the ethical concerns surrounding structured risk assessment?

Assessing risk of violent recidivism can evoke ethical concerns and criticisms, mainly because of the potential harm done to offenders without justification in terms of the offender's welfare. Therefore, it is critical to consider the ethical conflicts emerging from the use of risk assessment procedures.

Naturally, predicting risk is a negative form of chance. It is defined by the probability that an adverse outcome will occur (Roychowdhury & Adshead, 2014). In terms of mental health, an assessment that produces a "high" risk level usually leads to an intervention that is intended to reduce the likelihood of the re-offense occurring. This intervention often takes the form of more intense treatment plans at the community supervision level or prolonged prison sentences. The possibility of implementing a risk assessment with poor predictive validity for offenders could lead to unnecessary restrictions fueled by high rates of false positives, which is a waste of resources (Large, 2014; Roychowdhury & Adshead, 2014).

Another key ethical consideration is the scientific validity of risk instruments, largely developed in North America. A large body of evidence points to the applicability of violence risk instruments to various populations around the world. Preliminary findings are also emerging on the African continent (Adjorlolo & Chan, 2019). The evaluation of instrument utility has been largely based on measures of their predictive accuracy. The "gold standard" for assessing predictive accuracy in violence risk research has been the Area Under the Curve (AUC) index that is generated using Receiver Operating Characteristics (ROC) analysis (Marzban, 2004; Vickers, Cronin, & Begg, 2011). One major advantage of ROC is their independence of base rates of violence in a given population (Mossman, 1994) as well as the possibility of creating cut-offs for violent categorization (Rice & Harris, 1995). Other measures of predictive accuracy that are commonly cited in violence risk assessment research include the positive predictive validity (PPV) and the negative predictive validity (NPV). Figure 6.1 shows the psychometric properties of commonly used risk assessment instruments. These statistics are derived from non-African populations and are mainly provided as indicators of the potential validity of these instruments in African settings.

The number needed to detain is the number of people assessed to be at risk who would need detention to prevent one future incident of violence while the number safely discharged calculates the number of people estimated to be of low risk who need to be discharged into the community before one future incident of violence occurs (Fazel, Trust, Singh, Doll, & Grann, 2012).

Taken together, these findings from validation studies and meta-analyses show that the predictive accuracy of widely used risk assessment instruments is largely satisfactory (AUC 0.70–0.80) (Sjöstedt & Grann, 2002).

On the whole, the poor to moderate values of the predictive accuracy of most of the instruments (Douglas et al., 2017; Fazel & Wolf, 2017; Singh et al., 2011)

Level of Service Inventory – Revised (LSI-R) (Andrews & Bonta, 1995)

- 54-item actuarial instrument predicting general recidivism
- Median AUC, PPV and NPV values of 0.67, 0.57, and 0.53 **(Singh et al., 2011).**
- Medium effect in predicting general (r = 0.29) and non-violent (r = 0.25) recidivism; small effect in predicting violent (r = 0.23) and sexual (r = 0.11) recidivism **(Olver et al., 2014)**

Violence Risk Appraisal Guide (VRAG) (Quinsey et al., 2006)

- 12-item actuarial instrument predicting violence in previously violent mentally disordered offenders
- AUCs of 0.74 – 0.75 in predicting violent recidivism among external validation samples of offenders **(Rice & Harris, 1995).**
- **(Singh et al., 2011)** - median values for AUC, PPV and NPV of 0.74, 0.66, and 0.74 in a meta-analysis.

The Psychopathy Checklist – Revised (PCL-R) (Hare, 2003)

- Actuarial instrument measuring psychopathy as a predictor of antisocial behaviour **(Leistico et al., 2008).**
- Meta-analysis shows median AUC, PPV and NPV values to be 0.66, 0.52, and 0.68 respectively **(Singh et al., 2011).**

The Historical, Clinical, Risk Management – 20 (HCR-20) (Douglas et al., 2014; Webster, Douglas, Eaves & Hart, 1997)

- 20-item SPJ instrument assessing violence in criminal justice, forensic and civil setting.
- Meta-analysis indicates median AUC, PPV and NPV of 0.70, 0.71, 0.67 **(Singh et al., 2011).** **AUC for violence prediction in psychopathy was 0.44 with a correct classification rate of only 38.6%* **(Coid et al., 2013)** *suggesting that it may not be better than chance in such populations.*

Spousal Assault Risk Assessment (SARA) (Kropp et al., 1999)

- 20-item SPJ instrument for predicting future violence in males arrested for spousal assault.
- AUC, PPV and NPV of 0.70, 0.53, and 0.79 respectively **(Singh et al., 2011)**.

The Static-99

- 10-item instrument for assessing long-term sexual recidivism among male sexual offenders **(Hanson & Thornton, 1999).**
- AUC, PPV and NPV of 0.70, 0.33, 0.82 respectively.

Structured Assessment of Violence Risk in Youth (SAVRY)

- 24-item SPJ instrument for violence risk assessment in adolescents **(Borum et al., 2003)**
- AUC values of 0.86 for summary risk rating and 0.80 for risk total score in predicting physical violence among incarcerated youth **(Lodewijks et al., 2008).** Meta-analysis shows more moderate AUC, PPV and NPV values of 0.71, 0.76, 0.76 **(Singh et al., 2011).**

Figure 6.1 Psychometric properties of commonly used risk assessment instruments.

has significant ethical implications in terms of the number of individuals that will be detained to prevent violence, the so-called "number needed to detain" (Fazel et al., 2012; Singh & Fazel, 2010). As opposed to the AUC, it depends on the base rate, sensitivity and specificity of violence risk assessment instruments and it rises as the prevalence (i.e., the likelihood) of violence falls. Consequently, since the sort of violence that detention seeks to prevent (serious violence) may be low (usually less than 4%), there is an increased potential for an increase in the number needed to detain. The high false positive rate represented by such increased numbers raises serious ethical questions with respect to delicate balancing of individual liberty with public safety as well as the attendant stigmatization and discrimination of those considered "high risk" (Douglas et al., 2017) or indeed deemed "dangerous" (Adshead, 2003; McMillan, 2003; Sayers, 2003; Szasz, 2003).

Are structured violence risk assessments being conducted in Africa?

Existing literature on Africa suggests that there are very few published studies involving the use or validation of structured violence risk assessment instruments. A recent comparative cross-sectional survey in Ethiopia by Tsigebrhan, Shibre, Medhin, Fekadu, and Hanlon (2014) compared the prevalence of violence and violent victimization between persons with severe mental illnesses (n = 201) and those without (n = 200). Lifetime and 12-month rates of violence and violent victimization were measured using an adapted version of the McArthur Violence Interview. It is relevant to note that the authors also utilized an adapted version of the HCR-20 in the study which included only three items from the HCR-20 that did not need clinician input. Lifetime and 12-month rates of violence were higher among patients (28.4% and 17.4%) than non-patients (15.0% and 8.5%). In both groups, being literate, male gender and violent victimization were associated with violence while being unmarried, exposure to stressful life events and non-response to medication were also associated with violence in the patient group alone.

In a fairly recent descriptive South African study, the Spousal Assault Risk Assessment Guide (SARA) was utilized in evaluating risk factors for ongoing intimate partner violence in a sample of 53 male respondents (Londt, 2017). Prevalent risk factors for spousal assault included criminal history (mainly previous assaultive behavior towards friends and family), poor psychological adjustment, psychiatric illness in the abuser, impulsivity and anger problems, history of spousal assault and presence of attitudes condoning spousal abuse. The study did not report on the psychometric properties of the SARA within a South African context but rather relied on the validity and reliability obtained from a Western sample.

Adjorlolo and Chan (2019) utilized a triangulation approach in a validation study of the HCR-20 version 3 by collecting data from prisoners, legal guardians/parents and prison officers in order to assess violence risk among incarcerated offenders in Ghana. Using general recidivism as the standard for estimating the discriminant property of the HCR-20v3, the results indicated positive and significant correlations between recidivism and HCR-20v3 scores ranging from 0.35 to 0.69. The AUC values ranged from 0.69 for the clinical presence ratings to 0.88 for the historical presence ratings. The sensitivity and specificity of the historical presence and relevance ratings were satisfactory at above 70%, while the clinical and risk management ratings suffered from either poor sensitivity or specificity. The total HCR presence score showed high sensitivity (93%) with marginal specificity (67%), while the HCR relevance score demonstrated a more satisfactory balance between sensitivity (78%) and specificity (85%).

In perhaps the only such study from Africa, Edelstein (2018) describes the development and validation of the Youth Violence Potential Scale, a locally derived instrument for the assessment of violence risk among South African youth. Using a sample of 12- to 14-year-olds (n = 318), exploratory and confirmatory factor analyses revealed a 19-item instrument with three factors consisting of deviant peers, pro-gangs' attitude and pro-violence attitude subscales. It showed high internal consistency (Cronbach's alpha = 0.91) as well as satisfactory discriminant and convergent validity among its subscales. Correlations with self-reported problem behavior and risk assessment by the maternal caregiver both supported its concurrent validity.

Apart from these four studies, the authors are not aware of any other African study that has used a structured instrument in assessing violence risk. In spite of this, an informal inquiry by Roffey and Kaliski (2012) in 2011 during a forensic psychiatry conference in South Africa revealed infrequency of routine use of SPJ tools in the country and there have been no documented attempts at validating these instruments. However, a pilot testing of the Short-Term Assessment of Risk and Treatability (START) was being undertaken at the Valkenberg Hospital in South Africa as early as 2010 (Roffey & Kaliski, 2012). The experience from the pilot testing suggests that the instrument demonstrates a lot of promise for obtaining comprehensive risk assessments as well as being "user-friendly." However, it is both time-consuming and manpower-demanding (it tends to require a multi-disciplinary team approach for its completion).

In Nigeria, very few psychiatrists use actuarial or SPJ tools and no published data are available yet. At a forensic psychiatry update course (West African College of Physicians, Faculty of Psychiatry 12–13 March 2013), one of the authors (AO) observed that only one psychiatrist among the participants had occasionally used the HCR-20 in conducting violence risk assessments, although he had no formal training. Apart from one of the authors (AO) who has had structured training in the HCR-20 versions 2 and 3, START and PCL-SV, the actual number of mental health practitioners who have had any experience with the use of structured risk assessment instruments in Nigeria is not reliably known. A recent personal communication with a leading Ghanaian psychiatrist (Osei, *personal communication*) suggests a similar picture of instrument non-use among psychiatrists in Ghana. Usually, assessment of violence risk is still being actualized based on unstructured clinical judgment based on clinical history, and mental state examination findings.

A literature search on North Africa yielded only one publication on the status of forensic psychiatry in the sub-continent (El Hamaoui, Moussaoui, & Okasha, 2009) without any mention of research on or practice of structured violence risk assessment.

A medico-legal view of violence risk assessment

To underscore the increasing importance of violence risk assessment, it is instructive to note that a cardinal criterion for civil commitment legislations in many parts of the world, including African countries, is the presence of risk of harm to oneself or to others (see for example, Mental Health Act, 2007; Lagos State Mental Health Law, 2018; Mental Health Care Act, 2002; Mental Health Act, 2012). Despite this reality, the predictability of violence has been shrouded in mystery and contention (Large, Ryan, Singh, Paton, & Nielssen, 2011; Large & Ryan, 2012; Large, Ryan, Callaghan, Paton, & Singh, 2014; Ryan, Nielssen, Paton, & Large, 2010; Steadman & Cocozza, 1978). The much-cited work of Monahan (1981), *The Clinical Prediction of Violent Behavior*, perhaps illustrates the uncertainties regarding unstructured violence risk prediction more clearly in indicating that clinicians were only able to predict future violent outcomes in a third of cases (Jackson & Guyton, 2008). Earlier on, Quinsey and Ambtman (1979) had demonstrated that experienced psychiatrists did not fare better than laymen (in this case, teachers) in their accuracy of predicting violent behavior. In the 1980s, there were warnings against clinicians participating in unstructured violence risk prediction that were regarded as subjective and hardly reliable (Webster et al., 1997).

Apart from this emergent ethical distrust of clinicians' attempts at violence risk prediction, a complex semantic difficulty has also arisen in time, with the evolution of the term "dangerousness," which has been perceived as an unjustifiable social connotation of the psychologically constructed concept of violence risk (Szasz, 2003). Dangerousness has been described as "the perceived likelihood of harm to the public" and is often considered as a simple, static and global characteristic of an individual (Eastman, Adshead, Fox, Latham, & Whyte, 2012). It may be safe to say that while mental health practitioners are interested in violence risk assessment as both a clinical and a legal issue, the concept of predicting dangerousness is inevitably a socio-legal matter (Monahan & Silver, 2003) and one which commands ambivalence and understandable suspicion on the part of mental health practitioners (Adshead, 2003; McMillan, 2003; Sayers, 2003). An attempt to convert violence risk ratings to direct estimations or prediction of dangerousness is fraught with several ethical difficulties. First, it may amount to using medical techniques for a non-medical purpose which could influence legal sanctions such as sentencing. Second, risk assessment regarded as a surrogate for "proof" of dangerousness is not fool-proof since there is always a margin of error largely due to assessor- and data-related imperfections. Some reliable risk assessment instruments (which have been briefly commented upon) utilize "group membership" (i.e., characteristics without individual specificity) (Hart, 2003) or broad generalizations. On the contrary, judicial processes require application on an individual basis. Third, the medical concepts of risk are different from its legal construction. While the legal decisions with respect to violence risk relate to the categorical or dichotomous Shakespearean basis of "to be or not to be"; the psycho-legal viewpoint follows a continuum of risk probabilities or a dimensional framework hinged on the need for risk management. On the basis of these arguments, it has been a contentious matter for mental health professionals in Europe and North America to engage with some of the psycho-legal tensions inherent in violence risk assessment. It is reasonable to infer that similar disquiet must plague mental health practitioners in other parts of the world including Africa where violence risk assessment is even more likely to be highly subjective given the non-use of structured risk instruments in most parts of the continent.

Assessing levels of dangerousness in psychiatry and psychology was likely driven by the development of new legal procedures (Monahan, 2000). Legal precedents in the United States in the late 1960s up until the 1990s contributed to this drive (Jackson & Guyton, 2008). According to a review by Monahan (2000), four key law-related developments resulted in the evolution of the violence risk assessment field in the United States: (1) "dangerousness to others" became one of the vital criteria for involuntary admission in the 1960s, (2) courts imposed liability on clinicians who failed to predict their patients' violence (see Tarasoff v. Regents of University of California (1976)), (3) many states authorized involuntary admission for patients considered to be "dangerous" and (4) the Americans with Disabilities Act (1990) became a law that permitted employers to establish qualification standards that will exclude individuals regardless of disability who pose a direct threat to co-workers or customers. Another important factor that has played a critical role in establishing the field of violence risk assessment is the established relationship between serious mental disorders and violent offending. This relationship has been a highly politically charged issue with varying societal postures on the matter over the last three decades (Busfield, 2017; Eastman et al., 2012; Varshney, Mahapatra, Krishnan, Gupta, & Deb, 2016; Whiting & Fazel, 2020).

Legal factors

Violence risk assessment became a major aspect of mental health evaluation as a result of certain legal developments (Monahan, 2000). Two of those developments, namely: the inclusion of the presence of harm to self or others in the criteria for involuntary admission and the liability placed on clinicians when they fail to rightly discern the level of their patients' violence risk have been highlighted. While the presence of risk of harm to self or others has been explicitly stated as criteria for involuntary admission/treatment in recent mental health laws (as well as proposals) in some African countries (MHCA (South Africa), 2002; Mental Health Act (Ghana), 2012; Lagos State Mental Health Law, 2018 (Nigeria)), other African countries still follow outdated laws that do not specifically emphasize risk to self or others as the primary basis for involuntary hospitalization. Indeed, many countries in Africa face the challenge of anachronistic mental health legislation (Morakinyo, 1977; Ogunlesi, Ogunwale, De Wet, Roos, & Kaliski, 2012; Ogunlesi & Ogunwale, 2012). The relevance of mental health legislation to violence risk assessment lies in the fact that without clear statutory provisions requiring clinicians to assess the patient's/offender's risk of harm to self or others, they would lack the necessary impetus to conduct such assessments in objective ways. Critically, contemporary statutory provisions must highlight the signaling function of violence risk in initiating clinical intervention (e.g., involuntary hospitalization).

With respect to professional or legal liability, African societies do not appear to impose liability for negligent assessment of risk levels on clinicians. Consequently, the motivation on the part of clinicians to conduct rigorous and objective violence risk assessment does not appear to be strong. This is not the case in more developed countries in which liability may be imposed on a clinician who is negligent in assessing and managing a patient's violence risk. For instance, in 2012, French psychiatrist Danièle Canarelli was convicted of manslaughter and handed a one-year suspended prison sentence for failing to recognize the danger posed by her patient who committed murder (Jonas & Abou, 2013).

Socio-economic factors

Most African countries are developing (either low or middle income) with a variety of socio-economic and political challenges. About 77% of low-income countries and most of the least developed countries are in Africa. While a few countries like Nigeria and Ghana may be regarded as lower middle-income countries, only nations like South Africa, Algeria, Angola, Botswana, Mauritius and Equatorial Guinea are categorized as upper middle-income countries (United Nations, 2014). Within this context, many countries have significant shortfalls in funding and human resources in the health sector and in particular, mental health. Current World Health Organization (WHO) statistics suggest there is a median number of 1 mental health worker per 100,000 population in low-income countries compared with 72 in high-income settings. The median number of beds per 100,000 population also shows a severe variation of below 7 in low and lower middle-income countries to over 50 in high-income countries, while funding of mental health care is quite low in low- to middle-income countries (World Health Organization, 2018). Currently, there is roughly one psychiatrist per million persons in many African countries (Ogunlesi et al., 2012). Against this background, there appears to be an even greater lack of forensic mental health practitioners in most countries as it is considered a fledgling subspecialty (Njenga, 2006). This latter observation is relevant to the extent that the field of violence risk assessment would tend to be more important to mental health practitioners who work in the interphase between psychiatry and the legal system (Roffey & Kaliski, 2012).

The role of gender in violence

A further consideration in assessing violence within African countries is the role of gender in violent behavior. While most Western societies have embraced movements toward gender equality, many African countries still endorse male dominance within the society (Ajala, 2016; Bassey & Bubu, 2019; Vetten & Ratele, 2013). Beyond the relevance of this observation to psychosocial issues such as gender-based violence, it seems that male evolutionary tendency toward risk and violent behavior may also drive the occurrence of male-to-male violence (Seedat, van Niekerk, Suffla, & Ratele, 2014; Vetten & Ratele, 2013). This has significant implication for the current elucidation of risk factors for violence which seemed to have left the offender's gender out of the predicting models (Quinsey, Harris, Rice, & Cormier, 2006; Rice & Harris, 1995; Webster et al., 1997). In African settings, it may be important to test the validity of gender inclusion in models that seek to predict violent behavior and to empirically determine gender differences in terms of violence risk in native African samples. Research in Western populations suggests that there are gender differences in the predictive accuracies of risk assessment instruments (Coid et al., 2009; Singh & Fazel, 2010; Singh et al., 2011;2011), although there have also been arguments that despite the empirical support for the inclusion of gender as a risk factor in violence risk assessment models, it remains politically charged and possibly socially objectionable (Douglas et al., 2014).

Ethics of practice in mental health

Additionally, it is important to consider the practice ethics of health care practitioners in many parts of the continent. Generally, individual autonomy is not as strongly exercised in communitarian societies like Africa as in Western societies. As such, paternalism in health care settings seems to subsist in African societies (Rowe & Moodley, 2013). This paternalistic position is also evident in mental health settings (Ramlall, 2012) where clinical judgment in most cases (including violence risk assessment) will likely go unchallenged by patients or their relatives with little inclination to interrogate the validity or veracity of such conclusions. Overall, beneficent paternalism might have been responsible for the delay of African mental health practitioners in adopting standardized and structured approaches to the risk assessment process. It is probable that as Western liberal influence permeates the continent, the autonomy-driven perspective may be more prevalent such that non-standardized, subjective opinions on violence risk will cease to be commonly regarded as expert or professional opinions and may become open to greater challenge in increasingly litigious African societies (Roffey & Kaliski, 2012).

The future of violence risk assessment in Africa

Despite the fledgling state of forensic psychiatric services in Africa (El Hamaoui et al., 2009; Njenga, 2006; Ogunlesi et al., 2012), it appears that the existing facilities can provide the necessary opportunities for the development of violence risk assessment research and practice within the next few years. Currently, formally trained practitioners are very few, but the necessary research personnel capacity can be developed by organizing additional training within each country.

Training and capacity development must necessarily take cognizance of a variety of factors such as the parlous state of funding for mental health care, the absence of secure forensic services, as well as lack of manpower with attendant low clinician: patient ratios. In practical terms, online training programs from overseas could be accessed through webinars. Additionally, those practitioners who have been trained may provide a trainer-pool that may serve national as well as regional training needs. In regions with more established evidence-based forensic services, significant training time and expenses as well as man-hours (up to 16 hours in some cases) are expended in violence risk evaluation and documentation (Fazel et al., 2017; Tully, 2017). In contrast, untrained assessors may produce substandard reports that omit some important predictive items (e.g., personality disorder in HCR-20) (Tully, 2017). Thus, in resource-limited African settings, there could be a preference for brief, simple-to-use instruments which are no less valid to ensure that mental health service providers are not overburdened with paperwork.

In our view, the four strategic objectives in violence risk assessment in Africa should be:

i. Psychometric evaluation of assessment instruments to establish culturally appropriate norms.
ii. Cost-effective research designs in violence risk assessment.
iii. Due consideration for clinical utility and practical purposefulness.
iv. Legislative change to reflect the contemporary role of violence risk assessment.

Psychometric evaluation of the risk assessment instruments

The meta-analysis by Singh et al. (2011) suggests that cultural and sample-based variations may be present in the utilization of different risk assessment instruments. Other quantitative studies as well as reviews have highlighted similar concerns (see Shepherd, 2014). Thus, it becomes vital that the psychometric properties of these instruments should be tested in different settings (civil psychiatric settings, quasi-forensic settings and correctional contexts including in-prison psychiatric clinics). Key reliability indices will include internal consistency (as determined by the Cronbach's alpha), test–retest reliability and inter-rater reliability. The latter is of particular significance for SPJ tools that require subjective clinical decisions in the final or summary stage of determination of risk levels. Furthermore, the validity of these instruments will require formal testing, although the face validity of some of them would appear satisfactory. It is recommended that the construct validity of these instruments be assessed where possible by the process of factor analysis in order to examine their true factor structure in populations that are culturally different from those upon which the instruments were constructed. Another critical measurement is the predictive accuracy of the instruments using the frequently adopted Area Under the Curve parameter (ROC). Cross-validation studies will further strengthen the predictive claims of the investigated instruments.

In addition to these basic methodological approaches, future research should also focus on mediation analyses that could help to model causal mechanisms in violence and potentially rationalize the actual risk factors involved in violent conduct (Buchanan, 2008) in order to improve the efficiency of risk assessment. Previous research had shown that fewer items on risk assessment instruments actually predict future offendings, perhaps suggesting some level of redundancy in the items populating these tools (Coid, Ullrich, & Kallis, 2013; Fazel et al., 2017; Tully, 2017). Statistical weighting of items (e.g., based on standardized regression coefficients) has equally been suggested as a way of ensuring greater efficiency in these instruments (Fazel & Wolf, 2017; Witt, Lichtenstein, & Fazel, 2015). Furthermore, effect modification models (highlighting interaction among potential predictors such as grouping variables) could also help in identifying specific groups in which these tools have optimal performance (O'Shea, Picchioni, Mason, Sugarman, & Dickens, 2014; Szmukler, 2003).

It is also critical to examine the place of cultural factors in the elucidation of risk variables as well as the responsivity end of risk management. Some of these culturally nuanced factors have been highlighted to include, among others: intergenerational trauma, cultural engagement, perceived racism, religion and spirituality, communal support/family support, stigmatization and cultural identity (Shepherd, 2016). While it has been argued that there appears to be a uniformity of risk factors across cultures, it is nevertheless intuitive to consider the significant impact of culture on clinical interaction dynamics at the stage of risk formulation particularly within an SPJ framework (Shepherd, 2014). For example, a deeply cultural African patient who sees the risk evaluator as a symbol of paternalism and authority may unconsciously repress or consciously suppress the age at first incidence of violence because it would be socially undesirable for him to be perceived as "ill-mannered" or "wild." The sensitivity of the interviewer to such sensibilities would thus be of utmost importance in achieving a valid response on such an HCR-20 item.

Research designs

These should focus on cross-sectional designs where initial validation is the key item of interest. Retrospective designs with case-controls have the advantage of being quicker and less costly in terms of time and resources; these may be adopted in the early research effort. However, they are limited in terms of actual prediction since they mainly indicate group differences. Furthermore, it is important for the data infrastructure of psychiatric facilities and correctional services across the continent to be adequately developed in order to provide reliable data required for retrospective study designs. Prospective designs will be planned based on preliminary findings. It is expected that the time to outcome for these longitudinal designs will be based on the availability of resources and continued access to research participants. The time frame may also be determined by the assessment instrument involved (e.g., the START). With regard to data collection from different collateral sources who may be geographically dispersed, innovative electronic means such as telephony, video-conferencing and e-mails may be adopted (Adjorlolo & Chan, 2015, 2019).

Clinical utility

In view of the limited resources in terms of funding and manpower in African societies, Roffey and Kaliski (2012) seem to argue for the introduction of structured professional judgment tools like the HCR-20 that are less time-consuming and labor-intensive than others like the START. Automation of the risk assessment process by devising IT-enabled "risk calculators" has also been advanced as an efficient means of dealing with time constraint and work overload considerations (Fazel et al., 2016, 2017; Monahan et al., 2000). More recently, machine learning techniques have been developed with the aim of optimizing accuracy although these have not been without reservations as to the fairness of the underlying algorithms (Barabas, Dinakar, Ito, Virza, & Zittrain, 2018; Hamilton, Neuilly, Lee, & Barnoski, 2015; Menger, Spruit, van Est, Nap, & Scheepers, 2019; Tolan, Miron, Gómez, & Castillo, 2019).

That said, violence risk assessment tools in mental health settings serve a dual function – clinical assessment and research where indicated. However, it is expected that in time, a combination of risk assessment tools may be needed based on the legal question to be answered, the context of the evaluation and the extant availability of resources. Nonetheless, at the moment, it would appear that strictly actuarial tools or SPJ tools used "actuarially" (i.e., by using total scores for risk categorization instead of clinical judgment) will be quite relevant for research purposes in developing countries.

Legislative change

Given that slightly less than half of African countries have mental health legislation (World Health Organization, 2018), it is crucial that as legislative amendments or fresh enactments take place, the risk of violence to self or others should be emphasized clearly as a primary basis for involuntary hospitalization. This is expected to drive clinicians to seek more objectivity in their risk assessments and thereby potentiate the drive towards structured risk assessment procedures within the continent. Additionally, discharge or parole procedures ought to require the assessing clinician to determine that the mentally ill offender has little or no risk of causing violence upon discharge. This responsibility imposed by law will undoubtedly impel psychiatrists as well as psychologists to adopt a more objective approach to violence risk assessment in such cases in order not to expose themselves to undue professional and/or legal liability.

Conclusion

Violence risk assessment remains a crucial part of clinical evaluations particularly in forensic mental health settings. This is an emerging reality in many developing parts of the world including Africa, in view of their changing socio-cultural and legal landscapes. It is therefore of paramount importance to develop systems and human capacity related to contemporary and culturally appropriate violence risk assessment techniques in African countries in order to derive the individual and public safety advantages inherent in violence risk assessment and management while respecting the ethical boundaries between individual autonomy and the legitimate interests of society in violence prevention.

References

Adjorlolo, S., & Chan, H. C. (2015). Forensic assessment via videoconferencing: Issues and practice considerations. *Journal of Forensic Psychology Practice*, *15*(3), 185–204.

Adjorlolo, S., & Chan, H. C. (Oliver). (2019). Risk assessment of criminal offenders in Ghana: An investigation of the discriminant validity of the HCR-20V3. *International Journal of Law and Psychiatry*, *66*, 101458. https://doi.org/10.1016/j.ijlp.2019.101458.

Adshead, G. (2003). Commentary on Szasz. *Journal of Medical Ethics*, *29*(4), 230–232. https://doi.org/10.1136/jme.29.4.227.

Ajala, T. (2016). Social construction of gender roles and women's poverty in African societies: The case of the Nigerian woman. *International Journal of Gender & Women's Studies*, *4*(2). https://doi.org/10.15640/ijgws.v4n2a1.

Americans With Disabilities Act. (1990). Pub. L. No. 101–336, 104 Stat. 328.

Andrews, D. A., & Bonta, J. (1995). *LSI-R: The Level of Service Inventory-Revised*. Multi-Health Systems.

Andrews, D. A., Bonta, J., & Wormith, J. S. (2006). The recent past and near future of risk and/or need assessment. *Crime & Delinquency*, *52*(1), 7–27. https://doi.org/10.1177/0011128705281756.

Arseneault, L., Moffitt, T., Caspi, A., Taylor, P., & Silva, P. (2000). Mental disorders and violence in a total birth cohort. *Arch Gen Psychiatry*, *57*, 979–986.

Barabas, C., Dinakar, K., Ito, J., Virza, M., & Zittrain, J. (2018, July 14). Interventions over predictions: Reframing the ethical debate for actuarial risk assessment. *Proceedings of FAT Conference*. FAT Conference, New York. http://arxiv.org/abs/1712.08238.

Barefoot v. Estelle, 697 F.2d 593 (5th Cir. 1983).

Bassey, S. A., & Bubu, N. G. (2019). Gender inequality in Africa: A re-examination of cultural values. *Cogito Multidisciplinary Research Journal*, *XI*(3), 21–36.

Baxstrom v. Herold. (1966). 383 U.S. 107, 86 S. Ct. 760, 15 L. Ed. 2d 620.

Bonta, J., Law, M., & Hanson, K. (1998). The prediction of criminal and violent recidivism among mentally disordered offenders: A meta-analysis. *Psychological Bulletin*, *123*(2), 123–142. https://doi.org/10.1037/0033-2909.123.2.123.

Borum, R., Bartel, P., & Forth, A. (2003). *Manual for the structured assessment of violence risk in youth (SAVRY): Version 1.1*. Tampa, FL: University of South Florida.

Buchanan, A. (2008). Risk of violence by psychiatric patients: Beyond the "actuarial versus clinical" assessment debate. *Psychiatric Services*, *59*, 184–190.

Busfield, J. (2017). Psychiatric disorder and individual violence: Evidence and perceptions. In: A. Buchanan (Ed.), *Care of the mentally disordered offender in the community*. Oxford: Oxford University Press.

Coid, J., Yang, M., Ullrich, S., Zhang, T., Sizmur, S., Roberts, C., Farrington, D. P., & Rogers, R. D. (2009). Gender differences in structured risk assessment: Comparing the accuracy of five instruments. *Journal of Consulting and Clinical Psychology*, *77*(2), 337–348. https://doi.org/10.1037/a0015155.

Coid, J. W., Ullrich, S., & Kallis, C. (2013). Predicting future violence among individuals with psychopathy. *British Journal of Psychiatry*, *203*(5), 387–388. https://doi.org/10.1192/bjp.bp.112.118471.

Dahlberg, L., & Mercy, J. (2009). History of violence as a public health issue. *AMA Virtual Mentor*, *11*(2), 167–172.

de Vries Robbé, M., de Vogel, V., & de Spa, E. (2011). Protective factors for violence risk in forensic psychiatric patients: A retrospective validation study of the SAPROF. *International Journal of Forensic Mental Health*, *10*(3), 178–186. https://doi.org/10.1080/14999013.2011.600232.

de Vries Robbé, M., Geers, M., Stapel, M., Hilterman, E., & de Vogel, V. (2015). *SAPROF Youth Version: Guidelines for the assessment of protective factors for violence risk in Juveniles*. Utrecht, the Netherlands: Van der Hoeven Kliniek.

Douglas, K. S., Cox, D. N., & Webster, C. D. (1999). Violence risk assessment: Science and practice. *Legal and Criminological Psychology*, *4*(2), 149–184. https://doi.org/10.1348/135532599167824.

Douglas, K. S., Hart, S. D., Webster, C. D., Belfrage, H., Guy, L. S., & Wilson, C. M. (2014). Historical-Clinical-Risk Management-20, Version 3 (HCR-20V3): Development and Overview. *International Journal of Forensic Mental Health*, *13*(2), 93–108. https://doi.org/10.1080/14999013.2014.906519.

Douglas, T., Pugh, J., Singh, I., Savulescu, J., & Fazel, S. (2017). Risk assessment tools in criminal justice and forensic psychiatry: The need for better data. *European Psychiatry*, *42*, 134–137. https://doi.org/10.1016/j.eurpsy.2016.12.009.

Eastman, N., Adshead, G., Fox, S., Latham, R., & Whyte, S. (2012). *Oxford specialist handbooks in psychiatry: Forensic psychiatry* (1st ed.). New York: Oxford University Press Inc.

Edelstein, I. (2018). Development and validation of the youth violence potential scale. *Violence and Victims*, *33*(5), 789–812.

El Hamaoui, Y., Moussaoui, D., & Okasha, T. (2009). Forensic psychiatry in North Africa. *Current Opinion in Psychiatry*, *22*, 507–510.

Fazel, S., Buxrud, P., Ruchkin, V., & Grann, M. (2010). Homicide in discharged patients with schizophrenia and other psychoses: A national case-control study. *Schizophrenia Research*, *123*(2–3), 263–269. https://doi.org/10.1016/j.schres.2010.08.019.

Fazel, S., Chang, Z., Fanshawe, T., Långström, N., Lichtenstein, P., Larsson, H., & Mallett, S. (2016). Prediction of violent reoffending on release from prison: Derivation and external validation of a scalable tool. *The Lancet Psychiatry*, *3*(6), 535–543. https://doi.org/10.1016/S2215-0366(16)00103-6.

Fazel, S., Gulati, G., Linsell, L., Geddes, J. R., & Grann, M. (2009). Schizophrenia and violence: Systematic review and meta-analysis. *PLoS Medicine*, *6*(8), e1000120. https://doi.org/10.1371/journal.pmed.1000120.

Fazel, S., Psych, M. R. C., Grann, M., & Psych, C. (2006). The population impact of severe mental illness on violent crime. *American journal of psychiatry*, *163*(8), 1397–1403.

Fazel, S., Trust, W., Singh, J. P., Doll, H., & Grann, M. (2012). Use of risk assessment instruments to predict violence and antisocial behaviour in 73 samples involving 24 827 people: Systematic review and meta-analysis. *The BMJ*, *4692*(July), 1–12. https://doi.org/10.1136/bmj.e4692.

Fazel, S., & Wolf, A. (2017). Selecting a risk assessment tool to use in practice: A 10-point guide. *Evidence-based Mental Health*, *21*(2), 41–43. https://doi.org/10.1136/eb-2017-102861.

Fazel, S., Wolf, A., Larsson, H., Lichtenstein, P., Mallett, S., & Fanshawe, T. R. (2017). Identification of low risk of violent crime in severe mental illness with a clinical prediction tool (Oxford Mental Illness and Violence tool [OxMIV]): A derivation and validation study. *The Lancet Psychiatry*, *4*(6), 461–468. https://doi.org/10.1016/S2215-0366(17)30109-8.

Fujii, D. E. M., Tokioka, A. B., Lichton, A. I., & Hishinuma, E. (2005). Ethnic differences in prediction of violence risk with the HCR-20 among psychiatric inpatients. *Psychiatric Services*, *56*(6), 711–716. https://doi.org/10.1176/appi.ps.56.6.711.

Garner, B. A. (2001). Black's law dictionary (7th ed.). Minnesota: West Publishing Company.

Grisso, T., & Appelbaum, P. S. (1992). Is it unethical to offer predictions of future violence? *Law and Human Behavior*, *16*(6), 621–633. https://doi.org/10.1007/BF01884019.

Grove, W. M., & Meehl, P. E. (1996). Comparative efficiency of informal (subjective, impressionistic) and formal (mechanical, algorithmic) prediction procedures: The clinical-statistical controversy. *Psychology, Public Policy, and Law*, *2*(2), 293–323.

Hamilton, Z., Neuilly, M.-A., Lee, S., & Barnoski, R. (2015). Isolating modeling effects in offender risk assessment. *Journal of Experimental Criminology*, *11*(2), 299–318. https://doi.org/10.1007/s11292-014-9221-8.

Hanson, R., & Thornton, D. (1999). *Static-99: Improving actuarial risk assessments for sex offenders (User Report 99-02).*

Hare, R. D. (2003). *The hare psychopathy checklist-revised.* ON, Canada: Multi-Health Systems.

Harris, G. T., Rice, M. E., & Quinsey, V. L. (1993). Violent recidivism of mentally disordered offenders: The development of a statistical prediction instrument. *Criminal Justice and Behavior*, *20*(4), 315–335.

Hart, S. D. (2003). Actuarial risk assessment: Commentary on Berlin et al. *Sexual Abuse: A Journal of Research and Treatment*, *15*(4), 383–388.

Hart, S. D., Michie, C., & Cooke, D. J. (2007). Precision of actuarial risk assessment instruments: Evaluating the 'margins of error' of group *v.* individual predictions of violence. *British Journal of Psychiatry*, *190*(S49), s60–s65. https://doi.org/10.1192/bjp.190.5.s60.

Heilbrun, K., Brooks Holliday, S., & King, C. (2013). Evaluation of violence risk in adults. In: R. Roesch, & P. Zapf (Eds.), *Forensic assessments in criminal and civil law: A handbook for lawyers* (pp. 74–87). New York: Oxford University Press.

Hodgins, S., Alderton, J., Cree, A., Aboud, A., & Mak, T. (2007). Aggressive behaviour, victimisation and crime among severely mentally ill patients requiring hospitalisation. *British Journal of Psychiatry*, *191*, 343–350.

Jackson, R., & Guyton, M. (2008). Violence risk assessment. In *Learning forensic assessment* (pp. 153–181). New York: Routledge Taylor & Francis Group.

Jonas, C., & Abou, N. (2013). Psychiatric liability: A French psychiatrist sentenced after a murder committed by her patient. *Psychiatric Times*, *30*(4). https://www.psychiatrictimes.

com/forensic-psychiatry/psychiatric-liability-french-psychiatrist-sentenced-after-murder-committed-her-patient.

Kropp, P., Hart, S., Webster, C., & Eaves, D. (1999). *Spousal assault risk assessment guide (SARA)*. ON, Canada: Multi-Health Systems.

Krug, E. G., Mercy, J. A., Dahlberg, L. L., & Zwi, A. B. (2002). The world report on violence and health. *The Lancet*, *360*(9339), 1083–1088. https://doi.org/10.1016/S0140-6736(02)11133-0.

Lagos State Mental Health Law. (2018). Ikeja: Lagos State Government.

Large, M. (2014). Risk assessment and evidence-based medicine. *The Psychiatric Bulletin*, *38*(4), 196–196. https://doi.org/10.1192/pb.38.4.196.

Large, M., & Ryan, C. J. (2012). Sanism, stigma and the belief in dangerousness. *Australian & New Zealand Journal of Psychiatry*, *46*(11), 1099–1100. https://doi.org/10.1177/0004867412440193.

Large, M. M., Ryan, C., Callaghan, S., Paton, M., & Singh, S. (2014). Can violence risk assessment really assist in clinical decision-making? *Australian & New Zealand Journal of Psychiatry*, *48*(3), 286–288. https://doi.org/10.1177/0004867413498275.

Large, M. M., Ryan, C. J., Singh, S. P., Paton, M. B., & Nielssen, O. B. (2011). The predictive value of risk categorization in schizophrenia. *Harvard Review of Psychiatry*, *19*(1), 25–33. https://doi.org/10.3109/10673229.2011.549770.

Leistico, A. M. R., Salekin, R. T., DeCoster, J., & Rogers, R. (2008). A large-scale meta-analysis relating the hare measures of psychopathy to antisocial conduct. *Law and Human Behavior*, *32*(1), 28–45. https://doi.org/10.1007/s10979-007-9096-6.

Lindqvist, P., & Allebeck, P. (1990). Schizophrenia and crime. A longitudinal follow-up of 644 schizophrenics in Stockholm. *British Journal of Psychiatry*, *157*, 345–350. https://doi.org/10.1192/bjp.157.3.345.

Lodewijks, H. P. B., Doreleijers, T. A. H., De Ruiter, C., & Borum, R. (2008). Predictive validity of the structured assessment of violence risk in youth (SAVRY) during residential treatment. *International Journal of Law and Psychiatry*, *31*, 263–271. https://doi.org/10.1016/j.ijlp.2008.04.009.

Londt, M. P. (2017). Batterer risk assessment: The missing link in breaking the cycle of interpersonal violence. *Southern African Journal of Social Work and Social Development*, *26*(1), 93–116. https://doi.org/10.25159/2415-5829/2181.

Marzban, C. (2004). The ROC curve and the area under it as performance measures. *Weather and Forecasting*, *19*(6), 1106–1114. https://doi.org/10.1175/825.1.

McMillan, J. (2003). Dangerousness, mental disorder and responsibility. *Journal of Medical Ethics*, *29*(4), 232–235. https://doi.org/10.1136/jme.29.4.227.

McNiel, D. E., Gregory, A. L., Lam, J. N., Binder, R. L., & Sullivan, G. R. (2003). Utility of decision support tools for assessing acute risk of violence. *Journal of Consulting and Clinical Psychology*, *71*(5), 945.

Menger, V., Spruit, M., van Est, R., Nap, E., & Scheepers, F. (2019). Machine learning approach to inpatient violence risk assessment using routinely collected clinical notes in electronic health records. *JAMA Network Open*, *2*(7), e196709. https://doi.org/10.1001/jamanetworkopen.2019.6709.

Mental Health Act. (2007). London: HMSO.

Mental Health Act. (2012). Act 846 of the Parliament of the Republic of Ghana. Accra: Government Printer, Assembly Press Ltd.

Mental Health Care Act. (2002). Act No. 17 (South Africa). Pretoria: Department of Health.

Monahan, J. (1981). *Predicting violent behavior: An assessment of clinical techniques.* Beverly hills, CA: Sage Publications.
Monahan, J. (1996). Violence prediction: The past twenty and the next 20 years. *Criminal Justice and Behavior, 23*(1), 107–120.
Monahan, J. (2000). Violence risk assessment: Scientific validity and evidentiary admissibility. *Washington and Lee Law Review, 57*(3), 901–918.
Monahan, J., & Silver, E. (2003). Judicial decision thresholds for violence risk management. *International Journal of Forensic Mental Health, 2*(1), 1–6. https://doi.org/10.1080/14999013.2003.10471174.
Monahan, J., Steadman, H. J., Appelbaum, P. S., Robbins, P. C., Mulvey, E. P., Silver, E., Roth, L. H., & Grisso, T. (2000). Developing a clinically useful actuarial tool for assessing violence risk. *British Journal of Psychiatry, 176*, 312–319.
Morakinyo, V. (1977). The law and psychiatry in Africa. *African Journal of Psychiatry, 3*, 91–98.
Mossman, D. (1994). Assessing predictions of violence: Being accurate about accuracy. *Journal of Consulting and Clinical Psychology, 62*(4), 783–792. https://doi.org/10.1037/0022-006X.62.4.783.
Njenga, F. (2006). Forensic psychiatry: The African experience. *World Psychiatry, 5*(2), 97.
Ogunlesi, A., & Ogunwale, A. (2012). Mental health legislation in Nigeria: Current leanings and future yearnings. *International Psychiatry, 9*(3), 62–64. https://doi.org/10.1192/S1749367600003234.
Ogunlesi, A., Ogunwale, A., De Wet, P., Roos, L., & Kaliski, S. (2012). Forensic psychiatry in Africa: Prospects and challenges. *African Journal of Psychiatry, 15*(1), 3–7. https://doi.org/10.4314/ajpsy.v15i1.1.
Olver, M. E., Stockdale, K. C., & Wormith, J. S. (2014). 30 years of research on the Level of Service Scales: A meta-analytic examination of predictive accuracy and sources of variability. *Psychological Assessment, 26*(1), 156–176. https://doi.org/10.1037/a0035080.
O'Shea, L., Picchioni, M., Mason, F., Sugarman, P., & Dickens, G. (2014). Differential predictive validity of the Historical, Clinical and Risk Management Scales (HCR – 20) for inpatient aggression. *Psychiatry Research, 220*(1–2), 669–678. https://doi.org/10.1016/j.psychres.2014.07.080.
Quinsey, V. L., & Ambtman, R. (1979). Variables affecting psychiatrists' and teachers' assessments of the dangerousness of mentally ill Offenders. *Journal of Consulting and Clinical Psychology, 47*(2), 353–362.
Quinsey, V. L., Harris, G., Rice, M. E., & Cormier, C. A. (2006). *Violent offenders: Appraising and managing risk.* American Psychological Association. https://doi.org/10.1037/11367-000.
Ramlall, S. (2012). The Mental Health Care Act No 17–South Africa. Trials and triumphs: 2002-2012. *African Journal of Psychiatry, 15*(6), 407–410.
Rice, M., & Harris, G. (1995). Violent recidivism: Assessing predictive validity. *Journal of Consulting and Clinical Psychology, 63*(5), 737–748. https://doi.org/10.1037/0022-006X.63.5.737.
Roffey, M., & Kaliski, S. (2012). Forensic Forum: 'To predict or not to predict – that is the question' An exploration of risk assessment in the context of South African forensic psychiatry. *African Journal of Psychiatry, 15*(4), 227–233. https://doi.org/10.4314/ajpsy.v15i4.29
Rowe, K., & Moodley, K. (2013). Patients as consumers of health care in South Africa: The ethical and legal implications. *BMC Medical Ethics, 14*(1), 15. https://doi.org/10.1186/1472-6939-14-15.
Roychowdhury, A., & Adshead, G. (2014). Violence risk assessment as a medical

intervention: Ethical tensions. *The Psychiatric Bulletin*, *38*(2), 75–82. https://doi.org/10.1192/pb.bp.113.043315.

Ryan, C., Nielssen, O., Paton, M., & Large, M. (2010). Clinical decisions in psychiatry should not be based on risk assessment. *Australasian Psychiatry*, *18*(5), 398–403. https://doi.org/10.3109/10398562.2010.507816.

Sayers, G. (2003). Psychiatry and the control of dangerousness: A comment. *Journal of Medical Ethics*, *29*(4), 235–236. https://doi.org/10.1136/jme.29.4.227.

Seedat, M., van Niekerk, A., Suffla, S., & Ratele, K. (2014). Psychological research and South Africa's violence prevention responses. *South African Journal of Psychology*, *44*(2), 136–144. https://doi.org/10.1177/0081246314526831.

Shepherd, S. M. (2014). Finding color in conformity: A commentary on culturally specific risk factors for violence in Australia. *International Journal of Offender Therapy and Comparative Criminology*, *59*(12), 1297–1307. https://doi.org/10.1177/0306624X14540492.

Shepherd, S. M. (2016). Violence risk instruments may be culturally unsafe for use with Indigenous patients. *Australasian Psychiatry*, *24*(6), 565–567. https://doi.org/10.1177/1039856216665287.

Shepherd, S. M., & Spivak, B. L. (2020). Finding colour in conformity part II—Reflections on structured professional judgement and cross-cultural risk assessment. *International Journal of Offender Therapy and Comparative Criminology*, 0306624X20928025. https://doi.org/10.1177/0306624X20928025.

Singh, J. P., & Fazel, S. (2010). Forensic risk assessment: A metareview. *Criminal Justice and Behavior*, *37*(9), 965–988. https://doi.org/10.1177/0093854810374274.

Singh, J. P., Grann, M., & Fazel, S. (2011). A comparative study of violence risk assessment tools: A systematic review and metaregression analysis of 68 studies involving 25,980 participants. *Clinical Psychology Review*, *31*(3), 499–513. https://doi.org/10.1016/j.cpr.2010.11.009.

Sjöstedt, G., & Grann, M. (2002). Risk assessment: What is being predicted by actuarial prediction instruments? *International Journal of Forensic Mental Health*, *1*(2), 179–183. https://doi.org/10.1080/14999013.2002.10471172.

Steadman, H. J., & Cocozza, J. (1978). Psychiatry, dangerousness and the repetitively violent offender. *The Journal of Criminal Law and Criminology*, *69*(2), 226. https://doi.org/10.2307/1142396.

Swanson, J., Holzer, C., Ganju, V., & Jono, R. (1990). Violence and psychiatric disorder in the community: Evidence from the epidemiological catchment area survey. *Hospital and Community Psychiatry*, *41*, 761–770.

Szasz, T. (2003). Psychiatry and the control of dangerousness: On the apotropaic function of the term 'mental illness'. *Journal of Medical Ethics*, *29*(4), 227–230. https://doi.org/10.1136/jme.29.4.227.

Szmukler, G. (2003). Risk assessment: 'numbers' and 'values'. *Psychiatric Bulletin*, *27*, 205–207.

Tarasoff v. Regents of University of California, 551 P.2d 334, 17 Cal. 3d 425, 131 Cal. Rptr. 14 (1976).

Tolan, S., Miron, M., Gómez, E., & Castillo, C. (2019). Why Machine Learning May Lead to Unfairness: Evidence from Risk Assessment for Juvenile Justice in Catalonia. *Proceedings of the Seventeenth International Conference on Artificial Intelligence and Law - ICAIL '19*, 83–92. https://doi.org/10.1145/3322640.3326705.

Torrey, E. F., Stanley, J., Monahan, J., & Steadman, H. J. (2008). The MacArthur violence risk assessment study revisited: Two views 10 years after its initial publication. *Psychiatric Services*, *59*(2), 147–152.

Tsigebrhan, R., Shibre, T., Medhin, G., Fekadu, A., & Hanlon, C. (2014). Violence and violent victimization in people with severe mental illness in a rural low-income country setting: A comparative cross-sectional community study. *Schizophrenia Research, 152*(1), 275–282. https://doi.org/10.1016/j.schres.2013.10.032.

Tully, J. (2017). HCR-20 shows poor field validity in clinical forensic psychiatry settings. *Evidence-Based Mental Health, 20*(3), 95–96. https://doi.org/10.1136/eb-2017-102745.

United Nations. (2014). *2014wesp_country_classification.pdf.* https://www.un.org/en/development/desa/policy/wesp/wesp_current/2014wesp_country_classification.pdf.

Varshney, M., Mahapatra, A., Krishnan, V., Gupta, R., & Deb, K. S. (2016). Violence and mental illness: What is the true story? *Journal of Epidemiology and Community Health, 70*(3), 223–225. https://doi.org/10.1136/jech-2015-205546.

Vetten, L., & Ratele, K. (2013). Men and violence. *Agenda, 27*(1), 4–11. https://doi.org/10.1080/10130950.2013.813769.

Vickers, A., Cronin, A., & Begg, C. (2011). One statistical test is sufficient for assessing new predictive markers. BMC Medical Research Methodology, *11*, 1–7.

Wallace, C., Mullen, P. E., & Burgess, P. (2004). Criminal offending in schizophrenia over a 25-year period marked by deinstitutionalization and increasing prevalence of co-morbid substance use disorders. *American Journal of Psychiatry, 161*, 716–727.

Wallace, C., Mullen, P., Burgess, P., Palmer, S., Ruschena, D., & Browne, C. (1998). Serious criminal offending and mental disorder Case linkage study. *British Journal of Psychiatry, 172*, 477–484.

Webster, C. D., Douglas, K. S., Eaves, D., & Hart, S. D. (1997). *HCR- 20: Assessing risk for violence* (Version 2). Simon Fraser University, Mental Health, Law, and Policy Institute.

Webster, C. D., Martin, M. L., Brink, J., Nicholls, T. L., & Desmarais, S. L. (2009). *Manual for the Short Term Assessment of Risk and Treatability (START)(Version 1.1).*Coquitlam, Canada: British Columbia Mental Health & Addiction Services.

Whiting, D., & Fazel, S. (2020). Epidemiology and risk factors for violence in people with mental disorders. In B. Carpiniello, A. Vita, & C. Mencacci (Eds.), *Violence and mental disorders* (Vol. 1, pp. 49–62). Cham, Switzerland: Springer International Publishing. https://doi.org/10.1007/978-3-030-33188-7_3.

Witt, K., Lichtenstein, P., & Fazel, S. (2015). Improving risk assessment in schizophrenia: Epidemiological investigation of criminal history factors. *British Journal of Psychiatry, 206*(5), 424–430. https://doi.org/10.1192/bjp.bp.114.144485.

Witt, K., van Dorn, R., & Fazel, S. (2013). Risk factors for violence in psychosis: Systematic review and meta-regression analysis of 110 Studies. *PLoS ONE, 8*(2), e55942(1–15). https://doi.org/10.1371/journal.pone.0055942.

World Health Organization. (Ed.). (2018). *Mental health atlas 2017.* Geneva: World Health Organization.

7 Competency to stand trial evaluations in Africa

Samuel Adjorlolo and Kofi E. Boakye

Introduction

Competency to stand trial (CST, also known as fitness to stand trial, fitness to plead, and adjudicative competency) is a concept of jurisprudence allowing trials for defendants who cannot participate in the criminal process (due to mental incapacitation and intellectual disability) to be postponed. It is frequently and substantially raised more often than the insanity defense, with available data suggesting that about 60,000 adjudicative competence evaluations are requested in the United States annually, costing an estimated annual expenditure of $300 million (Zapf, Roesch, & Pirelli, 2014). Derived from old English common law, CST is one of the procedural requirements for upholding and maintaining due process rights, judicial sanctity and procedural fairness (Adjorlolo & Chan, 2017). Fundamentally, the posture of the law across jurisdictions is that no one should be tried when they cannot contribute meaningfully and satisfactorily to the criminal adjudication process. The essence of CST was summarized by Lord Edmund-Davies in *R v Podola* (1960) in Britain as "no man may be brought to trial upon any criminal charge unless and until he is mentally capable of fairly standing trial." The court is obliged to ensure that defendants are actively involved in criminal proceedings. When issues of incompetency are suspected and/or raised before or during the adjudication process, a request for a CST evaluation is normally made by the court. Forensic mental health professionals such as clinical psychologists and psychiatrists are invited to conduct CST evaluations. The evaluation report is intended to assist the court to decide whether proceedings should be continued for those found to be competent or discontinued for those declared incompetent to stand trial. The literature on CST has gained traction over the years because CST issues are raised substantially more than other psycholegal issues (e.g. insanity at the time of offense). However, relatively little information exists with respect to CST from Africa. To fill this important gap in the literature, the chapter focuses specifically on CST in African settings and is organized as follows; the first section will examine the history and definition of competency as used in the legal system. This will be followed by an overview of CST legislations across Africa and selected high-income countries. The third section will discuss the evaluation of CST, with a focus on the administration of competency evaluation instruments and collateral sources of data. The last section will focus on the disposition of incompetency and competency restoration of incompetent defendants.

Competency-to-stand-trial legislations

The concept of CST originated from the British judicial system (Rogers, Blackwood, Farnham, Pickup, & Watts, 2008). Historically, English common law has prevented defendants from being processed via the judicial system on the grounds that they are mentally incompetent to participate in their trials (Zapf et al., 2014). That is, the English common law primarily allowed for an arraignment, trial, judgment or execution of a defendant to be stayed until he or she is declared competent. Just like the insanity defense legislation, the English common law concept of CST has had significant influence on CST legislation across the globe, particularly countries constituting the Commonwealth of Nations and the United States (Zapf et al., 2014). Nevertheless, countries have formulated legislation for determining whether a defendant is competent or incompetent to stand trial. This is sometimes based on a landmark ruling that subsequently becomes the standard for CST.

In England and Wales, this is based on the professional interpretation of *Pritchard criteria* (1836), which defined CST as follows: (1) ability to plead, (2) ability to understand evidence, (3) ability to understand court proceedings, (4) ability to instruct a lawyer and (5) knowing that a juror can be challenged (Rogers et al., 2008). In the United States, CST standard was formulated in *Dusky v US* (1960) where CST is stated as follows: (1) the defendant must have sufficient present ability to consult with defense counsel with a reasonable degree of rational understanding and (2) a rational as well as factual understanding of the proceedings against him or her. Section 2 of the Criminal Code of Canada 1992 lists the essential ingredients of CST as abilities to (a) understand the nature or object of the proceedings, (b) understand the possible consequences of the proceedings and (c) communicate with counsel. In Australia, CST is determined on the basis of the *Presser criteria*, which comprise the following: (1) ability to understand the charge; (2) ability to plead to the charge and exercise the right to challenge; (3) understanding of the basic nature of the proceedings; (4) ability to follow the course of the proceedings in broad terms; (5) ability to understand the substantial effect of any evidence and be able to make a defense or answer to the charge, including the ability to instruct counsel and (6) have sufficient capacity to be able to decide what defense strategy will be relied upon and make this known to the court and counsel (White, Batchelor, Pulman, & Howard, 2012). In Hong Kong, a former British colony, the legal provision relating to CST is contained in section 75(1) of the Criminal Procedure Ordinance which states that an individual is not competent to stand trial if he labors "under any disability such that apart from this Ordinance it would constitute a bar to his being tried." Owing to the confusion associated with the terminology "under disability" the Hong Kong court in *R v Leung Tak-Choi* (1995) elaborated on the CST legislation by defining "under disability" as when the defendant lacks ability to understand the charges, instruct defense counsel,

Table 7.1 Indicators of competency to stand trial across jurisdictions

1	Ability to understand the arrest process
2	Ability to make decisions after receiving advice
3	Ability to understand the current legal situation
4	Ability to maintain a collaborative relationship with counsel and help plan legal strategy
5	Ability to understand the charges, both in nature and severity
6	Ability to understand relevant facts
7	Ability to follow testimony for contradictions or errors
8	Ability to understand the legal issues and procedures
9	Ability to testify relevantly and be cross-examined if necessary
10	Ability to understand potential legal defenses
11	Ability to challenge prosecution witnesses
12	Ability to understand the possible dispositions, pleas and penalties
13	Ability to tolerate stress at trial and while awaiting trial
14	Ability to appraise the likely outcome
15	Ability to refrain from irrational and unmanageable behavior during trial
16	Ability to appraise the roles of the defense counsel, prosecutor, judge, jury, witnesses and defendant
17	Ability to disclose pertinent facts surrounding the alleged offense
18	Ability to protect oneself and utilize legal safeguards available
19	Ability to identify witnesses
20	Ability to appraise the likely outcome of the case
21	Ability to relate to counsel in a trusting and communicative fashion
22	Ability to comprehend instructions and advice

challenge jurors, understand the evidence against him or her and give evidence in defense.

Despite differences in the wording of CST legislations, it is interesting to note similarity in the CST indicators across jurisdictions. As can be seen in Table 7.1, the discrete court-related functions that are indicative of CST are evident in the CST legislations or standards in England and Wales, the United States, Australia and Hong Kong (Adjorlolo & Chan, 2017).

Competency-to-stand-trial legislations in Africa

As noted previously, the CST provisions in several African countries are influenced by English common law. These provisions allow for arraignment, trial and judgment of defendants to be placed on hold if there are indications that the defendant is not competent to stand trial. The legal provision relating to CST in Ghana is contained in Section 133 (1) of Criminal and Other Offences (Procedure) Act, 1960 (Act, 30; henceforth Act 30) which states that "Where in the course of a trial or preliminary proceedings the Court has the reason to believe that the accused is of unsound mind and consequently incapable of making a defense, it shall inquire into the fact of such unsoundness by causing the accused to be medically examined and shall after the examination take medical and any other available evidence regarding the state of the accused's mind" (see Adjorlolo, Chan, & Agboli, 2016, p. 2). The CST in Nigeria is very similar to the CST provision in Ghana. More specifically, Section 223 of the Nigerian Criminal Procedure Act (1963) provides that when a judge or a magistrate holding a trial has reason to suspect that the accused is of unsound mind and as a result is incapable of making his defense, the court shall investigate it, either in the presence of the accused or in his absence if his presence would be against public decency or against his or other persons' interest. Section 77 of the South African Criminal Procedure Act (CPA) 51 of 1977 also states that "If it appears to the court at any stage of criminal proceedings that the accused is by reason of mental illness or mental defect not capable of understanding the proceedings so as to make a proper defense, the court shall direct that the matter be enquired into and be reported on in accordance with the provisions of section 79" (see Pillay, 2014, p. 49). The CST legislations in Africa and elsewhere have recognized essentially that only defendants who are competent to stand trial should be processed via the justice system. Compared with the legislations from outside Africa, it is evident that the African CST legislations are somewhat vague and ambiguous. With the exception of understanding trial proceedings that appear to resonate across the legislations, other specific indicators of whether a defendant is competent to stand trial or otherwise are not explicitly provided. Nevertheless, the processes involved in determining whether defendants are competent for trial proceedings, or otherwise, appear universal and they include the following: (1) raising the question and requesting for competency examination, (2) the CST evaluation stage, (3) judicial determination CST, (4) disposition and provision of treatment to incompetent defendants and (5) re-hearings on competency of incompetent defendants, or release of incompetent defendants (Adjorlolo et al., 2016). These are discussed briefly below under the broad heading of CST evaluations in accordance with the focus of this chapter.

Competency-to-stand-trial evaluations

CST is a legal, rather than a mental health concept, which means that the ultimate decision relating to the competency or otherwise of a defendant is the sole decision of the court. The decision-making process of the court is, however, aided by assessment reports relating to the defendant's mental states. Because mental health problems and intellectual disabilities are the major factors contributing to incompetence to stand trial, the courts tend to rely on mental health professionals for their expert opinion, which is contained in the assessment report. Issues relating to a defendant's CST can be raised by the defense and prosecution attorneys and sometimes the judge or magistrate. When the issue is raised by the defense or prosecution attorney, the court must be convinced or satisfied with the reasons or facts presented before a request for a CST evaluation can be made. To ensure due process rights and to uphold sanctity of the judicial system, the courts normally grant requests for CST evaluation. Yet, in some instances, such requests can be denied by the courts for several reasons, including the perception that raising issues relating to CST is a strategy to prolong the criminal adjudication process or the reasons proffered are not convincing.

This is illustrated by an ongoing high-profile case, *Republic vs. Daniel Aseidu* (2018) in Ghana where the defendant, Daniel Asiedu, was accused of murdering a member of parliament of Ghana. A request by the defense attorney during one of the court proceedings to have the defendant mentally examined for CST had been turned down by the sitting judge, following a brief interaction with the defendant (Adjorlolo, 2016). There are also instances where CST is not raised during the trial process, although the defendant's utterances and contemporaneous behaviors are suggestive of incompetency. This mostly happens when there is a lack of, or inadequate legal representation of, defendants from poor socioeconomic backgrounds because of the high cost of legal fees, thus, making it possible for their mental status to be overlooked during the adjudication. One such case, *Republic vs. Charles Antwi* (2016), that attracted public attention in Ghana involved Charles Antwi, who was accused of attempting to murder then sitting president, John Dramani Mahama. The defendant, after his arrest, made several exaggerated and illogical claims (e.g., the presidential seat belongs to him and was stolen by the president) suggestive of mental incapacitation. This incident was widely reported by both print and electronic media in Ghana. The defendant's mother also told local media that her son had mental health problems. However, neither the police nor the court referred him to a psychiatric hospital or requested a mental state examination (Adjorlolo, 2016). Last, although a defendant can waive the right by not asserting it, the court and the prosecution would fail in their duty of ensuring a fair trial if they did not raise the matter of CST when reasonable grounds exist (Afolayan & Onoja, 2017).

CST evaluation process

As stated previously, when the court is satisfied that CST is needed to aid the adjudication process, a request for CST evaluation is made. In Ghana and Nigeria, the request is directed to the head of any nearby public psychiatric hospital in the country. In South Africa, the referring court often appoints a panel of two or three psychiatrists if the alleged offense involved serious violence and the discretion to appoint a clinical psychologist as well (Swanepoel, 2015). In line with international practice, the referral letter must specify the kind of request needed and must contain other pertinent information to assist in the evaluation. This is because the assessment protocols appear to be specific to the psycho-legal question, which include mental state at the time of offense (insanity evaluation), mental state during criminal adjudication (CST evaluation) and mental capacity for custody (mental capacity to undertake custodian roles). In some African countries like Ghana, the request can be ambiguous. The letter does not explicitly inform mental health professionals on the kind of psycho-legal issue the court is interested in resolving with their professional help. Therefore, the kind and depth of assessment conducted is mostly guided by professional discretion, the facts of the case and experience with forensic assessments. Just like insanity evaluations, the CST evaluation is data driven. Data is obtained from different sources and carefully integrated to form an opinion. In addition to the review of past medical and social histories, psychiatric or psychological assessments are conducted to examine the defendant's mental state. The tests conducted are traditional, mainstream psychiatric or psychological tests that were designed as forensic mental health assessment tools. The major reason underpinning the continuous use of traditional psychiatric assessment measures to assess competency is the lack or limited number of forensic mental health professionals on the African continent (Mars, Ramlall, & Kaliski, 2012; Ogunlesi, Ogunwale, Roos, De Wet, & Kaliski, 2012). In Ghana, there are no mental health professionals with extensive training in forensic mental health issues, including assessment and rehabilitation. The usual practice, therefore, is to extend mainstream psychiatric or psychological practice to the forensic arena through experience. The practice is that the accused is often referred to a qualified and licensed psychiatrist for examination, although under some limited circumstances, clinical psychologists may be called upon to perform this assessment. The law recognizes clinical psychologists as experts on mental health issues, provided they document and demonstrate their expertise through training, practice and experience (Adjorlolo, Agboli, & Chan, 2016). In Western countries, specialized tests called competence assessment tools have been developed. Early tests include the Competency Screening Test, the Competency Assessment Instrument, the Interdisciplinary Fitness Interview and the MacArthur Competence Assessment Tool-Criminal Adjudication (Zapf et al., 2014). These assessment instruments are developed and validated on forensic samples and are intended to assess distinct but somewhat interrelated aspects of competency. For example, the MacArthur Competence Assessment Tool-Criminal Adjudication was developed to assess three main indicators of CST: understanding, reasoning and appreciation. The Interdisciplinary Fitness Interview, on the other hand, assesses both legal and psychopathological aspects of CST. Despite the debate over which of the assessment tools is best for CST evaluation, there is a general consensus that these tools are effective and have contributed significantly to clinical opinion formation in relation to CST (Pirelli, Gottdiener, & Zapf, 2011). However, the utility of these tests in the African context could be limited or raise several professional and ethical issues given that they are not standardized on African samples. This casts doubt on the extent to which they could accurately, reliably or validly address the psycho-legal questions, as the acceptance and utility of forensic assessments partly depend on the question of validity and reliability of the evaluations (Hilsenroth & Stricker, 2004). It is not uncommon for tests validated or developed on Western samples to be administered in African samples. However, given the implication of the assessment results on the integrity and sanctity of the judiciary, adherence to due process rights and upholding the fundamental human rights of defendants, assessment instruments that incorporate specific cultural nuances may appear more promising and practically useful. It is against this background that the Specialty Guidelines for Forensic Psychologists explicitly admonish forensic evaluators to "use assessment instruments whose validity and reliability have been established for use with members of the population assessed" (Adjorlolo & Chan, 2015).

Upon completion of the assessment, evaluators are expected to furnish the court with reports that are not excessively burdened with jargon and to summarize the method employed in gathering the relevant data, findings and observations. The report of the inquiry also includes a diagnosis of the defendant's mental condition. Information about the background of the evaluators may be provided, including training, qualifications, experience and competence. The courts usually accept mental health professionals' judgments about competency, particularly when a major psychiatric disorder has been diagnosed. Indeed, across several African countries, issues of competency are raised when there are indications that a defendant is not mentally sound (Adjorlolo et al., 2016; Swanepoel, 2015). Thus, a confirmation of unsound mind or mental disorders by a mental health professional and his or her conclusions regarding competency is usually accepted by the court without any detailed review as it is normally the case for assessment in insanity defense trials.

Difficulties with CST evaluations

In conducting CST evaluations, mental health professionals are faced with substantial challenges linking the assessment finding to the psycholegal issue. This difficulty arises mostly because of the nature of the CST legislations on the continent, as noted previously. For example, the key words in the legislations in Ghana and Nigeria are "unsound mind" and "incapable of making a defense." Clinical enquiries into "unsound mind" and its causal factors appear very broad and may not be restricted to only the presence of a mental disorder, but also other conditions such as physical illnesses and brain injuries. The inherent difficulty is linking the "unsound mind" to "incapable of making a defense." The phrase "incapable of making a defense" may seem imprecise, broad and ambiguous to psychiatrists and psychologists without the requisite training in forensic mental health professonals who are not familiar with forensic practices. The terminology may encompass several of the abilities enumerated in Table 7.1, such as (1) understanding the charges, and the nature of proceedings; (2) ability to instruct and consult with the defense counsel; (3) understanding the evidence, and also to challenge witnesses, and jurors and (4) understanding the roles of the judges, the prosecution and the defense counsel. Without insight into these specific indicators of CST, many mental health professionals would offer an opinion that the court may not find useful. Indeed, the mere presence of a mental disorder or evidence of unsound mind does not indicate incompetency unless it is linked to some agreed-upon indicators. According to the Criminal Code of Canada (1992) clinicians, for instance, can formulate their clinical opinion based on whether the defendant can "(a) understand the nature or object of the proceedings, (b) understand the possible consequences of the proceedings, or (c) communicate with a counsel." On this basis, others have argued for a revision to be made to the legislations to include some salient indicators of CST to help streamline the assessment and opinion formation processes (Adjorlolo et al., 2016). Another important consideration relates to whether "incapable of making a defense" encompasses competency to waive counsel, and competency to plead guilty. This concern has also been raised in Canada about whether competency is a unitary construct, or whether there should be different thresholds of competencies for different offenses (Adjorlolo, Chan, et al., 2016). Although these have not been resolved conclusively, there is some understanding and agreement, at least among researchers, that the evaluation and the opinion formation are guided by the specific demands and circumstances of each referral question (see Grisso, 2003; Zapf et al., 2014). Therefore, the courts in Africa must indicate the specific competency abilities required in each case.

Across the continent, there is a significant backlog of individuals referred for CST or insanity evaluations, putting pressure on mental health facilities and the courts. These backlogs are mostly due to: (1) examinations requested directed mainly to psychiatrists, (2) the limited number of psychiatrists, (3) limited number of forensic mental health facilities in the country and (4) limited follow-up by the referring court (Adjorlolo, 2016; Pillay, 2014). In 2012, a position statement by the South African Society of Psychiatrists (SASOP) noted with concern that there were only ten units in the country designated to conduct CST examinations (van Rensburg, 2012). The complexity of the case at hand and variations in the assessments across institutions appear to contribute to delays. Whereas some facilities use a multidisciplinary team approach, others rely on the services of a sole professional. There are notable consequences of having long lists of defendants awaiting assessments. These include the (1) potential for harm such as suicide, self-harm, and victimization given that symptoms of mental illness worsens in the absence of treatment; (2) overcrowding of jails and mental health facilities and (3) increase financial costs to taxpayers. Obviating these challenges calls for several interventions, including expanding the pool of evaluators (e.g., including more psychologists), increasing the number of evaluation facilities and screening and triaging of referred cases (Gowensmith & Robinson, 2017).

Disposition of incompetent-to-stand-trial defendants

Defendants declared incompetent to stand trial would have the charges stayed or proceedings postponed, while they are committed to treatment for competency restoration (Adjorlolo, Chan, et al., 2016; Afolayan & Onoja, 2017; Swanepoel, 2015). In this regard, the Criminal Procedure of Act of Ghana (Act 30) theoretically provides two routes (i.e., government commitment and self-commitment to treatments) to competency restoration; however, practically, incompetent defendants are committed to treatment by the government at a psychiatric hospital or any other place designated by the court. This is explicitly exemplified in Section 76 of the Mental Health Act (2012; Act 846) of Ghana which states that "an offender assessed and found not fit to stand trial shall have the charges stayed while undergoing treatment." When a defendant is in custody, he or she shall be deemed to be in the lawful custody of the person or the authority in whose custody he or she was at the time of such committal (Swanepoel, 2015). During the course of treatment in Ghana, the head of the psychiatric institution has the obligation to notify the state attorney on whether a defendant is (1) capable of making a defense, and/or (2) fit to be discharged unconditionally. If the state is not interested in pursuing the case further by invoking the jurisdiction of the referral court, the defendant is discharged unconditionally (i.e., absolute discharge). This practice is similar to the practices in several common law and Commonwealth countries such as England and Wales (Rogers et al., 2008). Analysts have noted that the state decision to discontinue criminal proceedings is influenced by several factors, including (1) the type and severity of the offense, (2) the type and the nature of the mental illness, (3) public interest in and the media coverage of the case, (4) lack of evidence to sustain a conviction and (5) lack of requisite resources (Adjorlolo, Chan, et al., 2016). In other African countries such as Nigeria and South Africa, however, the defendants declared competent to stand trial are taken back to court for proceedings to continue (Afolayan & Onoja, 2017; Swanepoel, 2015). As stated previously, the criminal provisions require that mental illness or mental defect must be present before the question of whether the accused is competent to stand trial is raised (Adjorlolo, 2016; Swanepoel, 2015). Therefore, the critical first stage is to determine whether the defendant is suffering from a mental illness or psychological or psychiatric factors that are associated with the request for assessment (Swanepoel, 2015). It is, therefore, unsurprising that Section 138 (1 and 2) of the criminal procedure Act of Ghana Act 30, states that the court shall proceed with preliminary proceedings or trials in the event that the defendant is not insane but simply cannot be made to understand the proceedings. However, in the event that the defendant is tried by a lower court, the decision reached regarding the culpability or otherwise of the defendant shall be forwarded to high court to make an appropriate determination (Adjorlolo, Chan, et al., 2016). This procedure raises the possibility that some defendants are only physically present in the law court but mentally absent.

Conclusion and recommendations for research

This chapter examined an important criminal procedural issue, competency to stand trial, in the judicial systems of particular African countries. Defendants have the right to fully participate in any criminal proceedings that involve them. The adversarial nature of the criminal justice system across the continent means that the ability of defendants to assist their attorneys by providing them with relevant information about the case and locating witnesses is extremely important. Despite the importance of CST in ensuring due process rights and judicial integrity in a continent known for human rights abuses, scholarly interest in this psycholegal issue is low, compared with the insanity defense. With the exception of South Africa, Ghana and Nigeria, there is a general paucity of empirical literature on CST on the African continent. This observation calls for increased scholarly interest in this topical issue. Among the areas in need of scholarly attention are the base rates of competency, legal and extra-legal factors affecting competency decision making, a comparative analysis of CST across countries in Africa, the characteristics and demographic backgrounds of defendants who have utilized the CST legislation and how competency registration is undertaken.

On the question of base rate, it would be helpful to identify the number of defendants declared as CST from the total number of defendants who have raised the competency issues and have been referred for assessment. A low base rate would indicate that the majority of people referred for assessment are not found to have mental health condition that affect their competency to stand trial, whereas a high base rate would suggest that more defendant are declared incompetent to stand trial because of presence of mental disorder. Insight into decision making relating to CST is important to ensure that the fundamental human rights of defendants with respect to fair trials are not truncated by personal biases, stigmatization of mental illness, negative attitudes, stereotypes and prejudice against defendants standing trial. Since jurors have instrumental roles in the criminal adjudicative process, it is important to understand their decision-making process, including the impacts of judges' instructions on their decision making. Likewise, research into the characteristics of defendants found to be incompetent to stand trial would help forensic mental health professionals to profile defendants raised for CST evaluation. Competency restoration is another crucial research area. Based on the authors' experience with the mental health system in Ghana, there is no special CST restoration program beyond improving the behavioral repertoire of the defendants via the psychopharmacological agents and sometimes with psychotherapy. It would be interesting to unearth the practices in other African countries and, more importantly, to trace how defendants who have been declared competent participate in the trial process by assisting their attorneys and their understanding or demonstration of the discrete court-related functions.

As noted previously, clinical opinion and reports regarding a defendant's CST is largely based on the outcome of the assessment process. This means that issues relating to the validity and reliability of the assessment tools should be prioritized. The majority of the existing forensic assessment instruments developed for assessing CST are based on samples from Western countries. Given the sociocultural and geopolitical differences between Western and African countries, it follows that measures developed in the former may have little utility in the latter. This observation calls for studies to develop and validate measures to assess for CST in the African context. In doing so, efforts should be made to address gender invariance of the measures to ensure that the assessment measures or scores are not biased (i.e., under- or overestimated) for one group. Furthermore, the role and involvement of mental health professionals in the assessment process and decision making in relation to CST should be investigated. For example, it would be useful to understand how assessment of CST is carried out in different jurisdictions across Africa, and whether more considerations are given to some factors than others and why. Also important is understanding the decision-making model utilized to link the vague and ambiguous psycholegal construct of insanity to the clinical findings of mental disorder.

References

Adjorlolo, S. (2016). Diversion of individuals with mental illness in the criminal justice system in Ghana. *International Journal of Forensic Mental Health, 15*(4), 382–392.

Adjorlolo, S., Agboli, J. M., & Chan, H. C. (2016). Criminal responsibility and the insanity defence in Ghana: The examination of legal standards and assessment issues. *Psychiatry, Psychology and Law, 23*(5), 684–695.

Adjorlolo, S., & Chan, H. C. (2015). Forensic assessment via videoconferencing: Issues and practice considerations. *Journal of Forensic Psychology Practice, 15*(3), 185–204.

Adjorlolo, S., & Chan, H. C. (2017). Determination of competency to stand trial (fitness to plead): An exploratory study in Hong Kong. *Psychiatry, Psychology and Law, 24*(2), 205–222.

Adjorlolo, S., Chan, H. C. O., & Agboli, J. M. (2016). Adjudicating mentally disordered offenders in Ghana: The criminal and mental health legislations. *International Journal of Law and Psychiatry, 45*, 1–8.

Afolayan, A., & Onoja, E. (2017). The plights of mentally ill persons under the criminal justice system in Nigeria. *Ajayi Crowther University Law Journal, 1*(1), 1–36.

Gowensmith, W. N., & Robinson, K. P. (2017). Fitness to stand trial evaluation challenges in the United States: Some comparisons with South Africa. *South African Journal of Psychology, 47*(2), 148–158.

Grisso, T. (2003). Evaluating competencies: Forensic assessments & instruments (2nd ed.). New York: Kluwer, Academic/Plenum.

Hilsenroth, M. J., & Stricker, G. (2004). A consideration of challenges to psychological assessment instruments used in forensic settings: Rorschach as exemplar. *Journal of Personality Assessment, 83*(2), 141–152.

Mars, M., Ramlall, S., & Kaliski, S. (2012). Forensic telepsychiatry: A possible solution for South Africa? *African Journal of Psychiatry, 15*(4), 244–247.

Ogunlesi, A., Ogunwale, A., Roos, L., De Wet, P., & Kaliski, S. (2012). Forensic psychiatry in Africa: Prospects and challenges.*African Journal of Psychiatry, 15*, 3–7.

Pillay, A. L. (2014). Competency to stand trial and criminal responsibility examinations: Are there solutions to the extensive waiting list? *South African Journal of Psychology, 44*(1), 48–59.

Pirelli, G., Gottdiener, W. H., & Zapf, P. A. (2011). A meta-analytic review of competency to stand trial research. *Psychology, Public Policy, and Law, 17*(1), 1.

Rogers, T., Blackwood, N., Farnham, F., Pickup, G., & Watts, M. (2008). Fitness to plead and competence to stand trial: A systematic review of the constructs and their application. *The Journal of Forensic Psychiatry & Psychology, 19*(4), 576–596.

Swanepoel, M. (2015). Legal aspects with regard to mentally ill offenders in South Africa. *Potchefstroom Electronic Law Journal/Potchefstroomse Elektroniese Regsblad, 18*(1), 3237–3258.

van Rensburg, B. J. (2012). The South African Society of Psychiatrists (SASOP) and SASOP State Employed Special Interest Group (SESIG) position statements on psychiatric care in the public sector. *South African Journal of Psychiatry, 18*(3), 16.

White, A. J., Batchelor, J., Pulman, S., & Howard, D. (2012). The role of cognitive assessment in determining fitness to stand trial. *International Journal of Forensic Mental Health, 11*(2), 102–109.

Zapf, P. A., Roesch, R., & Pirelli, G. (2014). Assessing competency to stand trial. In I. B. Weiner & R. K. Otto (Eds.), *The handbook of forensic psychology* (4th ed., pp. 281–314). United States: Wiley.

Statutes cited

Dusky v United States (1960) 362 US 402.
R v Leung Tak-Choi (1995) 2 HKCLR 32
R v Podola [1960] 1 QB 325

8 Malingering assessments in African forensic settings

Olanrewaju Sodeinde

Introduction

Malingering is as ancient as human history and has found expressions in both classical literature and biblical accounts (Wessely, 2003). From King David (1 Samuel 21:12–14) to Ulysees, illustrations of illness simulation abound in human life. It has even been suggested that the history of forensic psychiatry is somewhat linked to malingering by the investigative discovery of the feigned madness of the Roman General Cincinnatus in order to escape military service (Gutheil, 2005). In its clinical essence, malingering is neither a psychopathology nor a clinical diagnosis but a socio-medico-legal term commonly used in clinical-forensic and correctional settings. Generally, it denotes intentional fabrication or magnification of mental or physical symptoms in order to attract secondary gain or external benefits such as seeking undue attention, avoiding military or work responsibilities, evading criminal prosecution, escaping deserved prison sentence or obtaining medication. This chapter provides an overview of malingering by focusing on definitional and theoretical issues. It will also examine the assessment of malingering while highlighting crucial challenges in this regard with reference to African forensic settings.

Overview of malingering

Definitional issues

The (American Psychiatric Association, 2013) in the fifth edition of the Diagnostic and Statistical Manual of Mental Disorders (DSM-5) defined malingering as the 'intentional production of false or grossly exaggerated physical or psychological problems, motivated by external incentives such as avoiding military duty, avoiding work, obtaining financial compensation, evading criminal prosecution, or obtaining drugs." This definition is instituted in the DSM-5 section V65.2, which consists of other conditions that may be a focus of clinical attention as they could possibly influence the diagnosis, course, prognosis or treatment of psychological disorder.

The World Health Organization (WHO, 2019) in the eleventh edition of International Classification of Disease (ICD-11) equally defined *malingering* as "feigning, intentional production or significant exaggeration of physical or psychological symptoms, or intentional misattribution of genuine symptoms to an unrelated event or series of events when this is specifically motivated by external incentives or rewards such as escaping duty or work, mitigating punishment, obtaining medications or drugs or receiving unmerited recompense such as disability compensation or personal injury damages award."

Malingering is often misconstrued and synonymously referred to as a factitious disorder. This is a misconception as factitious disorder is a deceptive behavior that can occur in the absence of external rewards when people present themselves to others as ill, impaired or injured. Factitious disorder involves the falsification of physical or psychological signs or symptoms, or induction of injury or disease, associated with identified deception. This is in contrast to malingering, in which obvious external rewards or incentives motivate the behavior. Malingering is also distinguished from conversion disorder and somatic symptom-related mental disorders by the deliberate production of symptoms and associated obvious external incentives. Definite evidence of faking is suggestive of malingering if obtaining an incentive is the main objective unlike factitious disorder in which the apparent aim is to assume a sick role.

Etiology

Malingering has no precise cause, but often results from a complex interaction of several factors including psychological, social and economic factors. Theodore Beck in his 1823 "Elements of Medial Jurisprudence" identified anxiety, shame or the hope of gain as the three major contexts that have explained malingering throughout the course of human history (Beck, 1823). He rightly noted that those who undertake assessments in situations where illness might be feigned have a "double duty … to guard the interests of the public … and also those of the individual, so that he be not unjustly condemned." Scientific evidence has further lent credence to these assertions in finding that individuals feign illness in order to avoid criminal responsibility, trial and punishment as well as social responsibility, occupational engagements or to acquire controlled drugs, facilitate transfer from prison to hospital or as a result of anti-social and histrionic personality traits or disorders (Sequeira, Fara, & Lewis, 2018; Lanska, 2018).

Epidemiology

Malingering is a common general medical practice phenomenon. The prevalence is however higher in medico-legal (10–20%) and forensic settings (32%) compared to civilian settings (1%), military service (5%) and emergency situations (13%) (Hickling et al., 1999). Furthermore, out of the 33,531 of the cases seen by the American Board of Clinical Neuropsychology during a one-year period, an estimated 30% likely malingered and symptom exaggeration was found in the disability evaluation – 29% in personal injury evaluation, 19% in criminal evaluation and 8% of medical cases (Mittenburg, Patton, Canyock, &

Condit, 2002). Additionally, females simulated medical symptoms about two-fold compared with males, but males had greater proportions with cognitive deficits (22.7%) than female coequals (6.4%). Likewise, there was an 8% prevalence rate of malingering among clinical defendants referred for evaluation of criminal responsibility in a pre-trial outpatient evaluation compared to 11% prevalence among 1710 federal pre-trial defendants. Defendants charged with kidnapping and robbery had higher malingering rates (23% and 17%, respectively), while those charged with murder had 4%. In another study, approximately 17% of individuals considered incompetent to stand trial were also found to be malingering (Cochrane, Grisso & Frederick, 2001; Rogers, Salekin, Sewell, Goldstein, & Leonard, 1998; Cornel & Hawk, 1989).

Subtypes of malingering based on theoretical models

Though it is important to understand the assessment techniques of malingering, it is first pertinent to understand the motivation for malingering. Malingering is often considered on a continuum in terms of degree of intentionality and symptom exaggeration involved, as well as the degree of actual impairment. This appears preferable to its formulation as a dichotomous variable or condition that is either present or absent. Consequently, different subtypes of malingering have been theoretically constructed.

Resnick model

This model was originally postulated by Garner (1965) Garner and later revised by Resnick (1997). It is based on the idea of varying levels of malingering. Three subtypes of malingering are proposed under this model: pure, partial and false imputation malingering.

a. Pure malingering involves complete or total fabrication of symptoms when the condition does not exist at all.
b. Partial malingering involves deliberate exaggeration of existing symptoms.
c. False imputation involves intentional attribution of symptoms to an unrelated cause.

The prevalence of these subtypes is uncertain as there are inadequate empirical studies. Partial malingering, however, appears to be the most common pattern (Resnick, 1998).

Roger model

This model proposed by Rogers, Salekin, Sewell, Goldstein & Leonard (1998), is an extension of Tversky & Kahneman (1974)'s decision theory. He asserted that the motivation to malinger is product of three factors: pathogenic, criminological and adaptational factors. According to him, malingering, in the pathogenic sense, could be regarded as a product of underlying psychopathology in which the malingerer exaggerates pre-existing symptoms. The criminological variant is thought to arise from the malingerer's attempt to seek reprieve from legal consequences. The adaptive form typically represents an adaptive response to adverse or stressful circumstances during which the malingerer seek to maximize their chances of success in whatever manner they wish to define it, although the end result may be to the contrary. Malingering could therefore be perceived as a poor or maladaptive coping skill.

Lipian and Mills model

Lipian and Mills model classified malingering into positive, negative, data tampering, false imputation, staging events and misattribution subtypes. This classification is based based on the degree of intentionality, symptom exaggeration and actual impairment.

a. Positive malingering implies that the malingerer is feigning the symptoms of an illness.
b. Negative malingering implies that the malingerer is hiding or misreporting the symptoms.
c. Data tampering involves altering diagnostic instruments, data or record, so as to influence the results of an examination or test.
d. Staging events means carefully planning, orchestrating and executing events, which might result later in an injury or an explanation for a feigned disability.
e. False imputation involves ascribing actual symptoms to a cause consciously understood to have no relation to the symptoms.
f. Misattribution implies ascribing actual symptom to a cause erroneously believed to have given rise to them.

Assessment of malingering in forensic settings

An overview

As noted earlier, motivations to malinger are higher in the forensic settings than other settings (Hickling et al., 1999; Mittenburg et al., 2002) as many criminal offenders often want to avoid criminal responsibility and punishment for their misbehavior. Motivation also depends on whether the evaluation is performed in a criminal or a civil setting. In the criminal setting, evaluation is often requested in order to ensure that the rights of an accused are not violated or during fitness assessment to determine if an accused is fit to stand trial. It may also be relevant in cases involving the insanity defense. Some accused persons often exaggerate or fabricate symptoms of illness to achieve plea-bargaining and for mitigation or application of lesser sentences in case of conviction. In civil cases, on the other hand, malingering usually occurs when petitioners falsely claim that they are suffering from a physical or emotional trauma or damage as a result of perceived negligence of other parties all in a bid to secure financial benefit or gain.

The assessment of malingering is therefore a very demanding task, as faulty assessments can lead to non-detection of malingering or errors in disposal of cases within the criminal justice system. Rosenhan (1973) in his classic study demonstrated the problem of malingering detection when his phony patients feigning hallucinations were all admitted to the psychiatric department of 12 different highly specialized hospitals but only one of them who was diagnosed as having a bipolar disorder received a clinical diagnosis of full-blown schizophrenia. Rosen, Mulsant, Bruce, Mittal, and Fox (2004) likewise reported that seasoned psychiatrists distinguished between actors and depressed patients during a clinical interview with a chance level accuracy. They further rated their confidence level in their diagnoses as 6.5 out of 10 in the case of patients and 7.1 in the case of actors, denoting that they were equally convinced of their right and wrong diagnoses. The results of these studies emphasized the need for a comprehensive assessment in malingering detection.

Assessment of malingering in African settings

A Nigerian example: Clinical assessment at Neuropsychiatric Hospital, Aro, Abeokuta, Nigeria

The Neuropsychiatric Hospital, Aro, Abeokuta is the foremost psychiatric hospital in Nigeria. Its forensic unit runs a prison in-reach service in selected federal prisons within Ogun state, Nigeria. It also cares for offenders who are referred by the police or transferred from prison based on court orders.

Assessment of malingering at the forensic unit is conducted by the multidisciplinary management team members made up of psychiatrists, psychiatric nurses and clinical psychologists. Most of the patients referred are males. They are usually referred for fitness to plead evaluation or assessment of mental state for the purpose of evaluating the validity of an insanity defense. Both are typically conjoint. Assessment and management are based on inpatient or outpatient basis, depending on the level of severity of the illness and the crime as well as the availability of security measures and funding for hospitalization. The author is not aware of any empirical studies that have been conducted to systematically test standardized assessment instruments for malingering in Nigeria.

Empirical studies in South Africa

In 2003, a study was conducted at the Sterkfontein Hospital in Gauteng, South Africa, among 94 pre-trial forensic patients to examine the utility of MMPI-2 in predicting criminal responsibility. As part of the report on the MMPI-2 profiles, malingering was described based on the "faking bad" scale. There was clear elevation of both F and Fb indices, thereby suggesting that malingering levels may be high among forensic patients (du Toit, 2003). A study by Wong (2008) determined the normative cut-off values of four malingering assessment instruments – Test of Memory Malingering (TOMM), Rey 15-item memory test, the digit span sub-test of WAIS-III and the trail making test – among a black, Xhosa-speaking population. It showed that the validated cut-off values for TOMM obtained in Western samples could be used among such a non-Western sample with the participants performing comparably with non-malingerers from other cultures. However, the performance of the study participants on the digit span sub-test of WAIS-III was quite below that of normal Western populations and essentially similar to malingerers in a Western sample. Similar findings were observed, with the trail-making test (poorer performance was noted in trail A but not B). Overall, the research evidence suggests that among non-Western populations such as those in Africa, it may be required to make necessary adjustments to cut-off values on standardized malingering assessment instruments.

Psychological assessment

As a result of the inherent danger of assessment errors, a high index of suspicion for malingering is maintained in all cases referred for forensic evaluation (Vitacco, Rogers, Gabel, & Munizza, 2007). This is particularly so in relation to cases of exaggerated, bizarre or ridiculous symptoms in excess of objective findings or observation, cases of marked discrepancy between the claimed stress or disability, and those demonstrating lack of cooperation during the diagnostic evaluation as well as compliance with the prescribed treatment regimen. Suspicions are also raised by cases demonstrating apparent environmental incentive for simulation of illness such as obtaining drugs or avoiding work. Possible voluntary control over symptoms is equally identified when symptoms worsen during observation, especially among individuals with a diagnosis of antisocial personality disorder. This is in accordance with DSM-5 and ICD-11 (American Psychiatric Association, 2013; WHO, 2019). The following sections detail subjective, objective and projective techniques of psychological assessment that are usually employed in the determination of malingering under the aforementioned circumstances.

Subjective technique

Subjective techniques involve periodic and detailed clinical interviews as well as behavioral observation. Comprehensive clinical interviews provide valuable information about the client for the purpose of generating appropriate clinical impression and management plan. The interview is often very exhaustive. Open-ended questions are asked, and clients are encouraged to elaborate where necessary without the examiner raising clues as to their suspicions. Detailed clarifications about the information obtained are also made while the accuracy of the information is verified in a non-threatening way. A non-judgmental approach is key to arriving at informed and accurate conclusions. Clients' appearance, grooming, gesture, facial expression, speech, mood, affect, thought process, perceptual and cognitive processes are also noted. Daily unobtrusive observation is also carried out by ward nurses to verify discrepancy between what is observed and claimed psychopathology. Besides information about onset of symptoms, past history of mental and behavioral disorders, previous history of conduct disorder, arrests by law enforcement agencies and substance-use disorder are obtained from significant collateral sources where possible. Information from family members may not always be entirely reliable as such individuals may conceal information that they consider damaging to the cause of the client.

Objective techniques

Objective techniques involve the administration of objective psychological tests. Assessments based on clinical interviews are usually the first step in malingering evaluations and they are hardly sufficient in arriving at confident conclusions. Interview outcomes may be affected by manipulative behavior put up by some clients, some of whom have admitted that their responses were based on "coaching" by their defense attorney. Moreover, inexperienced mental health professionals may miss important malingering clues. To ensure objectivity, therefore, psychological tests are administered as crucial adjuncts to the clinical interviews. There are various objective psychological instruments used for the assessment of malingering. These include the Minnesota Multiphasic Personality Inventory (MMPI; Butcher, Dahlstrom, Graham, et al., 1989), Test of Memory Malingering (TOMM; Tombaugh, 1976), Miller Forensic Assessment Symptoms Test (M-FAST; Miller, 2001); Structured Inventory of Malingered Symptomatology (SIMS; Smith & Burgen, 1997a, b), Structured Interview of Reported Symptoms (Rogers et al., 1992), Personality Assessment Inventory (PAI; Morey, 1991), M-Test (Beaber et al., 2000) and Rey's memory tests (Rey, 1964), among others. At the Aro Neuropsychiatric Hospital in Nigeria, the MMPI is the most widely used psychological instrument for the detection of malingering.

Minnesota Multiphasic Personality Inventory (MMPI-2)

The MMPI-2 is a 567-item self-report inventory developed by Hathaway and McKinley (1943) to assess personality traits and psychopathology. It is the most widely researched and most widely used personality inventory and may be regarded as the gold standard in personality testing. The test has gone through various revisions, with the latest in 1989 (Butcher, Dahlstrom, Graham, Tellegen, and Kraemmer, 1989). Test items reflect a range of psychiatric, medical and neurological disorders, gender role characteristics and style of self-presentation, among others. It has two sets of scales: validity and clinical scales, each of which have other subscales.

The validity scales are designed to evaluate a client's test-taker's attitude, including any attempts to exaggerate symptoms. The scale contains three types of validity measures: those designed to detect non-responding or inconsistent responding (Cannot Say Scale (? Scale), Variable Response Inconsistencies (VRIN) and True

Response Inconsistencies (TRIN); those designed to detect whether a client is over-reporting or exaggerating psychological symptoms: Infrequent Scale (F-Scale), Infrequent back (Fb), and Infrequent Psychopathology (Fp)) and those designed to detect whether a test-taker is under-reporting or downplaying psychological symptoms: (Lie Scale (L Scale), Correction Scale (K Scale), and Superlative self-presentation (S Scale)). These scales will now be briefly considered in turn.

- **Cannot Say Scale (? Scale):** This measures the number of omitted items. Clients are encouraged to respond to all the test items. The test is considered invalid when 30 or more items are not answered.
- **Variable Response Inconsistencies (VRIN):** This scale consists of 47 pairs of items with either similar or opposite content designed to measure tendency to respond inconsistently to MMPI items.
- **True Response Inconsistencies (TRIN):** This scale is designed to identify individuals who respond inconsistently to items by giving true or false responses to items indiscriminately.
- **Lie Scale (L Scale):** This is designed to detect a deliberate and rather unsophisticated attempt by the respondent to "fake good" or present self in a favorable light.
- **Infrequent Scale (F-Scale):** This may be regarded as the malingering index, designed to detect deviant or atypical test taking attitude (i.e., faking or bad). This scale is a very useful indicator of degree of psychopathology and also helpful in generating inference about other behavioral characteristics of the test-taker. Infrequent back (Fb) and Infrequent Psychopathology (Fp) are F-Scale supplementary scales designed to identify infrequent responding.
- **Correction Scale (K Scale):** This is an effective index for detection of test-taker's defensiveness, evasiveness or denial of psychopathology. This scale validates the clinical scales.
- **Superlative self-presentation (S Scale):** This scale is designed to assess tendency of test-takers to present themselves as highly virtuous, responsible individuals devoid of psychological problem, have no moral flaws, content with life and relate well with people.

The synchronization of a low L scale, a high F-scale and a low K scale on the MMPI-2 is suggestive of malingering. MMPI-2 can also detect malingering by experts despite test-takers' information symptoms (Bagby, Nicholson, Buis, et al., 2000). A South African study among pre-trial forensic patients indicated that there was clear elevation of both F and Fb indices, thereby suggesting that malingering levels may be high among forensic patients (du Toit, 2003). This tendency to malingering may arise from some degree of psychological stress due to confrontation with the legal system (du Toit, 2003; Peay, 2019). Overall, while MMPI-2 appears to be very helpful in identifying malingerers, it is not infallible. Klotz Flitter et al. (2003) found that F-scale scores were high among victims of childhood sexual abuse, while Pelfrey (2004) found that higher intelligence and knowledge of MMPI-2 tend to produce realistic patterns that are hard to detect.

The use of the subjective approach alone or in combination with MMPI-2 is illustrated by three clinical vignettes that have been developed from actual clinical experience with Nigerian cases involving malingered psychiatric symptomatology.

Case 1

A 34-year-old female charged with the murder of a business partner who suddenly developed a mental illness in prison characterized by talking irrationally, talking to unseen people in clear consciousness and shouting inappropriately. She was court-referred for psychiatric evaluation to determine fitness to plead. She was managed as an inpatient and was on 24-hour surveillance by the prison guard since the hospital was not a secure facility. She was physically restrained to the bed by the prison authorities to prevent escape. At the ward round, she came in naked, behaved as a deaf mute and did not respond to any of the questions asked. Her family members claimed that the client's psychological illness was recurrent. Nurses were instructed to keep close observation. When she noticed that she was being carefully observed by staff, she would pick and eat feces from the toilet. However, when she felt she was left unattended, she tried to remove her leg cuff in the night in order to escape.

When she was confronted, she confessed that she was coached by a fellow prisoner while in prison and some family members to feign mental illness in order to escape justice. Apart from the eventual confession, there was inconsistency in the disorganized behavior that depended largely on whether the client was being observed or not and the clearly "organized" attempt at escape was equally not in keeping with a psychotic state, which was the malingered condition.

Case 2

This is a case of a 23-year-old single unemployed male court referral with a background history of conduct disorder as well as substance abuse and prior criminal conviction in adulthood. He fatally stabbed his mother when he was alone in the house with her. He denied recollection of the events surrounding his mother's death but he had a vivid memory of other events that occurred on the day. Though he had initially confessed killing his mother to the police, he later claimed that he did so under duress. He had been remanded in prison for three years. When he was transferred to the hospital for assessment, he did not demonstrate any extensive loss of memory for any other event or circumstances except his mother's murder. His clinical evaluation revealed intact cognition, anti-social personality disorder (MMPI-II) and psychopathy (PCL-RV score = 31).

His highly selective memory loss is not consistent with any clear ICD-10 diagnosis (e.g., dissociative amnesia). His clinical profile also suggests an individual who may adopt deception as a strategy under his delicate circumstances. In this case, there is a high likelihood of malingering fueled by an admixture of anti-social tendencies and the prospect of secondary gain (i.e., avoiding the mandatory death penalty that his crime of homicide must attract).

Case 3

A 29-year-old single, unemployed young man who dropped out of school referred by the court to determine his competency to stand trial on account of killing his father and dismembering him. He denied the allegation, claiming that he could not remember ever killing anyone, and least of all, his father. He had a background history of illicit drug use and association with deviant peers. He denied drug use around the time of the crime. There was no personal history of mental illness prior to the killing. His recollection of events on the day before the murder and thereafter did not reveal any significant gaps. He later confessed to killing his father with a kitchen knife before cutting him into pieces for easy disposal using a bag. He also described cleaning up all the blood stains in order to destroy the evidence. He admitted lying about the killing because he did not wish to be jailed.

As with case 2 above, his memory loss for the killing was highly selective and certainly not in keeping with any clear ICD-10 diagnosis (e.g., dissociative amnesia). His clinical profile also suggests an individual who may adopt deception as a defensive strategy given the fact that he had been arrested for murder. In this case, there is a high likelihood of malingering fueled by an admixture of anti-social tendencies and the prospect of secondary gain (i.e., avoiding the mandatory death penalty that his crime of homicide must attract).

Projective techniques

This involves the use of projective tests such as the Rorschach Inkblot Test, sentence completion test and draw a person test (DAP). The projective techniques are a very effective tool for detecting malingering as it is very difficult to fake. The technique tends to divert test-taker's attention away from self, thereby reducing embarrassment and undue defensiveness. Besides, it also offers little or no threat to respondent's prestige or self-esteem since any response given is "right." Projective techniques have also been found to overcome the limitation of culture barriers since some projective techniques, including the Draw-A-Person test, are especially useful for children, illiterates and persons with language difficulties.

Rorschach inkblot test

The Rorschach is the most famous and most widely utilized projective technique developed by Herman Rorschach in 1921. The test consists of ten cards, each containing a bilaterally symmetric inkblot design which vary in color and complexity. Five of the inkblot designs are black and gray, two contain black, gray and red and the remaining three cards contain poster colors of various shades. Each of the ten cards are presented twice during administration and the test-taker is asked what it looks like. The response is recorded verbatim. The first phase of administration is the free-association phase while the second is the inquiry phase. The Rorschach is, however, to be used with caution as studies till date are inconclusive about the utility of the Rorschach in detecting malingering. Perry and Kinder (1990) found no specific malingering pattern with the Rorschach, while Ganellen, Wasyliw, Haywood and Grossman (1996) reported that malingerers give less emotion-laden and more dramatic responses on Rorschach. They also recommended the combined use of MMPI-2 and Rorschach as a powerful psychometric technique.

Sentence Completion Test (SCT)

This technique consist of a stem which is the beginning of a sentence such as: "I like …….."; "The happiest time ….."; "I wish ……."; "My greatest worry……"; "I need ……."; "The future ….", etc. There are different versions of the test, with the Rotter's Incomplete Sentence Blank (College form) by Rotter and Rafferty (1950) consisting of 40 sentence stems being the most commonly used. The sentence stem provides the word or phrase which the respondent fills with words that best fit the incomplete sentence. Consequently, they "project" their thoughts, feelings and other inner desires that they would not ordinarily express. Interpretation is based on the response analysis.

Draw a person (DAP)

The use of drawing in psychological evaluation was first popularized by Good enough (1926). This technique is based on the widely believed assumption that creative works, especially in the fine arts, and handwritings, drawings and paintings in particular, reflect the personality of the artists. DAP is a paper and pencil performance technique in which the respondent is provided with a blank white sheet of paper and pencil and instructed to "draw a person," after which s/he is then instructed to draw a person of the opposite gender. Artistic ability is irrelevant. The clinician however takes note of whether the client accepts the task with hesitation, reluctance, complete refusal or appears apologetic about their drawing. The time taken to draw, the frequency of erasure (and what is erased) and the gender drawn first are also noted. Client's "free-association" and other vital information about the model drawn are equally obtained. Interpretation is essentially based on the diagnostic handbook (Wenck, 1997). Bizarre details are suggestive of schizophrenia. Erasures are suggestive of restlessness, anxiety and possibly neurotic tendency. Drawing with aggressive content such as knife or gun is suggestive of delinquent or anti-social tendency. Drawing of a small figure is suggestive of poor self-concept while drawing with hard solid lines, absence of erasure and encompassing the entire page may be used to infer that the subject is self-assured. With regard to the detection of malingering, it has been noted that DAP is susceptible to deliberate distortion by test-takers but its validity is improved by interpreting the drawings along with cognitive skill scores (Carmody & Crossman, 2011). Malingerers were found to demonstrate lower cognitive skills scores in drawings based on malingered emotions. These authors have further argued that situations in which cognitive ability based on the drawing scores is lower than that obtained from an independent test of cognitive ability could potentially signal malingering.

Overall, it would appear that the best approach to the assessment of malingering is to adopt a combination of tests while ensuring a clear focus on significant contextual factors. A helpful injunction in this regard by Rey (1958) is approvingly recalled by Frederick (2002; p. 22):

> We see how it is possible to suspect the exaggeration and the simulation by using appropriately a battery of tests. It is sufficient to know the degree of intrinsic difficulty of each test well. However, the tests must be numerous in order to accumulate the suspicious signs: We will not be able to arrive at a conclusion on a single sign. Besides, it is always necessary to attribute these signs to the particular problem of the individual, to the traits of his personality, and to establish clearly what interests he may have in simulating disorders of a psychological nature.
>
> (Rey, 1958; p. 123)

Challenges of malingering assessments in African forensic settings

There are crucial challenges to the assessment of malingering given the peculiarities of African settings and the investment of time and human resources involved. These challenges relate to the availability of trained personnel and validity of malingering assessment instruments.

Mental health human and other resources

Available data suggest that there is 1 psychologist to 1 million citizens in Africa as a WHO region (World Health Organization, 2018). This meager number has to provide services across different mental health sub-specialties. Thus, there are few hands available for forensic assessments including malingering evaluation. Currently, there are few psychological instruments available for the assessment of malingering in African settings (as evidenced by existing empirical research data) and the extent of training in many parts of the continent on the use of some the testing instruments is still largely uncertain. The need for structured training in forensic psychology has been noted in South Africa (Pillay, Gowensmith, & Banks, 2019) and this is likely to be similar to the state of affairs in other African nations. Evidently, the use of assessment measures by inadequately trained examiners raises critical methodological, ethical and legal questions.

Validity of malingering assessment instruments

The validity of structured assessment instruments in the detection of malingering has been largely determined for Western samples while such information with regard to African populations appears insufficient and largely unavailable. The administration of malingering assessment scales developed in one culture to defendants from another culture in which the reliability and validity of such scales have not been interrogated may result in measurement inaccuracies and potentially, miscarriage of justice. To deal with such situations, less culture-biased and non-verbal assessment scales for such measurements (e.g., the dot counting test) have been suggested (Weiss & Rosenfeld, 2010). Another important usefulness of non-verbal tests is that they may lend themselves easily to the use of interpreters without doing great injury to utility value (Wagoner, 2017). It must be noted however, that an instrument such as the dot counting test has been found to have very poor sensitivity (Frederick, 2002; Weiss & Rosenfeld, 2010). Furthermore, the non-verbal scales may not be entirely culturally unbiased since they are likely to have been constructed based on images that may be differently perceived in dissimilar cultures.

Getting more specific, while MMPI-2 appears to be very helpful in identifying malingerers, it is not fool-proof. Its susceptibility to effects of childhood sexual abuse (Klotz Flitter, Elhai, & Gold, 2003) as well as higher intelligence and knowledge about it (Pelfrey, 2004) requires that it should be used with caution. Moreover, instruments such as MMPI-2 and sentence completion tests are sensitive to literacy and may have limited application in some African settings in which the defendants to be tested are illiterate.

Similarly, projective tests such as the Rorschach inkblot test and DAP, though fairly available, appear questionable when used alone. The need for additional assessment instruments further stretches the already over-burdened manpower in many African forensic mental health settings. Additionally, the "standardized" interpretation of such projective measures is likely to be culturally nuanced and the extent of their direct application to cultures in which they were not originally developed needs to be further determined by empirical research.

Conclusion

Malingering is not a psychopathology or diagnosis but a focus of clinical attention that can affect diagnosis. Even though many medical conditions may be faked under various clinical circumstances, malingering is more prevalent in the medico-legal setting as offenders often feign or exaggerate psychological symptoms in order to appear non-culpable for their actions or to mitigate their punishment. Malingering is usually difficult to detect in many cases as there is no fool-proof method or gold standard for its assessment. Besides, there are few psychological instruments for it and training in many parts of the continent is still inadequate. This raises complex methodological, ethical and legal questions. A systematic approach with inputs from the multi-disciplinary team members and the administration of appropriate combination of psychological tests utilized in a culturally appropriate context may be a useful means of identifying the condition. Given the considerable societal cost of malingering, it is essential that forensic and other mental health professionals pay due attention to the possibility of feigned symptoms in order to be better equipped to deal with them and avoid unfortunate misclassification of criminal defendants or civil litigants.

References

American Psychiatric Association (2013). Diagnostic and statistical manual of mental disorders (DSM 5) (5th ed.). Washington DC : American Psychiatric Association.

Bagby, R. M., Nicholson, R. A., Buis, T., & Bacchiochi, J. R. (2000). Can the MMPI validity scales detect depression feigned by experts? *Assessment*; *71*, 55–62.

Beaber, R. J., Martson, A., Michelli, J., Mills, M. J. (2000). A brief test for measuring malingering in schizophrenic individuals. *The American Journal of Psychiatry, 142*, 1478–1481.

Beck, T. R. (1823). The elements of medical jurisprudence (Vol 1). Albany, NY: Webster and Skinner.

Butcher, J. D., Dahlstrom, W. G., Graham, J. R., Tellegen, A., & Kaemmer, B. (Eds.). (1989). Minnesota Multiphasic Personality Inventory-2 (MMPI-2). Manual for administration and scoring. Minneapolis: University of Minnesota Press.

Carmody, D., & Crossman, A. M. (2011). Artful liars: Malingering on the draw-a-person task. *The Open Criminology Journal*, *4*(1), 1–9. https://doi.org/10.2174/1874917801104010001.

Cochrane, R. E., Grisso, T., & Frederick, R. I. (2001). The relationship between criminal charges, diagnoses and psycholegal opinions among federal pretrial defendants. Behavioral Sciences and the Law, *19*, 565–582.

Cornel, D. G., & Hawk, G. L. (1989). Clinical presentation of malingerers diagnosed by experienced forensic psychologist. *Law and Human Behavior, 13*, 375–383.

du Toit, E. (2003). *An evaluation of the MMPI-2 using South African pre-trial forensic patients: Prediction of criminal responsibility and assessment of personality characteristics* (Masters thesis). Rhodes University.

Frederick, R. I. (2002). A review of Rey's strategies for detecting malingered neuropsychological impairment. *Journal of Forensic Neuropsychology*, *2*(3–4), 1–25. https://doi.org/10.1300/J151v02n03_01.

Ganellen, R. J., Wasyliw, O. E., Haywood, T. W., & Grossman, L. S. (1996). Can psychosis be malingered on the Rorschach? An empirical study. *Journal of Personality Assessment, 66*, 65–80.

Garner, H. H. (1965). Malingering. Illinois Medical Journal, 128: 318–319.

Gutheil, T. G. (2005). The history of forensic psychiatry. *The Journal of the American Academy of Psychiatry and the Law, 33*(2), 4.

Hathaway, S. R. (1943). MMPI. Manual for administration and scoring. Minneapolis: University of Minnesota Press.

Hickling, E. J., Taylor, A. E., Blanchard, E. B., et al. (1999). Simulation of motor vehicle accident related PTSD: Effects of coaching with DSM-IV criteria. In E. J., Hickling, & E. B., Blanchard (Eds). The international handbook of road traffic accidents and psychological trauma: Current understanding, treatment and law (pp. 305–320). New York: Elsevier.

Klotz Flitter, J. M., Elhai, J. D., & Gold, S. N. (2003). MMPI-2 F scale elevations in adult victims of child sexual abuse. *Journal of Trauma Stress*, *16*, 269–274.

Lanska, D. J. (2018). The dancing manias: Psychogenic illness as a social phenomenon. *Frontiers of Neurology and Neuroscience*, *42*, 132–141.

Miller, H. A. (2001). Miller-forensic assessment symptoms test: Professional manual. Odessa, FL: Psychological Assessment Resources.

Mittenburg, W., Patton, C., Canyock, E. M., & Condit, D. C. (2002). Base rates of malingering and symptom exaggeration. *Journal of Clinical and Experimental Neuropsychology*, *4*, 1094–1102.

Morey, L. C. (1991). Personality assessment inventory: Professional manual. FL, USA: Psychological Assessment Resources Inc.

Peay, J. (2019). *Legal malingering: A vortex of uncertainty*. LSE Law, Society and Economy Working Papers 10/2019.

Pelfrey, W. V. Jr. (2004). The relation between malingerers' intelligence and MMPI-2 knowledge and their ability to avoid detection. *International Journal of Offender Therapy and Comparative Criminology*, *48*, 649–663.

Perry, G. G., & Kinder, B. N. (1990). The susceptibility of the Rorschach to malingering: A critical review. *Journal of Personality Assessment*, *54*, 47–57.

Pillay, A. L., Gowensmith, W. N., & Banks, J. M. (2019). Towards the development of a forensic psychology training curriculum in South Africa. *South African Journal of Psychology*, *49*(4), 536–549. https://doi.org/10.1177/0081246319879291.

Resnick, P. (1997). The malingering of posttraumatic disorders. In R. Rogers (Ed.) Clinical assessment of malingering and deception (pp. 84–103, 2nd ed.). New York, NY: Guildford Press.

Resnick, P. (1998). Malingered psychosis. In R. Rogers (Ed.). Clinical assessment of malingering and deception. New York: The Guilford Press.

Rey, A. (1958). L'examen clinique en psychologie (The psychological examination). Paris: Universitaires de France.

Rey, A. (1964). L'examen clinique en psychologie (Clinical testsin psychology). Paris: Presses Universitaires de France.

Rogers, R., Bagby, R. M., & Dickson, S. E. (1992). Structured Interview of Reported Symptoms (SIRS) and professional manual. Odessa: Psychological Assessment Resources.

Rogers, R., Salekin, R. T., Sewell, K. W., Goldstein, A., & Leonard, K. (1998). A comparison of forensic and non-forensic malingerers: A prototypical analysis of explanatory models. Law and *Human Behavior*, *22*, 353–367.

Rosen, J., Mulsant, B. H., Bruce, M. L., Mittal, V., & Fox, D. (2004). Actors' portrayals of depression to test interrater reliability in clinical trials. *The American Journal of Psychiatry* *161*, 1909–1911.

Rosenhan, D. (1973). On being sane in an insane place. Science, *179*, 250.

Rotter, J. B., & Rafferty, J. E. (1950). The Rotter incomplete sentences blank. *Journal of Consulting Psychology*, *14*, 333.

Sequeira, A. J., Fara, M. G., & Lewis, A. (2018). Ethical challenges in acute evaluation of suspected psychogenic stroke mimics. *Journal of Clinical Ethics*, *29*(3), 185–190.

Smith, G. P., & Burgen, G. K. (1997a). Detection of malingering: Validation of the structured inventory of malingered symptomatology (SIMS). *Journal of the Academy of Psychiatry and the Law*, *25*, 180–183.

Smith, G. P., & Burgen, G. K. (1997b). Detection of malingering: Validation of the structured inventory of malingered symptomatology (SIMS). *Journal of the Academy of Psychiatry and the Law*, *25*, 183–189.

The World Health Organization (WHO) (2019). International Classification of Disease and related health problems (11th ed.).

Tombaugh, T. N. (1976). The test of memory and malingering (TOMM): Normative data from cognitively intact and cognitively impaired individuals. *Psychological Assessment*, *9*, 260–268.

Tversky, A., & Kahneman, D. (1974). Judgement under uncertainty: heuristics and biases. Science, 185, 1124–1131.

Vitacco, M. J., Rogers, R., Gabel, J., & Munizza, J. (2007). An evaluation of malingering screens with competency to stand trial patients: A known-groups comparison. *Law and Human Behavior*, *31*(3), 249–260.

Wagoner, R. C. (2017). The use of an interpreter during a forensic interview: Challenges and considerations. *Psychiatric Services*, *68*(5), 507–511. https://doi.org/10.1176/appi.ps.201600020.

Weiss, R., & Rosenfeld, B. (2010). Cross-cultural validity in malingering assessment: The dot counting test in a rural Indian sample. *International Journal of Forensic Mental Health*, *9*(4), 300–307. https://doi.org/10.1080/14999013.2010.526680.

Wenck, L. S. (1997). House-tree-person drawings: An illustrated diagnostic handbook. Los Angeles: Western Psychological Services.

Wessely, S. (2003). Malingering: Historical perspectives. In P. W. Halligan, C. M. Bass, & D. A. Oakley (Eds.), *Malingering and illness deception*. Oxford University Press.

Wong, A. J. (2008). *Normative indicators for a Black, Xhosa speaking population without tertiary education on four tests used to assess malingering* (Masters thesis). Rhodes University.

World Health Organization. (2018). *Mental health atlas 2017*. Geneva: World Health Organization.

9 Not guilty by reason of insanity (NGRI): Adjudication, clinical outcomes and rehabilitation

Kofi E. Boakye and Samuel Adjorlolo

Introduction

In several jurisdictions across the globe, criminal liability generally is a function of two essential factors. There is a requirement that a person actually commit or attempted to commit a crime (actus reus) and that the person had and/or had acted on the requisite rational intent, knowledge and free will (mens rea). The general presumption is that any individual charged with any offense is deemed to have the necessary mens rea. At the same time, an argument can be advanced that mens rea was impaired or that a defendant lacks the necessary mens rea at the time the offense was committed. The two major considerations in this regard are whether mental disorder contributed to the defective or irrational mens rea and, consequently, whether the insanity defense is appropriate. Invoking the insanity defense law essentially means that there is no contention about the commission of the offense. Instead, the adjudication and disposition processes would be centered on the mental element or mens rea of the defendent at the time the offense was committed. The disposition associated with a successful insanity defense plea is Not Guilty by Reason of Insanity (NGRI). The insanity defense plea and its associated disposition have dominated the attention of researchers, criminal justice practitioners and sometimes the public over the years. However, there is a dearth of literature on these constructs from Africa. This chapter fills this void by examining NGRI, taking into consideration the adjudication process, clinical outcomes and rehabilitation of individuals who have raised the insanity defense or acquitted based on the defense.

This chapter is organized as follows. The first section provides a brief overview of the insanity defense law and its origins, and how the insanity defense law has been applied in selected African countries. The second section examines the criminal adjudication process involving the insanity defense plea and dispositions associated with a successful insanity defense plea. We then evaluate clinical outcomes of defendants invoking the insanity defense and rehabilitation of insanity acquittees. The chapter concludes by offering some recommendations for future research into the insanity defense in Africa.

Insanity defense legislation in Africa

Contemporary insanity defense legislation and practices are strongly linked to the case involving Daniel M'Naughton, who mistakenly shot and killed the private secretary of the Prime Minister of England, Edward Drummond (Syed, 2019). M'Naughton was acquitted of the murder charges brought against him by prosecutors because the court, based on a psychiatric assessment report, reasoned that M'Naughton was mentally incapacitated at the time the offense was committed (Allnutt, Samuels, & O'driscoll, 2007). To quell public tension and controversies surrounding the acquittal, the judges of the Queen's Bench made two seemingly important proclamations (Yeo, 2008). First, they opined that the insanity plea can be raised if it is proven that (a) the party accused was laboring under such a defect of reason, from a disease of the mind, as not to know the nature and quality of the act being committed or (b) that he or she did not know that the act was wrong. The judges also stated that a person under insane delusion who commits an offense could be exculpated.

These proclamations, termed as the M'Naughton Rules, have influenced the insanity defense legislations of commonwealth African countries and former colonies of Britain. As the first country to have gained independence from the British in Africa, Ghana's insanity defense legislation retain essential elements of the M'Naughton Rules. Section 27 of the Criminal Offences Act, 1960 (Act 29; henceforth Act 29), which is termed "special verdict in respect of an insane person," states that insanity plea can be claimed (a) if that person was prevented, by reason of idiocy, imbecility, or a mental derangement or disease affecting the mind, from knowing the nature or consequences of the act in respect of which that person is accused or (b) if that person did the accused act under the influence of an insane delusion of a nature that renders that person, in the opinion of the jury or of the court, an unfit subject for punishment in respect of that act at the time of the crime is applicable (Adjorlolo, Chan, & Agboli, 2016).

The insanity legislations in Commonwealth countries in Eastern and Central Africa, namely Botswana, Kenya, Tanzania and Uganda, have similar wordings; "A person is not criminally responsible for an act or omission if at the time of doing the act or making the omission he is, through any disease affecting his mind, incapable of understanding what he is doing, or of knowing that he ought not to do the act or make the omission…" (Yeo, 2008, p. 243). In South Africa, the insanity defense legislation is contained in the Criminal Procedure Act 51 of 1977 ("the Act"). Section 78(1) of the Act states "A person who commits an act or makes an omission which constitutes an offence and who at the time of such commission or omission suffers from a mental illness or mental defect which makes him or her incapable—(a) of appreciating the wrongfulness of his or her act or omission; or (b) of acting in accordance with an appreciation of the wrongfulness of his or her act or omission, shall not be criminally responsible for such act or omission" (Stevens, 2015). Section 28 of the Criminal Code of Nigeria contains the insanity plea provisions. The Section states that for an insanity defense to be raised, it must be proven that "(A) The Accused person suffers from disease of mind/natural mental infirmity at the relevant time which deprived him of the capacity to understand what he was doing, control his action or know that he ought not to do an act or make an omission" (B) "A person whose mind at the time of his doing/omitting to do an act is affected by delusions on some specific matter(s), but who is not otherwise entitled to the benefit of the foregoing provisions of this section, is criminally responsible for his acts/omissions, to the same extent as if the real state of things had been such as he was induced by the delusions to believe to exist" (Ogunwale & Oluwaranti, 2020).

The insanity defense legislations are characterized by two important elements: biological/pathological and psychological elements. The biological element requires that a person suffers from mental disorder or defect of reasoning at the time the offense was committed. The defect of reason should be a product of disease of the mind which is a legal, not medical, concept. That is, what qualifies as a disease of the mind is primarily determined by courts of competent jurisdiction. The relevant legal provisions in Ghana and many African countries are silent on the exact constituents of the biological element. In the case of South Africa, this was clarified in State v Stellmacher (1983), where the court made a finding that basically defines the criteria for a mental illness/disorder: that it must be pathological, and it must be endogenous; that is, not as a result of external stimuli (Mosotho, Timile, & Joubert, 2017). The psychological component requires that the person lacks the requisite mental capacity to appreciate the wrongfulness of the act (Stevens, 2015). The mere presence of a mental disorder of any sort is necessary but not sufficient for the defense to be raised successfully. Instead, it should be demonstrated that the mental disorder significantly impairs the psychological and mental capacity of the accused such that they are unable to appreciate the wrongfulness of the act. For instance, in the case involving Helegah vs The Republic of Ghana (1973), the court reasoned that amnesia does not constitute insanity. The essential ingredient is that the defect in reasoning resulting from mental disorder should cause an individual not to know the nature and quality of the act or the act is wrong. More importantly, the nature and quality of an act refers to the physical, and not moral, element. Similarly, the wrongfulness of an act is defined in the sense of legal, and not moral, interpretation.

As with the provision in many African countries, the insanity defense legislation in Ghana has been criticized on several grounds, including being redundant and containing outmoded terminologies. Adjorlolo, Chan, et al. (2016) argued that it is needless for the second part of the legislation to focus exclusively on delusions. This is because delusions are a major part of mental disorders, either as symptoms or distinct disorders. Second, the emphasis on congenital cognitive disabilities resulting in "idiocy" and "imbecility," mental derangement arising from disease or natural degeneration, and disease of the mind as the conditions that can impair an individual's knowledge of criminal acts is needless. These conditions, particularly those relating to congenital mental retardations and terminologies such as "idiocy" and "imbecility," apart from their pejorative overtone, also convey the notion that the mind must be in total deprivation for the insanity defense to be raised (Adjorlolo, Chan, et al., 2016). When jurors, for instance, are directed to consider this narrowed interpretation of the defense during the criminal adjudication process, the tendency that some individuals will be denied the defense may be high. The authors, therefore, propose the term *mental disorder* or its variant as a suitable replacement for all the aforementioned conditions. The Canadian insanity plea used to contain these outmoded terms such as "natural imbecility" "insanity," "disease of the mind," "idiocy" and "lunacy" (Zhao & Ferguson, 2013). When the legislation was revised in 1992, mental disorder was introduced to subsume all the previous descriptors. Canadian Criminal Code Section 16(1) now reads: "No person is criminally responsible for an act committed or an omission made while suffering from a mental disorder that rendered the person incapable of appreciating the nature and quality of the act or omission or knowing that it was wrong" (Zhao & Ferguson, 2013). In the United States, United Kingdom and across several European countries, the insanity legislation makes reference to "mental illness," "mental disorder" and "mental defect" (Bal & Koenraadt, 2000).

One other commonality in the insanity legislation across jurisdictions is the lack of a definition of mental illness or mental disorder (Adjorlolo, 2016; Mosotho et al., 2017; Ogunwale & Oluwaranti, 2020). Thus, the criminal law may consider adopting the term "mental disorder" not only because other jurisdictions have done so, but also because it will conform to the definition used in Ghana's Mental Health Act 846. Act 846 (2012) defines mental disorder as "a condition of the mind in which there is a clinically significant disturbance of mental or behavior functioning associated with distress or interference of daily life and manifesting as disturbance of speech, perception, mood, thought, volition, orientation or other cognitive functions to such a degree as to be considered pathological but excludes social deviance without personal dysfunction" (pp. 4–42). The Mental Health Act of Zimbabwe (Act No 23 of 1976) also defined mentally disordered or mentally defective as "suffering from mental illness, arrested or incomplete development of mind, psychopathic disorder or any other disorder or disability of the mind" (Menezes, Oyebode, & Haque, 2009, p. 430). The proposal for an updated definition of mental disorder or illness by the criminal laws and mental health legislation is particularly attractive given the indication that the definition of mental illness as contained in the Mental Health Act in South Africa is not binding on the determination of criminal responsibility during the adjudication process (Mosotho et al., 2017).

Insanity defense and criminal adjudication process

In general, trials involving the mental state at the time of offense (insanity plea) have some essential elements, including the following: (1) raising the question about mental state at the time of offense, (2) request for mental state examination, (3) mental state evaluation stage, (4) judicial determination of appropriateness of insanity plea and (5) disposition of insanity acquittees and commitment to treatment (Adjorlolo, Agboli, & Chan, 2016; Adjorlolo, Chan, et al., 2016). Every accused is presumed not to suffer from a mental incapacitation and so is criminally liable, unless the issue is raised otherwise. Although, in principle, the insanity defense can be raised by either the defense or prosecution, in practice the defendant mental state at the time of offense is mostly raised by the defense attorney who has the burden of proof (Adjorlolo, Agboli, et al., 2016; Adjorlolo, Chan, et al., 2016; Swanepoel, 2015).

To ensure due process prevails and that the rights of defendants are not violated, the trial court normally requests a retrospective assessment of the defendant's mental state at the time of the offense. The court can refer an accused at any stage of the trial for a psychiatric or psychological assessment of his or her mental state (Swanepoel, 2015). Defendants referred for assessments are mostly committed to a psychiatric hospital or to any other place designated by the court.

Consistent with practices elsewhere, the assessments are conducted by mental health professionals. A major challenge is that because the majority of African countries lack trained forensic psychiatrists and/or forensic psychologists, mental state examinations are often undertaking by "general" psychiatrists and psychologists with little or no training in forensic assessment and issues. These mental health professionals mostly conduct interviews and collect third-party information, such as collateral reports, witness statements, police reports, crime scene information and other demographic, biopsychosocial, medical and psychiatric histories (Mosotho et al., 2017; Ogunwale & Oluwaranti, 2020; Stevens, 2015).

Another source of data involve the administration of traditional/forensic assessment instruments. However, because the majority of forensic assessment instruments are not validated or standardized on local samples, others have questioned the validity and reliability of the assessment results (Adjorlolo, Agboli, et al., 2016; Adjorlolo & Chan, 2019; Mosotho et al., 2017). Likewise, the use of neuroimaging techniques such as computed tomography scans for mental state assessment for criminal responsibility decisions have been questioned (Mosotho et al., 2017). The court is then furnished with the assessment reports to assist in determining the defendant mental state at the time of offense. When one or all the parties contesting a case is/are not satisfied or convinced with the assessment result, the medical officer is called in open court and cross-examined. During this cross examination, issues such as qualification, experience, assessment methods, procedures and findings are thoroughly probed (Adjorlolo, Agboli, et al., 2016). In providing their expert opinion, mental health professionals are prohibited from commenting on the criminal responsibility of the defendant based on the assessment report, the so-called ultimate issue (Stevens, 2015). The court in Ghana, for instance, addressed the ultimate issue in Kwadwo Mensah vs. The Republic (1959) when it stated that the determination of insanity at the time of the offense is the sole preserve of the trial court (judge/jury) in view of all the available evidence. The court in the State vs. Van As (1991) in South Africa also noted that it is not the responsibility of the mental health professionals to take over or replace the function or duties of the court in deciding on the culpability of the defendant.

For trials involving jurors, the presiding judge has the sole responsibility of directing the jurors on the facts to consider in order to determine the culpability or otherwise of the defendant. In the case involving Abugiri Frafra vs Republic of Ghana (1974), the defendant was accused of murder, and the psychiatrist who testified diagnosed the defendant with paranoid schizophrenia, which took the form of persecutory delusions. The trial court instructed the jurors to "ask themselves whether there is evidence from which they can infer that at the time of offence the mind of the accused was in a high degree of disorder and that he was incapable of controlling his conduct" (Adjorlolo, Chan, et al., 2016). Defendants found to be insane at the time of offense are traditionally rendered the special verdict of not guilty by reason of insanity (NGRI). However, for reasons such as to appease the public or victims, the NGRI has been reworded in such a manner to place some responsibilities on the accused. Countries such as Ghana and Zimbabwe prefer guilty but insane verdict (also known as guilty but mentally ill; GBMI) (Adjorlolo, Chan, et al., 2016; Menezes et al., 2009), whereas others such as South Africa and Nigeria still maintain NGRI (Kaliski, 2012; Ogunwale & Oluwaranti, 2020). The GBMI arguably makes Ghana's defense of insanity a partial defense, and therefore raised an interesting topical issue not only in Ghana but also in other jurisdictions rendering a similar verdict. In particular, it appeared to conflict with the underlying philosophy of the law that an insane person is not morally responsible because of the defective mind, and so cannot form mens rea or criminal intent (Adjorlolo, Chan, et al., 2016). Of particular interest is the pattern of utilization of the insanity plea on the continent. Though this topical issue has not been explored, a recent study found that the insanity plea has been successful in a modest number of cases in Nigeria (Ogunwale & Oluwaranti, 2020). The authors examined the judgments from appeal cases since 1948 and found that, out of 34 cases adopting the insanity plea, the rate of plea success was 26.5% ($n = 9$). It further emerged that the main factors contributing to a successful insanity defense plea is an inability of the accused to comprehend his/her action. Defendants who are not satisfied with the decisions of the trial courts can make an appeal to a higher court (e.g., the High Court, the Appeal Court, and the Supreme Court). In the case involving Collins vs The Republic of Ghana (1987–1988), the defendant, diagnosed with schizophrenia, was convicted of murder by the trial court. On appeal, the appellate court substituted the guilty verdict with GBMI on the ground that the trial court erred by failing to recognize and include the defendant's history of schizophrenia.

Disposal of insanity acquittees

Despite the variations in how the insanity defense verdict is worded, the arrangement and disposition of insanity acquittees across the continent appear to be the same. More specifically, the disposition associated with a successful insanity plea is commitment to treatment as prescribed by the criminal laws and Mental Health Acts of the various countries. Depending on factors such as the nature and seriousness of offense, the court will order the accused to be admitted to a psychiatric hospital, forensic psychiatric facility or even an outpatient facility, for further treatment and rehabilitation. Section 28 of the Mental Health Act No 23 of 1976 of Zimbabwe states that, "when an accused is found to be guilty but insane, the court will commit the accused to treatment and the president may give such directions as he deems fit as to the further detention, care, management and treatment of the patient concerned in an institution, special institution or other place, including a prison" (Menezes et al., 2009). Ghana, for instance, does not have forensic psychiatry hospitals or prisons. However, the psychiatric institutions have "forensic units" where all categories of offenders with mental illness (e.g., insanity acquittees, defendants who are incompetent to stand trial and prisoners who have been administratively transferred to the hospitals) are accommodated, catered for and treated. These individuals are brought together in the same unit because of their involvement in the criminal justice system without recourse to the nature of their crimes and mental disorders. That is, extremely violent and aggressive offenders with severe mental disorders (i.e. psychosis with bizarre delusions and hallucinations) are housed in the same units with non-violent offenders with less severe mental disorders (Adjorlolo, Abdul-Nasiru, Chan, & Bambi, 2018).

In jurisdictions such as South Africa and Ghana, an insanity acquittee who committed a serious offense (e.g. murder, rape, and assault with the intent to do grievous bodily harm), is declared a state patient and will be discharged back to their community once they are stable (Houidi & Paruk, 2018). The purpose of the admission as a state patient is not punishment but rather treatment, care, and rehabilitation, while simultaneously monitoring and managing their potential risk to the community (Houidi, Paruk, & Sartorius, 2018). State patients may be discharged, conditionally or unconditionally, or reclassified as involuntary mental health care users (Marais & Subramaney, 2015).

Clinical characteristics of insanity acquittees

An earlier study in Ghana found that out of 138 insanity acquittees, 31% were diagnosed with schizophrenia, 20.2% with drug-induced psychotic disorder and 13.3% with non-specified psychosis (Turkson & Asante, 1997). Nearly half (48.6%) of the offenders charged with murder or attempted murder were diagnosed with schizophrenia. Data on 273 (males = 251) insanity acquittees from Zimbabwe revealed that the majority were diagnosed with schizophrenia (n = 195), whereas 11 (4.02%) had a diagnosis of substance misuse disorder, 6 (2.19%) had psychopathic personality disorder, 7 (2.56%) had mental impairment and 44 (16.11%) had other diagnoses (Menezes et al., 2009). In this sample, insanity acquittees diagnosed with schizophrenia committed homicide, compared with other violent and non-violent crimes. They also used different methods, namely blunt and sharp instruments, firearms and strangulation, to commit the crimes. In terms of demographics, the males comprised the bulk of patients (N = 251), with females in the minority (N = 22). Ages ranged from 17 to 59 years. More than half of the acquittees were not married.

Relatedly, a review of insanity acquittees admitted to a forensic unit in KwaZulu-Natal, a coastal South African province, from 2013 to 2016 revealed that 33 (36.26%) had a diagnosis of intellectual disability, 26 (28.57%) had diagnosis of schizophrenia and 52 (57.14%) had substance use disorder (Houidi & Paruk, 2018). Further analysis revealed that the majority of the acquittees had comorbid diagnoses (n = 70, 76.92%), with substance-use disorder, head injury and other general medical conditions emerging as the three most occurring comorbidities. In terms of demographics, males were overrepresented (*n* = 90, 98.90%). Although the ages of the insanity acquittees ranges from 15 to 45 years and above, it was observed further that the majority were within the age group of 15 to 35 years. The majority of the acquittees were unemployed (*n* = 89, 97.80%) and single (*n* = 89, 97.80%) (Houidi & Paruk, 2018). In yet another study from South Africa, Marais and Subramaney (2015) reported that psychotic disorders were commonly diagnosed among insanity acquittees and individuals declared unfit to stand trial. More specifically, 44% (*n* = 50) were diagnosed with schizophrenia and 20% (*n* = 23) with psychosis. A total of 34 patients were diagnosed with mental retardation (*n* = 18), organic brain syndrome (*n* = 6), dementia (*n* = 5) and epilepsy (*n* = 5). The majority of patients committed offenses against persons such as murder and rape (*n* = 103, 68%). Property offenses were committed by 25% of the patients (*n* = 38). In terms of demographic characteristics, the majority of patients were males (*n* = 99, 87%). The age of the patients also ranged from 10 to 69 years; however, individuals aged between 20 and 49 years old were overly represented. The majority of the patients were single (*n* = 91, 80%), unemployed (*n* = 89, 78%) and had less than 12 years of formal education (*n* = 88).

In summary, emerging studies from Africa have revealed that the majority of insanity acquittees are diagnosed with schizophrenia and other psychotic spectrum disorders. Acquittees were also likely to be males, young adults, unemployed with low or no educational background. In terms of offense history, the majority of acquittees committed violent acts, including murder and rape. These preliminary findings are largely consistent with extant literature from Western countries. Adjorlolo, Chan, and DeLisi (2019) observed that the most common diagnosis among insanity acquittees is schizophrenia. Males were also found to dominate the insanity acquittees' population across jurisdictions. Lastly, the authors found that violent crimes dominated the crimes committed by insanity acquittees.

Rehabilitation of insanity acquittees

Once at treatment centers within forensic institutions, insanity acquittees are expected to undergo rehabilitation. Rehabilitation has two principal elements. The first relates to the provision of treatment to restore sanity. In this context, insanity acquittees are put on treatment regimens and supervised by health professionals. Psychopharmacological management, involving the administration of psychotropic medications, is the dominant management practice across the continent. Due to the financial and logistical challenges besetting the provision of mental health on the continent, typical (e.g., haloperidol and chlorpromazine) rather than atypical antipsychotic (e.g., clozapine and olanzapine) medications are often used in the treatment and management of insanity acquittees and other patients with mental illness (Adjorlolo et al., 2018). These medications not only prolong the treatment period but also induce unpleasant side effects, prominent among which are the extra-pyramidal symptoms such as Parkinson disease. These symptoms generally make it difficult for patients to adhere to treatment while on admission and after discharge, thus adversely affecting the outcome of treatment, both in the short and long term.

The limited use of psychotherapy and other psychosocial interventions to complement the pharmacological treatment is another notable issue (Adjorlolo, 2015). The second phase of rehabilitation, following a reduction in and stabilization of the symptoms of mental disorders, is occupational therapy. Here, the insanity acquittees are taken through vocational training to enable them to acquire skills in basic vocations such as basket weaving, bead making and carpentry. The effectiveness of the occupational program is mostly hampered by limited resources. Thus, most insanity acquittees are not able to acquire the requisite skills that could set them on independent pathways from their caregivers after they have been discharged from the psychiatric institutions (Adjorlolo, 2016). In Ghana and perhaps other jurisdictions, it is not uncommon for insanity acquittees to escape from treatment centers. This observation may have fueled the conception that the insanity defense is abused, or those pleading insanity at the time of the offense are not truly insane, culminating in negative attitudes toward the insanity defense (Adjorlolo et al., 2018). The aforementioned challenges have created situations where insanity acquittees and patients with mental disorders in general spend longer times at the treatment centers than they would have serving their prison terms.

Conclusion and future directions

The question of how to deal with crime and dispense justice fairly has been a perplexing issue for all societies. This question is even more pertinent when it comes to how the criminal justice system handles its most vulnerable in society. The M'Naughton Rule established the foundational principle for safeguarding the fundamental rights of one of the most vulnerable groups of people in society, mentally disordered offenders. In this chapter, we examined the laws and legal safeguards afforded to offenders laboring under some form of mental disorder and the varied forms these insanity clauses operate in Africa. We reviewed and compared the adjudication processes in relation to cases involving suspected offenders with mental disorders. The varied disposal options available to the courts in different juridictions on the continent were also examined. Finally, we reviewed the clinical characteristics of insanity acquittees and effectiveness of rehabilitation regimes across jurisdictions in Africa.

With regard to the law, it is clear that much of what passes as an insanity legislation in African jurisdictions are colonial inheritances which have seen very little reform. The evidence of this is seen, for example, in often pejorative and vague terminologies such as "idiocy," "imbecility" or "disease of the mind" within insanity legistlations in various jurisdictions. These terminologies inherited from the M'Naughton Rules of 1843 have been the subject of intense criticism (Bradley 2009; Law Commission, 2013; Syed, 2019). The often vague and varied interpretations these terminologies invoke in the minds of judges and juries could result in unfair verdicts. For example, as shown, the legal definition of insanity or disease of the mind is considered out of step with medical understanding of what consistutes a "disease of the mind" (Fennell, 1992; Law Commission 2013; Syed 2019). It is therefore important to research and interrogate these terminologies, their meanings and appropriateness in the jurisdictions such as Ghana where they continue to be used. This is particularly important given concerns about the stigmatizing effect of some of these terminologies.

The lack of qualified forensic mental health practitioners to support the adjudication process must be addressed to ensure justice delivery. While the determination of guilt or otherwise is the sole preserve of the judge/jury, it is important that verdicts are based on the most rigorous assessment and evidence. To achieve this, it is essential to develop culturally appropriate assessment tools informed by contextually relevant research into mental disorders. There is also the need for research into the charactersitics of insanity acquittees to understand better the category of mental disorders that increase the risk for offending, particularly serious violence. As the evidence from the limited research shows, mentally disordered offenders are likely to suffer from schizophrenia and psychosis (Adjorlolo et al., 2019; Ogunwale & Oluwaranti, 2020). The evidence also shows that young males are disproportionately represented in the mentally disordered offender population (Adjorlolo et al., 2019; Ogunwale & Oluwaranti, 2020). However, this finding confirms what we already know based on evidence from previous research. That is, there is gender disproportionality in offending population generally with young males more likely to offend whether it is violent (Boakye, 2020; Lauritsen, Heimer, Lynch, 2009) or non-violent offending (Boakye, 2013; Loeber, Farrington, Stouthamer-Loeber, & Van Kammen, 1998). Further research is needed that investigates multilevel factors to identify unique characteristics that distinguish mentally disordered offenders from other offenders in the normal population. To achieve this, longitudinal studies in different African countries are required to establish the etiology of mental disorders and to establish factors that explain offending among the mentally disordered population. There is a clear urgent need to address the lack of forensic psychiatric hospitals across Africa. However, the generally negative effect of institutionalization and the unique feature of a collective value system that characterize African societies present opportunities to explore effectiveness of community-based intervention programs, especially for low-level and non-violent mentally disordered offenders.

References

Adjorlolo, S. (2015). Can teleneuropsychology help meet the neuropsychological needs of Western Africans? The case of Ghana. *Applied Neuropsychology: Adult, 22*(5), 388–398.

Adjorlolo, S. (2016). Diversion of individuals with mental illness in the criminal justice system in Ghana. *International Journal of Forensic Mental Health, 15*(4), 382–392.

Adjorlolo, S., Abdul-Nasiru, I., Chan, H. C., & Bambi, L. E. (2018). Mental health professionals' attitudes toward offenders with mental illness (insanity acquittees) in Ghana. *International Journal of Offender Therapy and Comparative Criminology, 62*(3), 629–654.

Adjorlolo, S., Agboli, J. M., & Chan, H. C. (2016). Criminal responsibility and the insanity defence in Ghana: The examination of legal standards and assessment issues. *Psychiatry, Psychology and Law, 23*(5), 684–695.

Adjorlolo, S., & Chan, H. C. O. (2019). Risk assessment of criminal offenders in Ghana: An investigation of the discriminant validity of the HCR-20V3. *International Journal of Law and Psychiatry, 66*, 101458.

Adjorlolo, S., Chan, H. C. O., & Agboli, J. M. (2016). Adjudicating mentally disordered offenders in Ghana: The criminal and mental health legislations. *International Journal of Law and Psychiatry, 45*, 1–8.

Adjorlolo, S., Chan, H. C. O., & DeLisi, M. (2019). Mentally disordered offenders and the law: Research update on the insanity defense, 2004–2019. *International Journal of Law and Psychiatry, 67*, 101507.

Allnutt, S., Samuels, A., & O'driscoll, C. (2007). The insanity defence: From wild beasts to M'Naghten. *Australasian Psychiatry, 15*(4), 292–298.

Bal, P., & Koenraadt, F. (2000). Criminal law and mentally ill offenders in comparative perspective. *Psychology, Crime & Law, 6*(4), 219–250. doi: 10.1080/10683160008409805

Boakye, K. E. (2013). Correlates and predictors of juvenile delinquency in Ghana. *International Journal of Comparative and Applied Criminal Justice, 37*(4), 257–278

Boakye, K. E. (2020). Child abuse & neglect juvenile sexual o ff ending in Ghana: Prevalence, risks and correlates. *Child Abuse and Neglect, 101*. Retrieved from https://doi.org/10.1016/j.chiabu.2019.104318.

Bradley, K. J. C. B. (2009). *The Bradley Report: Lord Bradley's review of people with mental health problems or learning disabilities in the criminal justice system* (Vol. 7). London: Department of Health.

Fennell, P. (1992). The Criminal Procedure (Insanity and Unfitness to Plead) Act 1991. *The Modern Law Review, 55*(4), 547–555.

Houidi, A., & Paruk, S. (2018). Profile of forensic state patients at a psychiatric unit in KwaZulu Natal, South Africa: Demographic, clinical and forensic factors. *The Journal of Forensic Psychiatry & Psychology, 29*(4), 544–556.

Houidi, A., Paruk, S., & Sartorius, B. (2018). Forensic psychiatric assessment process and outcome in state patients in KwaZulu-Natal, South Africa. *South African Journal of Psychiatry, 24*(1), 1–6.

Kaliski, S. (2012). Does the insanity defence lead to an abuse of human rights? *African Journal of Psychiatry, 15*(2), 83–87.

Lauritsen, J. L., Heimer, K., & Lynch J. P. (2009), Trends in the gender gap in violence: re-evaluating NCVS and other evidence. *Criminology, 47*(2), 361–400.

Law Commission. (2013). *Criminal liability: Insanity and automatism: A discussion paper*. London: The Stationery Office.

Loeber, R., Farrington, D. P., Stouthamer-Loeber, M., & Van Kammen, W. (1998). *Antisocial behavior and mental health problems*. Mahwah, NJ: Lawrence Erlbaum.

Marais, B., & Subramaney, U. (2015). Forensic state patients at Sterkfontein Hospital: A 3-year follow-up study. *South African Journal of Psychiatry*, *21*(3), 86–92.

Menezes, S., Oyebode, F., & Haque, M. (2009). Victims of mentally disordered offenders in Zimbabwe, 1980–1990. *The Journal of Forensic Psychiatry & Psychology*, *20*(3), 427–439.

Mosotho, N. L., Timile, I., & Joubert, G. (2017). The use of computed tomography scans and the Bender Gestalt Test in the assessment of competency to stand trial and criminal responsibility in the field of mental health and law. *International Journal of Law and Psychiatry*, *50*, 68–75.

Ogunwale, A., & Oluwaranti, O. (2020). Pattern of utilization of the insanity plea in Nigeria: An empirical analysis of reported cases. *Forensic Science International: Mind and Law*, *1*, 100010. doi: https://doi.org/10.1016/j.fsiml.2020.100010

Stevens, G. P. (2015). Adjudicating pathological criminal incapacity within a climate of ultimate issue barriers: A comparative perspective. *International Journal of Law and Psychiatry*, *38*, 29–37.

Swanepoel, M. (2015). Legal aspects with regard to mentally ill offenders in South Africa. *Potchefstroom Electronic Law Journal/Potchefstroomse Elektroniese Regsblad*, *18*(1), 3237–3258.

Syed, H. (2019). Defence of insanity: 'Humpty Dumpty' law reform. *North America Academic Research*, *2*(3), 72–80.

Turkson, S., & Asante, K. (1997). Psychiatric disorders among offender patients in the Accra Psychiatric Hospital. *West African journal of medicine*, *16*(2), 88–92.

Yeo, S. (2008). Insanity defense in the criminal Laws of the Commonwealth of Nations. *Singapore Journal of Legal Studies.*, 241–263.

Zhao, L., & Ferguson, G. (2013). Understanding China's mental illness defense. *The Journal of Forensic Psychiatry & Psychology*, *24*(5), 634–657. doi: 10.1080/14789949.2013.830318

Statutes cited

AbugiriFrafra vs. The Republic (1974). 2 Ghana Law Review, 447, CA.

Kwadwo Mensah vs. The Republic (1959). Ghana law review. 309. CA.

State v. Stellmacher (2) SA 181 (SWA) (1983).

Sv Van As 1991 2 SACR 74 (W).

Helegah vs The Republic (1973). 2, Ghana law report 29, CA.

R. v. Luedecke, 2008 ONCA 716 (CanLII). Retrieved on 2015-05-13 from http://www.canlii.org/en/on/onca/doc/2008/2008onca716/2008onca716.html.

10 Best practices in expert testimony and report writing in Africa

Adegboyega Ogunlesi and Adegboyega Ogunwale

Introduction

History and purpose of expert psychiatric testimony

From antiquity, the significance of intention in shaping human conduct was already apparent. In Babylonian law as represented by the code of Hammurabi as well as in Judeo-Christian scriptures (e.g., Deuteronomy 19:1–5), it had been pointed out that the status of an offensive act ought to be judged by the intent of the actor (Prosono, 2003). Equally, Roman law recognized the lack of criminal responsibility on the part of those who did not show malicious intent. A 2nd century (AD 180) text by Macer, written during the time of Marcus Aurelius (Spruitt, 1998), seemed to broadly lay down the key elements of the expert witness role in criminal cases involving the mentally ill. These elements included careful assessment, consideration for the possibility of malingering, deferring to other authorities on the final determination of culpability and clinical management of risk to the defendant and others (Gutheil, 2005).

By the Middle Ages, the Justinian ("Corpus Iuris Civilis") as well as the Theodosian codes had recognized the non-culpability of "insane" persons and in essence, Roman law adopted the principle that an insane person could be likened to a seven- or eight-year-old child who was incapable of malicious intent as a result of lack of understanding (Eigen, 1983; Prosono, 2003). By the 13th century, English law began to observe the development of tests of legal insanity. For example, Bracton's "wild beast test" required that for the insane to be free of criminal responsibility, he must have the "wildness" of beasts, suggesting that in such a state, the insane were incapable of forming malicious intent (Allnutt, Samuels, & Driscoll, 2007).

During most of the medieval period, physicians were not particularly associated with expert witness roles except in cities like Bologna in Italy and Freiburg im Breisgau in Germany. The recognition of medical forensic expertise by legal authorities became observable at the beginning of the 16th century. Three cardinal factors could have been responsible for this development in forensic psychiatry in particular: (i) evolution of legal and medical theories regarding insanity, (ii) development of legal tests/criteria for the determination of insanity and (iii) evolution of putative treatments for mental disorders (Prosono, 2003).

The 18th century signaled the first documented psychiatric expert witness, John Munro, in the 1760 case of Earl Ferrers (Eigen, 1983). By mid-19th century (1843), the landmark case of Daniel M'Naghten's case crystallized the most "modern" test of legal insanity upon which many Anglo-Americans as well as other jurisdictions across the world have erected their judicial position on insanity with various adaptations. Essentially, the M'Naghten Rules indicate that an accused person lacks criminal responsibility if he suffers from a defect of reason arising from a mental disorder, which prevents him from recognizing the nature/quality of his action or the wrongness of such conduct (M'Naghten's case, 1843).

While the history of forensic medicine generally dates back to antiquity with roots in African (Egyptian) civilization (Kharoshah, Zaki, Galeb, Moulana, & Elsebaay, 2011), in many African jurisdictions, expert psychiatric witnesses came to the stage around the mid-1900s. This occurred against a background of evolving criminal legislations requiring psychiatric participation despite the availability of very few mental health services and abject lack of trained manpower across the continent (Milner, 1966). By 1963, few Sub-Saharan African countries had trained psychiatrists. Situating the utilization of psychiatric experts by the courts within this context of lacking human resources, Milner (1966) further argues that the existence of legal provisions for mental assessments at different stages of criminal trials largely reflected judicial idealism rather than practical reality. At the time, the small number of psychiatrists were torn between clinical and administrative duties with barely any time available to devote to forensic work. Whenever they could provide expert services, they did so in relation to courts within their locality and mainly in criminal cases involving murder or serious violence. Murder cases were given priority perhaps because psychiatric testimony was likely to be requested in such situations. Given the shortage of manpower, it became the norm that only one expert opinion would be before the court, thereby making a battle between experts a rarity in most African jurisdictions. This has remained the pattern in many African countries to date. Even in countries where two experts are nominated by the courts for the purpose of psychiatric evaluation in criminal cases, they are expected to issue a joint report (Touari, Mesbah, Dellatolas, & Bensmail, 1993).

Using Nigeria as an illustration, Bienen (1976) observed that by 1972, only three psychiatrists at the Aro Hospital for nervous diseases in Western Nigeria (now Federal Neuropsychiatric Hospital, Aro, Abeokuta) were handling all court referrals for psychiatric opinion. At the time, rebuttal expert opinions were not required, not all accused persons could be assessed and there were delays in getting such assessments. In addition, judges had full discretion as to calling expert evidence in cases involving the insanity defense and it was not improbable that the level of sympathy of each judge to psychiatric factors in offending played a major role in the frequency of utilization of expert opinions (Bienen, 1974). These observations by Bienen still effectively describe the current position of the courts regarding expert psychiatric testimony, although there are now more psychiatrists in the country who engage in forensic work.

On the whole, expert psychiatric testimony with its focus on mental health issues in offending offers much for defendants (and indeed the larger society) by way of therapeutic jurisprudence (Wren, 2010). This refers to an interdisciplinary approach to law that focuses on the psychological impact of the law on participants in the legal process. It also addresses the societal impact of the legal system. It is equally important to note that the psychiatric expert witness seeks to project the neutrality of opinion while balancing delicately between the forces of humane care for the "mad" and those of society's legitimate interest in the punishment of the "bad" (Mullen, 1993).

Psychiatric expert witnesses may be required to provide testimony (written and/or oral) within a fair number of civil and criminal matters (Buchanan & Norko, 2011; Eastman, Adshead, Fox, Latham, & Whyte, 2012; Rix, Eastman, & Adshead, 2015). These include but are not limited to:

- Examination of the state of mind of criminal defendants in relation to various legal tests or criteria (e.g., insanity defense, fitness to plead, etc.).
- Proffering opinion in the sentencing of offenders usually in the context of mental disorder (e.g., in the context of sex offending).
- Giving opinion on psychiatric injuries in personal injury litigation in civil proceedings.
- Providing opinion on allegations of negligence in psychiatric care.
- Child custody as well as advising on the risk of physical or emotional harm posed by parents with mental disorder towards their children.
- Competency to practice and licensing.
- Proffering opinion in the context of professional regulation in cases where the mental health of practitioners, or the professional conduct of psychiatrists is being investigated.
- Examination of the mental capacity of persons making different types of legal decisions (e.g., capacity to consent or withhold consent to treatment, testamentary capacity, etc.).

Who is an expert?

A most pertinent question then arises: who is an expert? A broad-based practical definition of an expert may be given as: a person who *"has sufficient knowledge of the subject acquired by study or experience; they may have professional qualifications in their subject but professional qualification does not necessarily confer 'expert' status. The test is one of 'skill'."* (Rix et al., 2015). Given differences across jurisdictions in terms of contextual definitions of experts, Box 10.1 provides exemplary interpretations of the term "expert" within legal statutes and jurisprudence of selected African countries.

In observing that the role of an expert is not determined solely by qualification, Eastman et al. (2012) have helpfully highlighted a number of other considerations that should also apply:

Box 10.1 Jurisdictional variations in the definition of experts

Nigerian Evidence Act (2011) section 68 (subsections 1 & 2)

"When the court has to form an opinion upon a point of foreign law, customary law, or custom, or of science or art, or as to identity of handwriting or finger impressions, the opinions upon that point of persons specially skilled in such foreign law, customary law or custom, or science or art, or in questions as to identity of handwriting or finger impressions, are admissible. Persons so specially skilled as mentioned in subsection (1) of this section are called experts."

South African Case Law

Menday v Protea Assurance Co Ltd 1976 (1) SA 565 (E), 569B-C

"In essence the function of an expert is to assist the Court to reach a conclusion on matters on which the Court itself does not have the necessary knowledge to decide. It is not the mere opinion of the witness which is decisive but his ability to satisfy the Court that, because of his special skill, training or experience, the reasons for the opinion which he expresses are acceptable."

Schneider NO & others v AA & another 2010 (5) SA 203 (WCC), 211J-212B

"An expert is not a hired gun who dispenses his or her expertise for the purposes of a particular case. An expert does not assume the role of an advocate, nor gives evidence which goes beyond the logic which is dictated by the scientific knowledge which that expert claims to possess."

Egyptian Perspective (Kharoshah et al., 2011)

The role of the expert witness is subsumed in the duties of the "forensic medical examiner" who is approved under Decree No. 96 of 1952 and appointed by the Forensic Medicine Authority. Specialists appointed by the authority are called "experts." The forensic examiner undertakes the forensic medical examination of living persons involved in criminal and civil cases.

- Whether a person without instruction or experience in knowledge or human experience would be able to form a sound judgment on the matter without the aid of a witness possessing such knowledge or experience.

- Whether the subject matter of the opinion forms part of a body of knowledge or experience that is sufficiently organized or recognized to be accepted as a reliable body of knowledge or experience.
- Whether the witness has acquired by study or experience sufficient knowledge of the subject to render his opinion of value in resolving the facts before the court.

Similarly, in Aguda's 1974 review of the law of evidence in Nigeria, it was suggested that *"a person can be regarded as an expert in a particular field even though he did not acquire his knowledge after a systematic tutoring in the particular field, provided that he has had, in the opinion of the court, sufficient practice in the particular field of knowledge as professional or as amateur, to make his opinion reliable."*

Principles guiding expert witness roles

In addition to the principles presented in Box 10.2, other attributes of the "good" or "excellent" mental health expert witness have been observed to be the ability

Box 10.2 Broad principles guiding expert witness roles (Eastman et al., 2012; Janofsky, Hanson, Candilis, Myers, & Zonana, 2014)

Experts should:

- Be impartial and unbiased in their evidence.
- Address the pertinent legal questions clearly.
- Provide reasons for their opinion and where necessary, reasons for rejecting alternatives.
- Cite evidence both for and against their opinion to provide a balanced view.
- Provide "conditional" opinions where their opinion would vary depending on the ultimate findings of fact by the court.
- Be ready to change their opinion if new information is made available.
- Acknowledge the limits of their expertise.
- Avoid taking on the posture of an advocate for either party to the suit.
- Appreciate the scope of their participation in the legal process.
- Strive for honesty and objectivity.
- Ensure confidentiality of information within the limits of the law.
- Obtain consent (or assent) as the case might require.

to tender firm conclusions, highlight relevant issues, exhibit clarity of language, write with good structure and display experience/credibility (Leslie, Young, Valentine, & Gudjonsson, 2007; Selemogwe, 2013).

Expert psychiatric testimony in practice: An African perspective

Studies on expert witness roles among mental health practitioners are scarce on the African continent. This may not be unconnected with the fledgling state of forensic mental health practice in most parts of Africa. It may also be due, in part, to the view of the courts that experts merely assist the courts in reaching "sound and just" conclusions such that they are required out of judicial discretion rather than statutory compulsion in many instances (Bienen, 1976; Milner, 1966). For example, the Justices of the Nigerian Supreme court have established a notion that: *"it is settled law that whether the accused person was sane or insane in the legal sense at the time when the act was committed is a question of fact to be determined by a jury, (Rex v Wangara 10 W.A.C.A 236; Walton v R. (1978) (66 Cr. App. R. 25) and not by a medical man however eminent (R. v. Riveth 34 Cr. App. R. 87) and is dependent upon the previous and contemporaneous act of the party, Rex. v Ashigufuwo 12 W.A.C.A 389)"* (Adesiyan, 1996). However, this is not the sole position in African settings. In Ghana, for instance, judges and magistrates are mandated by section 137 of the Criminal and other Offences (Procedure) Act, 1960 (Act 30) to request expert opinion on the mental state of a defendant when the insanity defense is invoked (Adjorlolo, Abdul-nasiru, Choon, Chan, & Bentum, 2017).

Be that as it may, several important studies across the continent have been conducted in the last three decades with a focus on the perceived role of mental health experts in the judicial process. These studies have focused on two critical areas: (i) the utility and credibility of expert witnesses and (ii) their relevance to the ultimate issue before the court. Ogunlesi and Sijuwola (1989) examined the views of Nigerian judicial officers on the usefulness of psychiatric reports provided for the courts. They found that nine out of ten of the magistrates and judges included in the sample had previously requested for psychiatric reports in their experience. Similarly, about nine out of ten respondents considered the reports to be quite useful in the process of adjudication. In particular, the study examined how frequently the respondents found some of the information in the reports useful and observed that comments on fitness to plead (100%), mental state examination as well as previous medical/psychiatric history (96%), personal history of the accused person including illness characteristics (92%) and the role of psychosocial factors in the illness (84%) were frequently found to be of utility.

A review of medical testimony (not specific to psychiatric testimony) in Nigerian courts two years later, (Ogunlesi, 1991) mainly detailed the nature of the Nigerian adversarial legal process, important sections of the evidence act relevant to expert opinions, preparations for a court appearance, challenges of "hearsay" as well as the risk of perjury while on the witness stand and a structural view of the stages involved in oral testimony. The paper concluded with the need for additional training for medical practitioners in order to improve the quality of their expert services to the courts. In a more recent quantitative study of reported criminal cases in Nigerian courts in which the insanity plea was raised, expert psychiatric witnesses were invited in only 32% of the cases and psychiatric opinion had no association with the direction of verdict by the court (Ogunwale & Oluwaranti, 2020).

In a study from South Africa examining the expectation and experience of judges, magistrates and lawyers (both defense and prosecution) with respect to whether psychologists as expert witness should address the ultimate issue, Allan and Louw (1997) observed that the respondents expected that psychologists would express their professional opinion of the ultimate issue in matters of criminal responsibility and child custody proceedings as well as sentencing. Consistently, prosecutors were less inclined than the other three groups to have this expectation. There were no significant differences between these expectations and the actual experience of the participants regarding the specific ultimate opinions except with respect to sentencing. The respondents considered that psychologists as expert witnesses were more inclined to address the ultimate issue related to sentencing than they were expected to. The authors suggested that a fair amount of uncertainty seems to exist in the legal arena as to whether experts should address the ultimate issue and that this state of uncertainty could be a reflection of judicial ambivalence or pragmatism towards the extant legal position of the ultimate issue question.

A Botswana study by Selemogwe (2013) examined criminal lawyers', judges' and magistrates' opinions about the skills and credibility of mental health professionals appearing as expert witnesses. She found that at least half of the respondents reported having used more than 20 mental health evaluation reports in their legal or judicial practice. The majority of the respondents (74.3%) suggested that the psychiatric or psychological reports were quite useful and that the mental health experts demonstrated adequate professional expertise. However, only roughly half of them indicated that the experts demonstrated adequate understanding of the legal criteria applicable to their mental health evaluations. One in three of the judges and half of the lawyers expected the expert to address the ultimate issue despite it being disallowed under Botswana law. Approximately four out of ten respondents agreed that mental health expert witnesses were credible and a little over half of all respondents noted that they were objective regardless of the fact that they could sometimes be retained by an attorney rather than being court appointed. The study equally found that the respondents described the qualities of an "excellent" mental health expert as impartiality (91.4%), ability to use simple, jargon-free language (88.6%) and capacity to provide evidence to support expert opinion/recommendation (100%). Some of these qualities had been highlighted in previous research assessing the opinion of criminal lawyers on mental health expert witnesses (Leslie et al., 2007).

The experience in Morocco suggests that expert psychiatric evaluations are conducted by general psychiatrists in the public sector and the reports are hardly detailed. The main area involving mental health expertise has to do with the determination of the mental state of an accused person at the time of an offense. Typically, the legal question also involves the determination of criminal responsibility although the court is not bound by the conclusion of the expert (El Hamaoui, Moussaoui, & Okasha, 2009). In a secondary data analysis of the archives of the Mental hospital of Berrechid in Morocco, these authors reported that 74 patients (33.8%) were referred for expert psychiatric evaluations during a seven-year period. An Algerian study examined 3984 expert psychiatric evaluations over a twenty-three-year period and found an increase in number of expert evaluations over time (Touari et al., 1993). This increase was as a result of optional psychiatric evaluations being sought for all types of crimes as well as increases in mandatory evaluations for less serious crimes in particular. Expert psychiatric evaluations were typically triggered by "patient-oriented" and "behavior-oriented" responses by the judiciary (Soothill et al., 1983). In Tunisia, a six-year analysis of expert psychiatric evaluations at the Sfax teaching hospital showed a total of 125 individuals (91.2% male) (Maalej, Zouari, Ben Mahmoud, & Zouari, 2005). The delay before evaluation was up to one month for about seven out of ten participants while roughly three out of ten of them experienced a delay of longer than one year before evaluation. This tardiness in conducting mental health expert assessments of offenders who raise the insanity plea had been reported within Africa (Bienen, 1974; Ogunwale & Oluwaranti, 2020) and beyond (Ramamurthy, Chathoth, & Thilakan, 2019); although this is not always the case, with one study documenting an interval between two and four months post-arrest (Touari et al., 1993).

Principles of writing the expert psychiatric report

Historically, oral psychiatric testimony predated the written expert report in psychiatric jurisprudence (Weiss, Wettstein, Sadoff, Silva, & Norko, 2011). Wills (2011) has suggested that writing a psychiatric report is *"an essential skill which involves accessing, examining, analysing, interpreting, prioritizing, and communicating clinical and other data that the psychiatrist will use to formulate opinions about legal questions ...."* In writing a psychiatric report, the expert must endeavor to meet the legal, ethical and professional obligations inherent in assuming the task. In doing this, it is crucial for the expert to understand the details of the case, the reasonable time limit imposed on the provision of the report and if there are ethical and/or legal conflicts that may arise with deciding to produce the report.

Preparation

Our conceptualization of preparation in this chapter relies heavily on the structure produced by Wills (2011) and essentially focuses on (i) initial contact, (ii) access to and examination of data, (iii) marshaling the evidence and (iv) communicating the opinion.

Initial contact with the case

At the first contact with the requesting attorney or a valid court order instructing the expert, it is important for the psychiatrist to understand the specific legal questions to be answered and whether they fall within the purview of standard forensic psychiatric practice within his/her jurisdiction of practice. It is equally important for the psychiatrist to determine if the case falls within the scope of his/her expertise or general practice (e.g., a general adult psychiatrist may find it more challenging to appear as an expert witness in a child custody proceeding). Furthermore, the expert witness will find it very helpful to clearly define the party that is inviting them to appear (when it is not the court). This is critical to navigating the challenge of neutrality. Carefully exploring these issues in the initial evaluation of the merit of the request will prevent future challenges in terms of adequate time for the task or difficulty with retaining objectivity as to make the position of the expert psychiatric witness untenable in the case. Given the complexity of the issues raised at this stage of the expert witness role, Wills (2011) has provided a simple acronym "**SLED-SOS**" that is aimed at helping the expert to recall the necessary things to consider in the initial contact. The acronym is fully rendered as follows: **S** – Schedule: checking schedule to see availability; **L** – Licensing requirements: to be sure that the expert has the required license/registration for the task being requested; **E** – Expertise: experience in the specific aspect of criminal/civil litigation; **D** – Duty: determining the task of the expert witness in the case; **S** – Stance: identifying the expected stance that the psychiatrist is expected to take in the case; **O** – Objectivity: identifying likely barriers to the expert witness' neutrality/objectivity/impartiality and **S** – Supplemental information: identifying any special arrangements to be made in order to achieve the expert task.

Accessing and examining relevant data

The accuracy of a forensic psychiatric report depends largely on the quality of the data and the process of analysis by the expert (Wills, 2011). When data collection is random, erratic or poorly coordinated, bias may be inadvertently introduced into the offered opinion and may also leave room for heightened scrutiny during cross-examination. Accessing data may involve both hard copies of documents as well as electronic information. The first stage of data analysis involves gathering, examining and organizing (e.g., tabulating) the relevant data. The process of data gathering and examination helps to flag missing but potentially useful information that may then be requested or sourced. A record of documents requested but not obtained should be kept so that this information may be added to the report as required (e.g., as qualifications on a particular finding or opinion). Apart from reviews of paper documents and electronic material, the expert usually will be expected to interview relevant parties in the case (e.g., retaining attorney, plaintiff, defendant, significant others in the life of the defendant or plaintiff and other witnesses). These interviews should take into consideration the peculiar needs of the interviewees and those of the expert as well. In particular, for evaluees who are in police custody or prison, the relevant local arrangements suitable for each setting must be made. These arrangements must be conscious of the schedule and internal cultural practices of each setting. It is also good practice to time each interview involved in the data gathering process as this would demonstrate that the opinion is not based on mere cursory or casual examination of facts but on adequate familiarity with the facts and/or persons upon whom the opinion is offered. During the interview, the expert must explain the peculiar nature of the interview to the evaluee stating that it is for the benefit of a third party and that it is not a typical clinical interview. The structure of the interview should be adapted to obtain specific information which is aimed at several things: (i) corroboration, (ii) clarification or (iii) contradiction of existing information. While some studies have suggested that in a criminal matter, the accused person's version of the alleged offense is not necessarily important to the courts (Ogunlesi & Sijuwola, 1989), such information might serve to satisfy any of these three aforementioned purposes of the interview.

The next stage involves identifying the specific evidence that supports the expert's position that has been framed by the initial information gathered. At the final stage, the expert considers supplementary information that was neither obtained during the paper or electronic review or during the interview. This may include existing scientific literature, laws, policies, etc.

It is relevant to note that within many African settings, these outlined processes meet with a number of practical impediments (Ogunlesi, Makanjuola, & Adelekan, 1988). Sometimes, by the time the expert is invited for an assessment, it might have been years after an alleged offense. This is largely due to the tardiness of the judicial process in many jurisdictions (Bienen, 1974; Mars, Ramlall, & Kaliski, 2012; Ogunwale & Oluwaranti, 2020; Ramamurthy et al., 2019). Furthermore, eyewitnesses may no longer be traceable in some cases, as well as some of them having difficulties with recall of events. In trials involving intra-familial homicide, the offender may be deserted by family members, thereby leading to the loss of contact with significant others who may provide helpful collateral history about the mental health of the accused person prior to the crime. Additionally, interview processes may be hampered by the persisting psychosis of the offender who may not have received any treatment due to lack of adequate mental health services in prison. Coupled with all of this may be the uncooperative attitude of correctional officers in planning and conducting the interview. Institutional factors within prisons may also occasion the lack of sufficient privacy in prison settings which may create difficulties with confidentiality. When accused persons are sufficiently ill to be transferred out of prison to non-secure psychiatric hospitals for observation/assessment and/or treatment, logistic constraints sometimes arise with respect to providing the necessary funding and 24-hour security arrangement. Such transfers are critical to reliable information gathering through the process of unobtrusive observation of the accused person by trained mental health staff over a substantial period which could be up to one month. With regard to having robust sources of information for the purpose of writing the report, the expert may need to approach the court to direct the prosecution to provide the necessary proofs of evidence especially when some agencies within the criminal justice system fail to cooperate with the expert for the purpose of producing a court report.

Marshaling the evidence

This aspect involves composing a preliminary opinion. Such an opinion must be "logical, relevant and valid" (Wills, 2011). Next, a hierarchy of supporting evidence is then constructed to establish the opinion. It is reasonable to present the strongest evidence first. The expert is then expected to examine the opinion and its grounds for possible weaknesses. These exposures are then dealt with by reevaluating the grounds for the opinion and removing those grounds that are considered weak or less logical. Additionally, concessions may be accommodated where no stronger arguments may be presented. This produces a more cogent opinion. These steps will be followed iteratively until the expert produces a logical opinion on solid ground with appropriate concessions granted where warranted.

Communicating the opinion

The expert witness in communicating the opinion should demonstrate the ability to tender firm conclusions in a clearly structured manner, exhibiting clarity of language devoid of confusing technical jargon which may be patently unhelpful to the court. In some cases, it may be necessary to discuss the findings and opinion with the attorney leading the expert in evidence. This may warrant some changes to the body of the report or the final opinion itself. The expert must exercise caution and avoid becoming a passionate advocate of any particular legal position and should only accommodate changes that are in keeping with the logic of the entire findings upon which the opinion is based.

Ethics

The ethics of forensic psychiatric practice have been robustly discussed over time (Appelbaum, 1997; Bailey, Scarano, & Varma, 2004; Niveau & Welle, 2018; Niveau, Godet, & Völlm, 2019). Against this backdrop, Bailey et al. (2004) have highlighted four crucial ethical priorities in forensic psychiatric evaluations as (i) respect for personal privacy and maintenance of confidentiality, (ii) the need to obtain informed consent from the individual before proceeding with forensic evaluation, (iii) possessing sufficient experience and qualifications, and (iv) adherence to the principles of honesty and striving for objectivity. With regard to confidentiality, the key step is to clearly notify the evaluee, collateral sources and other relevant third parties of the lack of confidentiality that applies to a report to be written for the court or the prosecution and the limits of confidentiality when the report is requested by the defense (Zonana, 2011). Informed consent is at the heart of psychiatric practice and the consent of a potential evaluee must be sought before proceeding with the forensic evaluation. Where the individual is unable to provide consent, it is sensible for the expert to follow the guidelines in place for such situations in their jurisdiction of practice (American Academy of Psychiatry and the Law, 2005). The possession of adequate education, training and experience as an expert witness improves role competence as well as impartiality (Heilbrun, Grisso, & Goldstein, 2009; Niveau et al., 2019). Ethics research seems to suggest that adherence to the principles of honesty and striving for objectivity have been viewed by forensic psychiatrists as being analogous to impartiality (Niveau et al., 2019). Impartiality serves the interest of justice as well as the ethical ideal of non-maleficence toward the evaluee since it more readily assists in securing "fairness" in the trial process (Niveau & Welle, 2018; Niveau et al., 2019). Perhaps one of the most frontal challenges to impartiality is the dual agency position in which the treating psychiatrist is called upon to serve as an expert witness. Several authorities advise against such dual roles on the basis of the risk of partiality while recognizing that exceptions may be made (Heilbrun et al., 2009). Others extend the argument into the disparities in the ethical approaches adopted by both roles (Appelbaum, 1997; Konrad & Opitz-welke, 2014; Niveau & Welle, 2018). However, in developing parts of the world like Africa with human resource shortages in forensic psychiatry, it is highly likely that such dual agency conflicts will arise and must be resolved by the individual expert on the basis of a keen awareness of the risk of bias and the determination to personally strive for honesty and objectivity by basing opinions on *all* available information (Cervantes & Hanson, 2013).

Writing a narrative

It has been argued that both the psychiatric court report and the oral testimony that flows from it are performative acts demanding both "cogent argumentation and artistry" (Griffith & Baranoski, 2007). The forensic report requires that experts organize information from a tapestry of sources and weave it into a coherent narrative (Griffith et al., 2011). While there is artistry involved in this task, the narrative of forensic reports is held to the highest standard of truth-telling and respect for the dignity of the person being reported upon. This notion of truth is significant to all parties in the legal arena and can best be served by the expert's attempt to use all available constructs (psychiatric, psychological, cultural, ethical, sociological and statistical, among others) to find the meaning to the observed phenomenon begging for truthful answers. In reporting the factual details of a person's life, striking a balance between writing a coherent story and telling the truth is to be sought carefully (Leach, 2004).

In order to achieve the foregoing, the forensic mental health expert must articulate the perspectives of all parties invested in the legal tussle by the use of what has been termed *expository narratives* (Griffith et al., 2011). This is done by capturing the voice of the person providing the information for the report. This ensures that the person is "heard" and their opinion acknowledged. It also protects the expert from being seen as "doctoring" the narrative to fit their own conclusion against all odds.

Another important factor to consider is the language of the narrative. Poor grammar and careless typographical errors diminish the effectiveness of a forensic report. Moreover, words that suggest incredulity such as "suspect," "possibly," etc. tend to weaken the premise of the report. Griffith et al. (2011) quoting

Resnick (2006) with obvious approval, highlight four principles of good writing regarding expert opinions: (i) clarity, (ii) simplicity, (iii) brevity and (iv) humanity. On the fourth principle, it is suggested that the use of direct quotations from the person "humanizes the subject of the narrative" and aids the author in their attempt to speak directly to the reader.

A most instructive element of the language of the forensic narrative is the challenge of avoiding the trap of lying which may occur in the process of artistic expression. Drawing heavily from the work of Hudgins (1996), a number of contextual lies in forensic narratives have been framed (Griffith et al., 2011):

i. The lie of narrative cogency in which the expert may leave out details to make the story simpler and avoid undue confusion by contradictory factual details. This may be in order to protect the dignity of the evaluee (e.g., leaving out embarrassing psychosexual history such as being a victim of rape that may not be relevant to the report), or to honor the request of a lawyer.
ii. The lie of texture in which there is embellishment and emphasis. This may be to fill in gaps of missing data, to enhance coherence or to humanize the subject. It may also be regarded as some form of "rhetorical exaggeration" when a position is over-stated in order to pursue coherence or consistency (Leach, 2004).
iii. The lie of emotional evasion in which the expert seeks to avoid a controversial subject such as religion, race, sexual orientation, etc. It may be in a bid to protect the personal dignity of the evaluee or to control the attention of the audience. This is what Hudgins calls the "sin of omission."

In addition to these, Hudgins also highlights the lie of interpretation which tends to "drive out other possibly valid interpretations and suppress ambivalence, ambiguity and chance" (Hudgins, 1996). While the forensic evaluation is frequently an exercise in interpretation, one way to avoid this trap is to be willing to consider alternative perspectives and be ready to make concessions as necessary. This will ensure transparency and striving for objectivity. The other safeguards that will ensure truthful narratives are comprehensive evaluation with attention to collateral sources and a focus on the formulation narrative which demonstrates reasons for rejecting alternative explanations while admitting the limits of the preferred narrative (Griffith et al., 2011).

Report structure

Buchanan and Norko (2011) have helpfully provided a simple structure for the psychiatric report which we adopt in this chapter. It is expected to cover the following areas:

- Preliminary and identifying information. This may include the name and date of birth of the evaluee, charges, court number, date of accident (if related to psychological injury). It may also include the author's credentials although there are those who prefer the author's details to be in the concluding material.

- Introduction. This includes the purpose of the report and legal questions to be addressed as well as dates and duration of interviews with the subject and others. It should also reflect the sources of information upon which the report is based and information regarding confidentiality given to the evaluee at the time of the interviews. A list of appendices should be added to the introduction.
- Body of the report. This will include background information, current events, circumstances surrounding those events and relevant follow-up events. Findings on examination as well as psychological and other laboratory results are included in the body of the report.
- Opinion section. There is no "hard and fast" rule on how to state the opinion. The conclusion may be stated first, and the reasoning presented thereafter, or the reasoning precedes the conclusion. None has been shown to be superior (Buchanan & Norko, 2011).
- Concluding material. This includes the signature of the author, name, qualifications, current post and the date of signing the report.

Incorporating psychological testing

Psychological testing is not mandatory in psychiatric court reports. However, they are frequently useful adjuncts to the psychiatric assessment (Baranoski, 2011). The psychological test to be utilized depends on the legal question that is to be answered. The use of appropriate psychological instruments administered by qualified personnel has significant advantages (Heilbrun et al., 2009). First, the tests are usually standardized such that their validity and reliability can be easily assessed, thus meeting the judicial standard for scientific evidence (Hamilton, 2011). Second, they assist in diagnostic formulation by sometimes helping to "make sense" of diverse symptoms that do not necessarily cluster under any or one diagnostic category. Third, some psychological tests can help to assess for feigning or malingering due to the available scales on those instruments. For instance, the Minnesota Multiphasic Personality Inventory-II (MMPI-II) has subscales that help to measure the validity of the responses as well as "faked" responses. In addition to these scales testing the validity of the scores, they can be used to indirectly assess malingering. That said, there are specific instruments that may be deployed for testing malingered symptoms. Fourth, in some cases whereby there is no clear-cut mental disorder but clear evidence of dysfunctional behavior, psychological tests such as structured personality assessments may help identify behavioral traits which could serve an explanatory function for the observed conduct.

More frequently, in African settings, psychiatrists rather than psychologists serve as expert witnesses although research suggests that judicial officers may not indicate any preference in some jurisdictions (Selemogwe, 2013). Where the psychological assessment is based upon a referral by the psychiatrist, Baranoski (2011) suggests that there are three common ways of incorporating the psychological assessment in the psychiatric report. First, the entire psychological report may be included. While it has the advantage of making the psychological report a helpful sub-section of the entire psychiatric report and allows for ownership by the psychiatrist, it has the disadvantage of holding the psychiatrist to account in defending the thinking and methods of another professional. On the stand, she/he may be asked minute details specific to the methods of the testing for which she/he may have no informed answer. Perhaps, a way to deal with this is for both the psychologist and psychiatrist to jointly sign the report and explain different aspects based on their expertise (Baranoski, 2011). However, this will require both appearing as experts.

Second, the psychiatrist may only include a jargon-free summary of the test report prepared by the psychologist. The advantage of this method is that it provides information that is relevant to the legal question and presents its main highlights clearly. It also cuts out technical aspects of the testing that the psychiatrist is not optimally competent to address. However, it suffers from the disadvantage that the psychiatrist may still be required to account for the wording adopted by someone else.

The third approach is for the psychiatrist to prepare a summary from the original rest report independently. In this way, the psychiatrist chooses information based on relevance and is able to couch the summary in his/her own words. The disadvantage of this method is that the psychiatrist's summary could be challenged as being selective as to what was included and what was left out. It may be reasonable to have a copy of the entire psychologist's report in this case in the possession of the psychiatrist at the time of offering testimony should it be required for clarification.

Whichever method is preferred by the expert witness, it has been suggested that the crucial points to note are these: history and clinical findings should correlate to psychological testing results, no single psychological test should form the sole basis for an expert's conclusion, standardized tests should be utilized and appropriate communication between the referring psychiatrist and psychologist should be ensured as this is crucial to the integration of the psychological test report into the expert opinion in a relevant and objective manner (Baranoski, 2011).

Legal tests for the validity of scientific evidence: Lessons from Frye and Daubert

While forensic mental health experts in Africa must be clearly guided by the evidentiary rules that govern the admissibility of their expert opinion in their jurisdiction of practice, there are important lessons to learn from two landmark judicial decisions in the United States that have been very crucial in defining the standards for the admissibility of scientific evidence in the courtroom (Heilbrun et al., 2009). In Frye v United States, 1923, the court held that admissible expert testimony of a scientific nature "must be sufficiently established to have gained general acceptance" in relation to the specific field to which it belongs. This became known as the "general acceptance standard" (Cheng & Yoon, 2005). About 70 years later, in *Daubert v. Merrell Dow Pharmaceuticals, Inc., 509 US 579—Supreme Court 1993*, the Frye general acceptance test was considered too restrictive and replaced by a slightly broader standard which required expert testimony to demonstrate the following: (i) empirical testability, (ii) evidence of being subjected to peer review, (iii) known or potential error rate and whether it is acceptable and (iv) general acceptability in the scientific community (Fradella, Fogarty, & O'Neill, 2003). Beyond the relevance and reliability of the expert opinion, it should be noted that the expectation of Daubert is that the methodology underlying the expert opinion must be based on scientifically valid techniques.

These standards are of significant implication for the forensic mental health arena in view of application of psychiatric/psychological instruments for such assessments as violence risk (Cunningham & Reidy, 2002) and dangerousness in sex offending (Hamilton, 2011), among others. It is the ethical duty of the expert witness under such circumstances to give careful attention to the validity and reliability of their methods (Hamilton, 2011). A consideration of the factors raised by Frye and extended in Daubert aids the expert witness in their pursuit of honesty and quest for objectivity that are fundamental ethical issues governing the expert witness role.

Oral testimony

Oral testimony in criminal and civil cases are typically adversarial with expert witnesses finding themselves in the "cross-fire" between two opposing interests while being expected to demonstrate neutrality in order to further the cause of justice. Ogunlesi (2005) has identified eight critical lessons to be remembered by the expert witness in achieving some level of comfort in dealing with the inherent pitfalls of oral testimony. First, the expert witness must carefully consider the reason or motive for the court appearance. Second, it is crucial to ensure that your review of the party upon whom the testimony is required is as recent as possible. Third, the expert must carefully review the copy of the report submitted to the court ahead of the appearance and cross-check this with the details contained in the relevant clinical notes or other documentary material. Fourth, it is quite helpful to hold a rehearsal of the oral testimony with the attorney who will be leading the expert in evidence. This is expected to highlight aspects of the testimony that may elicit rigorous interrogation by the opposing counsel. Fifth, the expert will have to deal with the reality of malingered symptoms that are intended to mislead him/her to arrive at an opinion that is at variance with actual facts. Sixth, it must be realized that the process of cross-examination is not one that suffers much professional courtesy. Seventh, the expert witness must not be intimidated or upset by cross-examination or perceive it as an affront to personal or professional dignity. It is the opinion of the expert that is under attack and not their person. Eighth, it is frankly realistic for the expert witness to accept that she/he would not have an answer to every possible question and to admit ignorance in such cases is truly a mark of sincerity.

Stages of expert testimony

Allowing for jurisdictional variations, the stages of oral testimony are usually divided into three (Evidence Act, 2011, section 215; du Plessis, 2012):

i. Direct examination. This is otherwise called "examination-in-chief" under Nigeria's law of evidence as well as under civil procedure rules in South African courts and it is described as "the examination of the witness by the party who calls him" (Evidence Act, 2011, section 214(1)).
ii. Cross-examination. This is the examination of the witness by any party other than the party who calls him (Evidence Act, 2011, section 214(2)).
iii. Re-examination. This is the examination of a witness by the party who called him after he/she had been cross-examined (Evidence Act, 2011, section 214(3)).

Both the examination-in-chief and the cross-examination must relate to relevant facts but the cross-examination may not be confined only to facts raised during the examination-in-chief. According to the Nigerian Evidence Act (2011), section 223, the purpose of cross-examination is to:

a. Test the witness' accuracy, veracity, or credibility.
b. Discover who the witness is and his position in life.
c. Shake his credibility by injuring his character.

Hearsay rules

Legally, hearsay refers to out of court statement(s) which may be offered to prove the truth of a claim asserted. In some cases, the evidence provided by a medical or psychological expert during a trial may invariably include things which the parties to the case or others have told the psychiatrist or psychologist (e.g., details of previous care received from a traditional or spiritual healer). This would ordinarily amount to hearsay if presented to the court by the expert. However, since it forms part of the information upon which the expert formed their opinion, it would be admissible. In one unreported case in which the second author appeared, the court was minded to agree that information obtained from other people about an accused person's abnormal behavior while in prison formed part of "collateral information" rather than hearsay. Also, judges in Nigeria have observed in the past that expert comments on previous care received from traditional or spiritual healers could have some utility value beyond hearsay (Bienen, 1976; Ogunlesi & Sijuwola, 1989). Nevertheless, this treatment of the hearsay rule may be conceptually problematic since the court must accept information that is essentially hearsay as relevant to the expert opinion but ignore it as evidence or proof of any other matter in the trial (i.e., it remains hearsay in any other respect).

Addressing the ultimate issue

The ultimate issue refers to the final decision before a court of competent jurisdiction (Eastman et al., 2012) and is termed "fact in issue" in Nigerian law (Evidence Act, 2011). There are jurisdictional variations with regard to whether the expert witness should address the ultimate issue or not (Buchanan & Norko, 2011; Selemogwe, 2013). For example in South Africa, the expert witness is typically expected to address the ultimate legal question (Allan & Louw, 1997) while in Botswana, the expert is precluded from doing so (Selemogwe, 2013). In Ghana, the position of the law as set out in *Kwadwo Mensah vs. The Republic (1959)* is that it is not in the place of the expert witness to address the ultimate issue in insanity cases (Adjorlolo et al., 2017). In Nigeria, the position is more flexible as the expert is at liberty to choose whether or not to address the ultimate issue (Evidence Act, 2011) with the proviso that the expert's opinion is non-determinative since it is one upon which the trier of facts must yet form an independent opinion (Ogunwale & Oluwaranti, 2020). This position of judicial independence in the presence of expert opinion on the ultimate issue is equally observable in South African jurisprudence (Allan & Louw, 1997) as well as in Morocco (El Hamaoui et al., 2009). A more interesting perspective emerges from Algeria in which the expert opinion is basically regarded as "consultative" but the weight attached to it by the courts as "decisive" (Touari et al., 1993). The Algerian position has been interpreted as one permitting the expert witness to address the ultimate issue of criminal responsibility. Despite the variations in the prevailing legal provisions, research has shown that a good number of lawyers and judges in jurisdictions where the expert is barred from addressing the ultimate issue would still prefer the expert to address it, thereby introducing uncertainties into judicial expectations of the expert witness (Selemogwe, 2013). This could potentially lead to ambiguity on the part of experts in stating their opinions in writing or during oral testimony.

In any case, Eastman et al. (2012) have provided a number of guidelines which will help the expert witness to avoid inadvertently addressing the ultimate issue in jurisdictions that preclude such conduct. These guidelines include (i) obtaining detailed judicial instructions and clarification (from court or the relevant lawyer) where legal rather than psychiatric questions are raised, (ii) ensuring that every statement made as an opinion is based firmly on evidence earlier highlighted in the report/oral testimony, (iii) avoiding undue assumptions and value judgments, (iv) using medical or psychological terms rather than legal terminology especially when addressing specific legal tests/criteria, (v) distinguishing between your psychiatric opinion and the legal implications of that opinion in the relevant section of your report and (vi) ensuring that the report is expressed in a way that can help the court to translate your psychiatric diagnosis or formulation into the relevant legal tests rather than expressing your opinion on whether the tests are met or not. It suffices to say that, in addition to these useful tips, it is sensible for the expert to be *au fait* with the relevant laws under which she/he is offering the oral testimony.

Critical challenges to expert testimony

Given the obvious complexities of expert psychiatric testimony, some key challenges have been highlighted (Selemogwe, 2013):

- Accepting roles that are not within expert's scope of practice. This may invariably question the validity and reliability of the expert's opinion. As a matter of credibility and legitimacy, it is good practice to stay within one's expertise (Heilbrun et al., 2009).
- Accepting dual roles (e.g., acting as both treating clinician and expert witness). The challenge of dual agency with its implication on independence (Royal Australian and New Zealand College of Psychiatrists, 2015) as well as objectivity has been examined under the section on ethics.
- Emotional involvement in the legal outcome: This is a common pitfall in psychiatric/psychological testimony (Wills, 2011). It must always be remembered that it is not the expert who is on trial but the parties to the case. Thus, the entertainment of bias is unethical (Heilbrun et al., 2009). Undue emotional involvement in the outcome for whatever reason may lead to contextual lying in the expert's construction of the narrative (Griffith et al., 2011) in order to achieve a preconceived outcome.
- Moral values of the expert: Research has shown that one of the key opponents of impartiality is personal beliefs such as moral convictions (Niveau et al., 2019). Experts must be aware of this influence on their value judgments and must strive to maintain objectivity under the weight of such convictions.
- Presence or absence of guidelines and/or code of ethics to guide practice: Guidelines relevant to different aspects of expert witness roles are helpful in standardizing practice. In this regard, some professional bodies such as the World Psychiatric Association, Royal Australian and New Zealand College of Psychiatrists and the American Academy of Psychiatry and the Law have issued ethical guidance for the practice of forensic psychiatry generally (American Academy of Psychiatry and the Law, 2005) and expert witness roles specifically (Janofsky et al., 2014; Mossman et al., 2007; Royal Australian and New Zealand College of Psychiatrists, 2015). Yet, these should be developed to provide flexibility and a range of possible approaches to the given task (Buchanan & Norko, 2011). They should not be regarded as "one size-fits-all" documents (Janofsky et al., 2014; Mossman et al., 2007) as they may not necessarily represent customary practice in many instances (Howard Zonana, 2008).

Such codes of ethics guiding expert witnesses in psychiatry or psychology are scarcely available in African jurisdictions. However, general direction on the conduct of the medical expert may be found in some national codes of medical ethics. For example, the Medical and Dental Council of Nigeria Code of Medical Ethics provides specific guidelines against contingency fees for expert testimony while allowing for reasonable payments for such services on a non-contingent basis but it offers no other guidance (Medical and Dental Council of Nigeria, 2008). The current state of practice in the arena of expert testimony in African countries highlights the urgent need for such ethical guidelines.

Conclusion

Expert witness roles in the frame of oral testimony and psychiatric court reports remain integral to the practice of clinical and legal forensic psychiatry in African countries. The focus of expert psychiatric testimony on mental health issues in offending offers much for defendants (and indeed the larger society) by way of therapeutic jurisprudence. The participation of the expert also stretches into civil matters such as opinions on psychiatric injuries in personal injury litigation, child custody issues, as well as mental capacity assessments in relation to different types of legal decisions, among others. While the expert brings significant skill and experience to the assistance of the court, there exist subtle jurisdictional variations in the way the courts perceive the weight of the expert opinion in the context of the ultimate issue. Apart from such legal considerations, the ethical challenges of the expert witness position such as a pragmatic approach to confidentiality, the need to obtain informed consent from potential evaluees, adherence to the principles of honesty and striving for objectivity and possessing sufficient experience and qualifications are no less obvious to the African forensic mental health specialist despite the peculiar challenges of resource constraints, manpower shortages leading to the dual agency of expert witness/treating physician and lack of structured forensic mental health training in most parts of the continent. In spite of these, a practical approach to the examination of the principles of writing psychiatric reports shows a careful focus on the steps to be taken in presenting the written narrative as a logical opinion founded on solid ground with appropriate concessions granted where warranted. Moreover, a critical review of the different stages of oral testimony using exemplars from African jurisdictions throws up several important lessons for the potential mental health expert in the witness box. Finally, a number of crucial challenges in the course of the expert witness role suggest the need for individual familiarity with local evidentiary rules as well as practice/ethical guidelines for expert testimony and report writing which will help in no small way to standardize practice at least within each jurisdiction.

References

Adesiyan, D. (1996). *An accused person's rights in Nigerian criminal law*. Heinemann Educational Books (Nigeria).

Adjorlolo, S., Abdul-nasiru, I., Choon, H., Chan, O., & Bentum, F. (2017). Attitudes toward the insanity defense: Examination of the factor structure of Insanity Defense Attitude-Revised (IDA-R) scale in Ghana. *International Journal of Forensic Mental Health, 16*(1), 33–45. https://doi.org/10.1080/14999013.2016.1235628

Allan, A., & Louw, D. (1997). The ultimate opinion rule and psychologists: A comparison of the expectations and experiences of South African lawyers. *Behavioural Sciences & The Law*, *15*, 307–320.

Allnutt, S., Samuels, A., & Driscoll, C. (2007). The insanity defence: From wild beasts to M'Naghten. *Australasian Psychiatry*, *15*(4), 292–298. https://doi.org/10.1080/10398560701352181

American Academy of Psychiatry and the Law. (2005). *Ethics guidelines for the practice of forensic psychiatry*. Adopted May, 2005.

Appelbaum, P. S. (1997). A theory of ethics for forensic psychiatry. *Journal of the American Academy of Psychiatry and the Law*, *25*(3), 233–247.

Bailey, R., Scarano, V., & Varma, S. (2004). The practice of forensic psychiatry: Is it the practice of medicine?. *American Journal of Psychiatry*, *25*, 1–9.

Baranoski, M. (2011). Incorporating psychological testing. In A. Buchanan & M. Norko (Eds.), *The psychiatric report: Principles and practice of forensic writing*. Cambridge University Press.

Bienen, L. (1974). Criminal homicide in Western Nigeria 1966–1972. *Journal of African Law*, *18*(1), 57–78.

Bienen, L. (1976). The determination of criminal insanity in western Nigeria. *The Journal of Modern African Studies*, *14*(2), 219–245.

Buchanan, A., & Norko, M. (2011). *The psychiatric report: Principles and practice of forensic writing* (1st ed.). Cambridge University Press.

Cervantes, A. N., & Hanson, A. (2013). Dual Agency and ethics conflicts in correctional practice: Sources and solutions. *The Journal of the American Academy of Psychiatry and the Law*, *41*(1), 7.

Cheng, E., & Yoon, A. (2005). Does Frye or Daubert matter? A study of scientific admissibility standards. *Va. L. Rev.*, *91*, 471.

Cunningham, M., & Reidy, T. (2002). Violence risk assessment at federal capital sentencing: Individualization, generalization, relevance, and scientific standards. *Criminal Justice and Behavior*, 29(5), 512–537. https://doi.org/10.1177/009385402236731

Daubert v. Merrell Dow Pharmaceuticals, Inc., 509 US 579—Supreme Court 1993, (1993).

du Plessis, H. L. M. (2012). The divergent approaches of English and South African courts, when considering actuarial expert testimony in the matter of an award for damages for future loss of earnings after a damage-causing event. *Annals of Actuarial Science*, *6*(1), 5–22. https://doi.org/10.1017/S1748499511000285

Eastman, N., Adshead, G., Fox, S., Latham, R., & Whyte, S. (2012). *Oxford specialist handbooks in psychiatry: Forensic psychiatry* (1st ed.). Oxford University Press Inc.

Eigen, J. P. (1983). Historical developments in psychiatric forensic evidence: The British experience. *International Journal of Law and Psychiatry*, *6*, 423–429.

El Hamaoui, Y., Moussaoui, D., & Okasha, T. (2009). Forensic psychiatry in North Africa. *Current Opinion in Psychiatry*, *22*, 507–510.

Evidence Act (2011).

Fradella, H., Fogarty, A., & O'Neill, L. (2003). The impact of Daubert on the admissibility of behavioural science testimony. *Pepperdine Law Review*, *30*(3), 403–444.

Frye v. United States. (1923). *Frye v. United States, 293 F. 1013—Court of Appeals, Dist. Of Columbia 1923.*

Griffith, E. E. H., & Baranoski, M. V. (2007). Commentary: The place of performative writing in forensic psychiatry. *The Journal of the American Academy of Psychiatry and the Law*, *35*(1), 5.

Griffith, E., Stankovic, A., & Baranoski, M. (2011). Writing a narrative. In A. Buchanan & M. Norko (Eds.), *The psychiatric report: Principles and practice of forensic writing* (pp. 68–80). Cambridge University Press.

Gutheil, T. (2005). The history of forensic psychiatry. *The Journal of the American Academy of Psychiatry and the Law, 33*(2), 259–262.

Hamilton, M. (2011). Public safety, individual liberty and suspect science: Future dangerousness assessments and sex offender laws. *Temp. L. Rev*, 83(c), 697.

Heilbrun, K., Grisso, T., & Goldstein, A. (2009). *Foundations of forensic mental health assessment*. Oxford University Press Inc.

Hudgins, A. (1996). An autobiographer's lies. *The American Scholar, 65*(4), 541–553.

Janofsky, J. S., Hanson, A., Candilis, P. J., Myers, W. C., & Zonana, H. (2014). AAPL practice guideline for forensic psychiatric evaluation of defendants raising the insanity defence. *Journal of the American Academy of Psychiatry and the Law, 42*(4), s3–s76.

Kharoshah, M. A. A., Zaki, M. K., Galeb, S. S., Moulana, A. A. R., & Elsebaay, E. A. (2011). Origin and development of forensic medicine in Egypt. *Journal of Forensic and Legal Medicine, 18*(1), 10–13. https://doi.org/10.1016/j.jflm.2010.11.009

Konrad, N., & Opitz-welke, A. (2014). The challenges of treating the mentally ill in a prison setting: the European perspective. *Clinical Practice, 11*(5), 517–523.

Leach, L. (2004). Lying, writing, and confrontation: Mary McCarthy and Lillian Hellman. *Literature Interpretation Theory, 15*(1), 5–28. https://doi.org/10.1080/10436920490278465

Leslie, O., Young, S., Valentine, T., & Gudjonsson, G. (2007). Criminal barristers' opinions and perceptions of mental health expert witnesses. *The Journal of Forensic Psychiatry & Psychology, 18*(3), 394–410. https://doi.org/10.1080/14789940701256229

Maalej, M., Zouari, L., Ben Mahmoud, S., & Zouari, N. (2005). Forensic psychiatric expertise: About 125 cases. *J Me'd Le' Gale Droit Me'd, 48*, 47–56.

Mars, M., Ramlall, S., & Kaliski, S. (2012). Forensic telepsychiatry: A possible solution for South Africa? *African Journal of Psychiatry, 15*(4), 244–247. https://doi.org/10.4314/ajpsy.v15i4.31

Medical and Dental Council of Nigeria. (2008). *The code of medical ethics in Nigeria*. Medical and Dental Council of Nigeria.

Milner, A. (1966). M'Naghten and the witch-doctor: Psychiatry and crime in Africa. *University of Pennsylvania Law Review, 114*(8), 1134–1169.

M'Naghten's case. (1843). *UKHL J16.*

Mossman, D., Noffsinger, S. G., Ash, P., Frierson, R. L., Gerbasi, J., Hackett, M., Lewis, C. F., Pinals, D. A., Scott, C. L., Sieg, K. G., Wall, B. W., & Zonana, H. V. (2007). AAPL practice guideline for the forensic psychiatric evaluation of competence to stand trial. *Journal of the American Academy of Psychiatry and the Law, 35*(4), s3–s72.

Mullen, P. (1993). Care and containment in forensic psychiatry. *Criminal Behaviour & Mental Health, 3*(4), 212–227.

Niveau, G., Godet, T., & Völlm, B. (2019). What does impartiality mean in medico-legal psychiatry? An international survey. *International Journal of Law and Psychiatry, 66*, 101505. https://doi.org/10.1016/j.ijlp.2019.101505

Niveau, G., & Welle, I. (2018). Forensic psychiatry, one subspecialty with two ethics? A systematic review. *BMC Medical Ethics, 19*, 25.

Ogunlesi, A. (1991). Medical testimony in Nigerian courts. *Nigerian Medical Journal, 21*(3 & 4), 119–122.

Ogunlesi, A. (2005). Court appearance, cross examination and cross-intimidation?: A personal experience and lessons learnt. *Annual General Meeting and Scientific Conference of the Association of Psychiatrists in Nigeria*, 2–13.

Ogunlesi, A., & Sijuwola, O. (1989). Psychiatric reports for Nigerian courts: An analysis of the views of the bench. *West African Journal of Medicine*, *8*(2), 122–129.

Ogunlesi, A. O., Makanjuola, J. D. A., & Adelekan, M. L. (1988). Offenders admitted to the Neuro-Psychiatric Hospital Aro, Abeokuta: A 10-year review Ogunlesi, A. O., Makanjuola, J. D. A. and Adelekan, M. L. (1988). Offenders Admitted to the Neuro-Psychiatric Hospital Aro, Abeokuta: A 10-Year Review. *West African Journal of Medicine*, *7*, 129–135.

Ogunwale, A., & Oluwaranti, O. (2020). Pattern of utilization of the insanity plea in Nigeria: An empirical analysis of reported cases. *Forensic Science International: Mind and Law*, *1*, 100010. https://doi.org/10.1016/j.fsiml.2020.100010

Prosono, M. (2003). History of forensic psychiatry. In R. Rosner (Ed.), *Principles and practice of forensic psychiatry* (2nd ed., pp. 14–30). Boca Raton, FL: Taylor & Francis.

Ramamurthy, P., Chathoth, V., & Thilakan, P. (2019). How does India decide insanity pleas? A review of High Court judgments in the past decade. *Indian Journal of Psychological Medicine*, *41*(2), 150–154. doi: 10.4103/IJPSYM.IJPSYM_373_18

Rix, K., Eastman, N., & Adshead, G. (2015). Responsibilities of psychiatrists who provide expert opinion to courts and tribunals, College Report CR 193. The Royal College of Psychiatrists.

Royal Australian and New Zealand College of Psychiatrists. (2015). Developing reports and conducting independent medical examinations in medico-legal settings. Retrieved from https://www.ranzcp.org/Files/Resources/College_Statements/Practice_Guidelines/PPG-11-FFP-Developing-reports-and-conducting-indep.aspx. (Issue February, pp. 1–5).

Selemogwe, M. (2013). The skills and credibility of Botswana mental health expert witnesses: Opinions from the Botswana legal bench. *American International Journal of Contemporary Research*, *3*(6), 59–64.

Soothill, K. L., Adserballe, H., Bernheim, J., Dasananjali, T., Harding, T. W., Thomaz, T., Reinhold, F., & Ghali, H. (1983). Psychiatric reports requested by the courts in six countries. *Medicine, Science and the Law*, *23*(4), 231–241. https://doi.org/10.1177/002580248302300402

Spruitt, J. (1998). The penal conceptions of the Emperor Marcus Aure- lius in respect of lunatics: Reflections on D. 1,18,14. *International Journal of Law and Psychiatry*, *21*, 315–334.

Touari, M., Mesbah, M., Dellatolas, G., & Bensmail, B. (1993). Association between criminality and psychosis: A retrospective study of 3984 expert psychiatric evaluations. *Revue d Epidemiologie et de Sante Publique*, *41*, 218.

Weiss, K., Wettstein, R., Sadoff, R., Silva, J., & Norko, M. (2011). History and function of the psychiatric report. In A. Buchanan, & M. Norko (Eds.), *The psychiatric report: Principles and practice of forensic writing* (1st ed., pp. 11–21). Cambridge University Press.

Wills, C. (2011). Preparation. In A. Buchanan & M. Norko (Eds.), *The psychiatric report: Principles and practice of forensic writing* (pp. 22–34). Cambridge University Press.

Wren, G. (2010). Mental health courts: Serving justice and promoting recovery. *Annals of Health Law*, *19*(3), 577–594.

Zonana, H. (2011). Confidentiality and record keeping. In A. Buchanan & M. Norko (Eds.), *The psychiatric report: Principles and practice of forensic writing* (pp. 35–55). Cambridge University Press.

Zonana, H. (2008). Commentary: When is a practice guideline only a guideline? *The Journal of the American Academy of Psychiatry and the Law*, *36*, 302–305.

11 Mental health legislation and forensic practice in Africa

Adegboyega Ogunwale, Katrina I. Serpa, Michael Elnemais Fawzy, and Jibril Abdulmalik

Introduction

The link between mental health legislation and forensic practice is quite remarkable. Eastman, Adshead, Fox, Latham, and Whyte (2012) have suggested that forensic psychiatry as a discipline comprises two sub-disciplines – "clinical forensic psychiatry" and "legal psychiatry." While the former refers to the assessment and treatment of mental disorders that have been associated with offending behavior, the latter essentially focuses on mental health legislation and other relevant laws (criminal or civil) related to mental disorders (American Academy of Psychiatry and the Law, 2005; Buchanan, 2012; Eastman et al., 2012). Mental health legislation is aimed at addressing the promotion of mental health and prevention of mental disorders as well as ensuring access to basic mental health care. It equally focuses on mental health assessments in accordance with internationally accepted principles in addition to provision of the least restrictive type of mental health care, self-determination and the right to be assisted in the exercise of self-determination with due respect for the rule of law (World Health Organization, 1996).

Although mental health legislation has been a component of mental health systems in some countries for close to two centuries, a human rights-based approach seems to have gained prominence in the last six decades (Kelly, 2011). This has largely been on account of the development of several human rights–related documents. These include the Universal Declaration of Human Rights (United Nations, 1948), principles for the protection of persons with mental illness (United Nations, 1991) and closer to home, the African Charter on Human and People's Rights (Organisation of African Unity, 1986). This chapter focuses on the current state of mental health legislation across Africa comparing exemplars from different sub-regions. It also critically examines human rights and ethical issues in mental health legislation as well as matters related to the treatment of mentally ill offenders under mental health law and relevant criminal legislations.

The state of mental health legislation across Africa: Texts and sub-texts

Despite the obvious importance of mental health laws as highlighted, many countries all over the world lack satisfactory mental health legislation in terms of currency and content. At least 37% of WHO member countries have no stand-alone mental health legislation and only 40% have updated their laws since 2013 (World Health Organization, 2018). Similarly, only 44% of countries in the African region have mental health legislation compared with 77% in Europe (World Health Organization, 2018). Previously, it had been reported that only about 30% of mental health laws in Africa were enacted after 1990 with some dating back to the colonial era of the early 1900s (Morakinyo, 1977; Ogunlesi et al., 2012). In particular, Nigeria, the most populous African country, has a "lunacy" law that is over a century old and recent attempts at reform have been met with limited success with 1 out of its 36 states enacting a brand-new mental health law in January 2019.

A desk review of mental health legislations across the African continent was conducted between March and April 2020 specifically for the purpose of producing this book chapter. Data was obtained from the WHO World Mental Health Atlas, country profiles for 47 countries (World Health Organization, 2020) and this was supplemented with additional information available to the authors about mental health laws of each country which was not covered by the WHO document. As shown in Table 11.1, the findings revealed that 53.3% (24/45; data for two countries were not included in the Mental Health Atlas) of countries in the continent have some form of mental health legislation. The era of mental health legislations spanned from 1838 in Madagascar (East Africa) to 2019 in Zambia (Southern Africa) with 58.3% of the countries having 19th- or 20th-century legislations. Only 41.7% of the countries had enacted relevant legislation in the 21st century.

Using a grading of 0–5 to determine the level of compliance of each country's legislation with human rights provisions (data reported for 20 countries; 42.6% of the total), the WHO profiles indicated that 5% (n = 1) reported "0" human rights compliance, while 10% (n = 2), 35% (n = 7) and 50% (n = 10), respectively reported scores of 3, 4, and 5. In terms of independent oversight of human rights compliance (data reported for 22 countries; 46.8%), 59.1% (n = 13) of the countries had an independent body to oversee human rights protection under the mental health legislation.

Furthermore, in line with current realities regarding contemporary mental health legislation, in 2005, the WHO published guidelines for drafting of mental health laws applicable to all member countries. It also provided a checklist for ascertaining the coverage of crucial issues in mental health legislation with a decidedly human rights orientation. A summary of the extent of compliance of selected existing mental health laws in Africa with the WHO "Checklist on Mental Health Legislation" (World Health Organization, 2005) is provided in Table 11.2. Notwithstanding the relative depth of such an approach, it is not without its own limitations. First, the WHO checklist is only a guide and not an inviolable international convention regulating legislation. Second, its focus is on existence of law and not on implementation; research suggests that there is remarkable difference in the two realities (Doku, Wusu-Takyi, & Awakame, 2012).

Table 11.1 Mental health legislation profile across African countries*

Country	*Sub-continent*	*Year of legislation*
Algeria	North	1985
Angola	South	–
Botswana	South	1971
Burkina Faso	West	–
Burundi	East	–
Cameroon	Equatorial	–
Central Africa	Equatorial	–
Chad	West	–
Congo	Equatorial	–
Cote d'Ivoire	West	–
Egypt	North	2009
Equatorial Guinea	Equatorial	2010
Ethiopia	East	–
Gabon	Equatorial	2016
Gambia	West	1964
Guinea Bissau	West	–
Ghana	West	2012
Guinea	West	–
Kenya	East	1989
Lesotho	South	–
Liberia	West	2017
Libya	North	–
Madagascar	East	1838
Malawi	South	–
Mali	West	–
Mauritania	West	–
Mauritius	East	1998
Morocco	North	1959
Mozambique	South	–
Namibia	South	1973
Niger	West	–
Nigeria	West	1916
Rwanda	East	–
Sao Tome and Principe	Central Africa	–
Senegal	West	1975
Sierra Leone	West	2015
Somalia	East	–
South Sudan	East	–
South Africa	South	2002
Sudan	North	2016
Swaziland	South	1978
Tanzania	East	2008
Togo	West	–
Tunisia	North	2005
Uganda	East	1964
Zambia	South	2019
Zimbabwe	South	1996

Note

* Other countries in the African Union not included in the sample: Benin, Cabo Verde, Comoros, the Democratic Republic of Congo, Djibouti, Eritrea, Saharawi Arab Democratic Republic, Seychelles.

This has been observed as the distinction between the *content* and *demonstrated effect* of legislation by Kelly (2011).

That said, in spite of cultural and economic differences, many countries in Africa share a common legal heritage in being commonwealth jurisdictions and countries that are in the same sub-continental region may demonstrate some degree of mimetic tendencies in drafting legal provisions that mirror those of the other countries within their bloc. Thus, substantial similarities are bound to be observed in their legislative tendencies and challenges.

Human rights and ethical issues in mental health legislation

Human rights

All fundamental human rights as recognized in other laws are provided for in the more contemporary legislations such as the South African Mental Health Care Act (2002) (SAMHCA) the Ghanaian Mental Health Act (2012) (GMHA), the Nigerian Lagos State Mental Health Law (2018) (LSMHL), the Tunisian Mental Health Act (TUMHA), the Egyptian Mental Health Act (2009) (EMHA) and the Zambian Mental Health Act (2019) (ZAMHA). These rights include, among others, right to human dignity, privacy, consent, protection from unfair discrimination as well as protection from exploitation and abuse. Freedom from torture, cruelty, forced labor and other forms of inhuman treatment is also guaranteed. Additionally, rights of families or other carers (e.g., right to information (with the consent of the patient)) are guaranteed under some of these legislations. This rights-based approach is in keeping with recommendations for contemporary legislation (World Health Organization, 2005) as well as international standards on human rights of persons with disability generally (United Nations, 2006) or mental illness in particular (United Nations, 1991). Indeed, an above-average performance of the South African Mental Health Care Act (2002) in meeting key "autonomy-based" mental health care issues had been documented (Fistein, Holland, Clare, & Gunn, 2009). This is not altogether surprising because the MHCA was promulgated ten years into post-apartheid South Africa in which conversations around human rights violations were quite prominent.

Nevertheless, some countries with older legislation would be seen to adopt a "paternalistic" posture towards patients rather than an "autonomy-based" approach. This would certainly be understood from the standpoint of the socio-political contexts in which those laws were crafted over a century ago (see, for example, Nigerian lunacy ordinance of 1916); this was observed to be a feature of earlier legislation in South Africa (Ramlall, 2012). In Egypt for example, the real change in terms of the environment of mental hospitals followed the policy of allowing visitors, the press and international professional organizations, which all offered to support the work. However, in a culture that is essentially patriarchal, in a society that lived under a dictatorship, it is not surprising that a body of resistance built up among clinicians, who felt that the new Act, by empowering

Table 11.2 Comparative mental health legislation in selected African jurisdictions

Item	*Legislative Issue*	*West Africa*	*Southern Africa*	*East Africa*	*North Africa*
A	Preamble and objectives: This should focus on protection of the human rights of people with mental disorders, improved access to mental health services and an emphasis on a community-based approach (in the context of a "least restrictive" approach to treatment.	In the Ghanaian Mental Health Act (2012) (GMHA), these elements are subsumed broadly in the objectives and functions of the Mental Health Authority; clear emphasis on rights is noted; least restrictive approach adopted under involuntary admission in the GMHA s. 42. Covered by s. 6 of the Lagos State Mental Health Law (2018) (LSMHL) under the functions of the state's mental health service governing board.	The South African Mental Health Care Act (2002) (SAMHCA) focuses on the protection of mentally ill persons in the preamble as noted in objectives in the title of the act. Human rights are covered in the relevant section. Objectives of the act are clearly stated with some emphasis on the facilitation of community-based treatment. The Zimbabwean Mental Health Act (2000) (ZIMHA) does not clearly outline any objectives.	Uganda's Mental Health Act (1964) (UMHA) has no focus on human rights. The Tanzanian Mental Health Act (2008) (TANMHA) does not focus specifically on rights but addresses the need for access to mental health services by the provisions for the establishment of mental health facilities. The National Council on Mental Health set up under s. 30–31 of the Act also addresses "mental health promotion" with community participation.	Tunisian Mental health legislation (TUMHA) was enacted in 1992 and reviewed in 2004, which focuses on the conditions of hospitalization of individuals with mental disorders (from the most to the least restrictive care). Developing the Egyptian 2009 Mental Health Act (EMHA) and its code of practice promote public awareness of the rights of patients. Although this law has many positive aspects, it still has gaps that prevent it from completely fulfilling the Egyptian government's legal obligations with respect to mental health care.

(*Continued*)

Table 11.2 (Continued)

Item	*Legislative Issue*	*West Africa*	*Southern Africa*	*East Africa*	*North Africa*
B	Definitions: should focus on clear definition of mental disorder, mental incapacity and other key terms in the bill. This is to ensure consistency in the use of such terms throughout the document. This will also prevent ambiguity in the interpretations of the "interpretable terms" in the document.	Within the GMHA (under s. 97 "interpretation"), while definitions are provided for "incapacity," "mental retardation" and "personality disorder," no definition is supplied for mental disorder. The Nigerian Lunacy Law (1916) (NLL) given its very archaic state, does not provide a definition for any form of mental disorder. The Lagos State Mental Health Law (LSMHL) provides definitions for mental disorder-related terms such as "mental challenge," "mental disability" and "mental/psychological incapacity."	The SAMHCA provides a broad-based definition for mental disorder simply as "mental illness" being a "positive diagnosis of a mental health–related illness" based on acceptable diagnostic criteria. The ZIMHA (sections 2 and 226) provides definitions for "mentally disordered or intellectually handicapped" as referring to a person suffering from "mental illness, arrested or incomplete development of mind, psychopathic disorder or any other disorder or disability of the mind." Psychopathic disorder lies defined in s. 2 as well.	Uganda's Mental Health Act enacted in 1964. It offers no definition for mental disorder and essentially uses derogatory terms such "diot," "lunatic" and "imbecile" as descriptors. The TANMHA defines mental disorder under the term "medical disorder," which refers to mental and behavioral disorder as classified under ICD-10. It also defines mentally disordered offender. It fails to define mental incapacity.	The EMHA had clear definitions and distinguished between compulsory admission and compulsory treatment and established different criteria and procedures for each.
C	Access to mental health care: in terms of adequate provision	Under the Ghanaian legislation, these are largely covered under	These are covered under the objectives of the SAMHCA. Furthermore,	These are only indirectly addressed by the functions of the National	

	for funding, equivalence of care (with physical illnesses), balanced allocation of resources, integration of mental health into Primary Health Care, access to psychotropic medication, psychosocial rehabilitative approach and a legislative provision of access to health insurance for treatment of mental disorder.	the functions of the Mental Health Authority. Covered by s. 2 of the Lagos State Mental Health Law (2018) (LSMHL) under the objectives of the law.	time limitations are imposed on length of treatment (6 months) and admission (2 months) without recourse to oversight by Head of the mental health institution in which treatment and/ or admission is taking place. The ZIMHA does not directly address the issue of access to mental health care but mentions the receipt of patients into private dwelling homes, receipt of "temporary" patients into designated hospitals or nursing homes, etc.	Council on Health under s. 31 of the TANMHA.	
D	Rights of users of mental health services: human rights, confidentiality, right to judicial review when necessary, access to medical information private to them, protection from cruel and inhuman/ degrading treatment,	Some of these rights e.g. right to refuse consent and confidentiality, are covered under sections related to voluntary as well as involuntary treatment. Right to judicial review is noted (GMHA s. 44). Others are covered specifically under ss. 54–63 including right to non-	Rights provided in the SAMHCA (sections 7 to 17) include all rights in other laws as well as right to respect, human dignity, privacy, consent and protection from unfair discrimination, protection from exploitation and abuse, disclosure of information, knowledge of rights, etc.	Uganda's Mental health Act places no emphasis on human rights. These are not clearly addressed by the TANMHA. However, a patient's welfare board under the terms of s. 29(2) may entertain complaints from patients, relatives and interested third parties.	Addressed by the TUMHA. There is only one mental hospital in Tunisia and it has regular (between two to four times by year) inspections of human rights protection of patients. The EMHA includes the establishment of National Mental

(Continued)

Table 11.2 (Continued)

Item	*Legislative Issue*	*West Africa*	*Southern Africa*	*East Africa*	*North Africa*
	minimal conditions stipulated for mental health care facilities, forced or inadequately remunerated labor within health institutions, responsibility of health authorities to inform patients of their rights, involvement of patients/relatives in policy formulation or legislation development.	discrimination and basic human rights. Involvement of patients/relatives in policy/legislation formulation is provided for under the functions of the Ghanaian mental health authority.	Rights are not specifically mentioned under the ZIMHA.		Health Council (NMHC) and a regional subsidiary council in every governorate that has inpatient mental health care under the National Mental Health Council, to monitor the country's enforcement of the 2009 mental health legislation However, the current structure, regulated by law (Article 6), weighs heavily towards officials from or affiliated with the government. Moreover, the NMHC is chaired by the Minister of Health himself, who should, in fact, be monitored by the Council, so a changing in this structure should be considered

E	Rights of families or other carers: right to information (with the consent of the patient), involvement of carers in treatment plan, right to appeal involuntary or treatment decisions, right to apply for discharge, involvement in development of mental health policy, legislation and service planning.	Right to appeal also noted (GMHA)	Rights to appeals and information provided for under the SAMHCA. Under the ZIMHA, right of appeal to the Mental Health Review Tribunal against detention in private dwelling home, right of appeal against detention in a special hospital, among others. Appeals against the decision of the MHRT shall lie to the Supreme Court of Zimbabwe.	The right to appeal an order of involuntary admission is contained in section 15 of the TANMHA. The Mental Health Board under s. 17(1)(b) shall also entertain relatives' and patients' complaints with regard to welfare-related matters.	Rights of families or other carers: right to information (with the consent of the patient) are guaranteed under Tunisian Legislation.
F	Competence, capacity and guardianship	Sections 68–70 under the GMHA apply to this. Guardians are appointed by the courts and they may be limited in their functions to the aspect of the patient's incapacity. Guardianship may be reviewed. These issues are addressed in detail in section 63–66 of the LSMHL with procedures outlined for the appointment of guardians as well as the	Covered under sections 59–65 of the SAMHCA. The emphasis is on those with "mental illness or those with severe or profound intellectual disability." This introduces a complexity of terms since intellectual disability is a variant of mental illness with some emphasis on "nature" and "degree" in this case. Under the Act, an "administrator" is court-	Matters of competence, capacity and guardianship are covered under sections 19–26 of the TANMHA and they empower the court to appoint managers to oversee the property of the mentally ill person.	The term "mental capacity" has been defined clearly under the EMHA. Under the TUMHA, competence, capacity and guardianship are not directly addressed. Issues regarding competency, capacity and guardianship for the mentally ill are included in other common laws.

(Continued)

Table 11.2 (Continued)

Item	*Legislative Issue*	*West Africa*	*Southern Africa*	*East Africa*	*North Africa*
		scope and review of guardianship.	appointed to manage the affairs of the affected patient. Under the ZIMHA, issues of capacity and guardianship are addressed in sections 84–94. In the first instance, the spouse, children (>18 years) or other relatives of the incompetent patient may administer his/her property pending the appointment of a "curator" by a judge or a magistrate.		
G	Voluntary admission and treatment	This is covered in GMHA; sections 30–33 of the LSMHL provide for voluntary admission and treatment.	Covered under s. 25 of the SAMHCA. Sections 46–49 of the ZIMHA covers voluntary admission and treatment in the terms of "informal admission and treatment."	This is covered under section 4 of the TANMHA.	Under the EMHA patients can be admitted voluntarily if they have mental capacity to give informed consent. In most cases, a documentation review revealed that free and informed consent for

					treatment was obtained from all voluntary service users. But information obtained from patients revealed that few service users were aware that they had rights, and that they were entitled to ask for information about their rights. Tunisia is concerned by human rights protection, and other laws, official bodies and NGOs look after this issue.
H	Non-protesting patients: involves patients who are incapable of making informed consent about admission or treatment but are not refusing, issues of converting from *non-voluntary (unable to either refuse or consent)* to *involuntary (able to refuse or consent but refusing)*.	These patients are not covered by either the GMHA or the NLL. s. 36 of the LSMHL allows for the admission of such patients as "involuntary" patients based on applications by nearest relatives, medical social worker or "any other person."	This is covered under sections 26–31 of the SAMHCA and referred to as "assisted care." Application is to be made by relevant carer based on the age of the patient. Oversight of such admissions is undertaken the Mental Health Review Board with initial as well as annual reviews conducted. Upon recovery of capacity,	These patients are covered under sections 5 and 6 of the TANMHA. S. 6 allows for temporary treatment of patients who are unable to express or withhold consent if it is in their best interest to be treated.	Under the EMHA, the provisions of compulsory admission, with all the safeguards connected to it, are to be applied, unless the patient has a legally appointed guardian who can apply for voluntary admission. Most of the service users reported that their own preferences on treatment plan are

(Continued)

Table 11.2 (Continued)

Item	*Legislative Issue*	*West Africa*	*Southern Africa*	*East Africa*	*North Africa*
			patient may be converted to voluntary patient (s. 31(2)) or to involuntary patient (s. 31(4)). This is covered under section 50 of the ZIMHA in which such patients are liable to remain admitted in an authorized facility for not more than 28 days. The secretary (usually in the ministry of health) shall be furnished with the report of the patient's mental condition and further directives as to the conversion of the patient into an involuntary patient or fit for discharge shall be issued by the secretary.		not taken seriously by the doctors.
I	Involuntary admission	In the GMHA, involuntary admission is to be implemented by an application to the court; this is similar to the NLL but the LSMHL	Under the SAMHCA, section 33, applications for involuntary treatment are made to the head of the mental health institution in which care	UMHA does not regulate involuntary admission and treatment. Involuntary admission is covered under sections 11–15 of the TANMHA.	The EMHA distinguished between compulsory admission and compulsory treatment. The legal process now includes

	provides for an application to the medical director of the designated treating hospital in keeping with more modern approaches. Covered by s. 34 of the LSMHL and based upon the recommendation of two mental health professionals – "medical practitioner" and "medical social worker." Oversight to be provided by the Mental Health Review Committee.	is sought. It is based upon the recommendation of two "mental health practitioners" one of whom must be qualified to "conduct physical examinations." Appeals against involuntary treatment to be directed to the Mental Health Review Board; where it fails, the decision of the Review Board must be statutorily reviewed by the high court. Under sections 4–10 of the ZIMHA, a patient can be involuntarily admitted on the orders of a magistrate based on two medical recommendations. Where only one medical practitioner is available, a psychiatric nurse or psychiatric nurse practitioner or a clinical psychologist may provide the second recommendation. These occupational groups lie defined in the ZIMHA.	The recommendation for admission shall be made by "an approved medical officer" and "an approved mental health practitioner" with proper certificates issued under section 10. The certificates are directed to the resident magistrate or district court. Appeals against involuntary admission lie to the high court. The admission is to last for a maximum of 30 days in the first instance and may be extended by the court to a period not exceeding 90 days. Where there is no magistrate, recommendations for reception into a mental health facility may be directed to an "officer" who is either the regional or district administrative secretary.	notifying a judicial authority and a quasi-judicial body called the Council of Mental Health of the detention, in order to get an independent assessment within 7 days of admission. The patient's condition should be reviewed 2 days, 7 days and 1 month after their compulsory admission, as well as every month thereafter. Mechanisms to oversee the involuntary treatment practices and involuntary hospitalization exist under the TUMHA.

(Continued)

Table 11.2 (Continued)

Item	*Legislative Issue*	*West Africa*	*Southern Africa*	*East Africa*	*North Africa*
J	Involuntary Treatment (When separate from involuntary admission)	In the GMHA, as well as the NLL and the LSMHL, there is no separation of admission and treatment in terms of involuntary hospitalization.	No separation of involuntary treatment from involuntary admission under the SAMHCA. Involuntary treatment is not separated from involuntary admission under the ZIMHA.	There is no separation of involuntary admission and treatment under the TANMHA.	The EMHA distinguishes between compulsory admission and compulsory treatment and established different criteria and procedures for each. A regional human rights review body exists which has the authority to review involuntary admission and discharge procedures and review complaints investigation processes. The review body sends its reports to the Ministries of Health and Justice, which are the only ones to have the authority to impose the sanctions envisaged by law (including prison

					sentences). These reviews are mandatory.
K	Proxy consent	Permitted under the GMHA with regard to patients found incompetent; under s. 1 (interpretation) of the LSMHL, provisions are made for "substitute decision makers."	Permitted under s. 110A of the ZIMHA with respect to applying to a high court for an order authorizing sterilization of a mentally ill patient. This is also provided for under section 23 of the Zambian Mental Health Act (ZAMHA).	Proxy consent not expressly provided for under the TANMHA.	No information available
L	Involuntary treatment in community settings	Not addressed.	Not addressed	Not addressed.	Not available in Egypt. The Ministry of Social Affairs has its own review body in these settings.
M	Emergency situations: criteria, clear procedure, level of professionals to give emergency certificate, time limit, prohibition of certain treatments under emergency admission, etc.	Under GMHA, clear procedure and time limit of 72 hours stated (ss. 48 and 49). The NLL provides for a certificate of emergency covering seven days (s. 10) while the LSMHL allows for a certificate of urgency for 72 hours due to its more modern orientation.	s. 34 of the SAMHCA provides for a 72-hour assessment period after which decisions as to further involuntary care (or conversion to voluntary care) must be taken within the oversight of the Mental Health Review Board. Sections 11 and 14 of the ZIMHA permits the admission of patients as a	The TANMHA makes no clear provisions for emergency situations.	There are clear instructions and procedures in emergency situations but the country suffers from a crucial shortage of mental health professionals, especially the psychosocial workers. There is a total of human resource of 8

(Continued)

Table 11.2 (Continued)

Item	*Legislative Issue*	*West Africa*	*Southern Africa*	*East Africa*	*North Africa*
			matter of urgency based on an application accompanied by a medical certificate indicating the need for the urgent admission. An order is then made by a magistrate to this effect. This may not exceed 14 days.		per 100,000 populations
N	Determination of mental disorder	In the GMHA, this is to be based on two recommendations: one by a "medical practitioner" and the other by a "mental health professional." While mental health professional/mental health practitioner/ mental health worker may be used interchangeably to refer to any member of the multidisciplinary team, "medical practitioner" is not clearly defined but	The SAMHCA defines the terms "medical practitioner," "mental health care practitioner" and "mental health care provider." The latter includes the first two as they case might require. Each mental health practitioner profession is further interpreted under the Act giving little room for confusion as to which professional qualifications are required for the mentioned roles. Under the ZIMHA,	Under the TANMHA, the determination of mental disorder is based on the recommendation of "an approved medical officer" and "an approved mental health practitioner" with proper certificates issued under section 10. The two professional levels lie defined in the interpretation section of the Act.	No information available

		perhaps refers to "psychiatrist" who is defined under the interpretation section. Under the LSMHL, determination of mental disorder requiring involuntary admission is based upon the recommendation of two mental health professionals – "medical practitioner" and "medical social worker." Oversight to be provided by the Mental Health Review Committee.	determination of mental disorder is based on two medical recommendations. Where only one medical practitioner is available, a psychiatric nurse or psychiatric nurse practitioner or a clinical psychologist may provide the second recommendation. These occupational groups lie defined in the ZIMHA.		
O	Special treatments such as sterilization, psychosurgery, ECT and other medico-surgical procedures.	Under the GMHA (s. 71), these apply mainly to sterilization, abortion and ECT. Consent should be obtained from patient where capable or from representative or tribunal where incompetent. An involuntary patient shall not be subjected to psychosurgery (Ghanaian MHA, s. 45(2)). Section 67 of the	Treatments such as ECT and psychosurgery are not specifically mentioned in the SAMHCA. However, s. 66(1)(a and b) provides for ministerial regulation of medical and surgical therapeutic procedures. Under the ZIMHA, only a high court can authorize the sterilization of a mentally ill patient based on medical	These were not directly addressed by the TANMHA.	No information available

(Continued)

Table 11.2 (Continued)

Item	*Legislative Issue*	*West Africa*	*Southern Africa*	*East Africa*	*North Africa*
		LSMHL addresses the need for consent before conducting major medico-surgical procedures including sterilization and ECT. Where capacity is lacking, power is granted to the review committee to provide authorization. In emergencies, the head of a mental health institution is empowered to provide authorization while duly informing the review committee.	recommendation from two medical practitioners and this applies to only female patients. ECT and psychosurgery are brought under ministerial regulations under s. 125(h) of the ZIMHA. This is brought under s. 27 of the ZAMHA.		
P	Seclusion and restraint	This is covered under s. 58 of the GMHA and should be practiced under strict institutional guidelines and documentation. Not to be used for the punishment of patient or convenience of staff. Covered by s. 51 of the LSMHL with provisions	These are brought under ministerial regulations listed in section 66(1)(d) of the SAMHCA. These procedures are regulated under sections 113 (restraint) and 114 (seclusion) of the ZIMHA. Key features of these sections are the need for adequate	Not addressed in the UMHA. Not directly addressed in the TANMHA.	In Egyptian settings, chemical restraints are considered by the majority of staff as necessary to cope with involuntarily admitted service users contesting their admission, refusing treatment, and/or labeled "dangerous."

		on how to be deployed and the need for detailed documentation within the authorized facility	documentation and statutory reports to supervising ministry. This is covered under s. 27(2) of the ZAMHA and is subject to intermittent reviews, supervision by a psychiatrist and limited to 72 hours unless an application is made to the board.		Data concerning the use of restraints were insufficiently systematic or comprehensive. A separate record of the use of mechanical restraints was kept and recorded in the nursing diary.
Q	Clinical and experimental research	Not directly addressed by the GMHA and the NLL but the LSMHL	Not directly addressed by the SAMHCA.	Not directly addressed by the UMHA or the TanMHA.	Scientific experimentations are not conducted without the approvals from ethical committees.
R	Oversight and review mechanisms	Multi-level: Mental Health Authority, Mental Health Review Tribunal and Visiting committees are recognized under the GMHA. Visiting committees reporting annually are equally recognized under the NLL while a Mental Health Commission and a Mental Health Review Committee are provided for under the LSMHL as oversight bodies.	The SAMHCA provides for the establishment of Mental Health Review Boards (ss 18–24) to consider appeals against hospitals, involuntary admissions as well as transfers to high-security hospitals. s. 68 of the ZIMHA provides for the establishment of mental health boards and special boards to oversee mental health institutions where patients are cared for.	Under the TANMHA, oversight functions are provided by the Mental Health Board (sections 16–18) as well as the national council on mental health (sections 31–32).	Under the TUMHA, regional human rights review body exists which has the authority to review involuntary admission and discharge procedures and review complaints investigation processes. The review body sends its reports to the Ministries of Health and Justice, which are the only

(Continued)

Table 11.2 (Continued)

Item	*Legislative Issue*	*West Africa*	*Southern Africa*	*East Africa*	*North Africa*
			Sections 75–82 are concerned with the establishment and administration of the mental health review tribunal.		ones to have the authority to impose the sanctions envisaged by law (including prison sentences). The EMHA includes the establishment of National Mental Health Council and a regional subsidiary council in every governorate that has inpatient mental health care under the National Mental Health Council, to monitor the country's enforcement of the 2009 mental health legislation. However, the current structure, regulated by law (Article 6), weighs heavily towards officials from or affiliated with the

					government. Moreover, the NMHC is chaired by the Minister of Health himself.
S	Police responsibilities	Indirect allusion to police duties under s. 74 of the GMHA. This has to do with the execution of warrants to remove a person with mental disorder. s. 46(2) of the LSMHL directs the psychiatrist in charge or the head of the mental health facility to report absconding patients to the police for immediate arrest without warrant. Section 41 of the LSMHL empowers the ministry of the environment to collaborate with the police in removing mentally ill persons from public places. A key consideration is that such mentally ill persons must be deemed	Direct statements are made on police duties under s. 40. In s. 40(4), police officers are required by law to aid in apprehending those who have absconded from psychiatric care. In s. 13 of the ZIMHA, mentally disordered persons who are deemed a danger to themselves or others may be removed by police officers without warrant.	s. 9 of the TANMHA authorizes the police to remove mentally ill persons to mental health facilities.	Not addressed.

(Continued)

Table 11.2 (Continued)

Item	*Legislative Issue*	*West Africa*	*Southern Africa*	*East Africa*	*North Africa*
		dangerous to themselves or others.			
T	Mentally ill offenders/ "state patients"	**Treated in Table 11.2**			
U	Discrimination	Dealt with under right to non-discrimination under s. 52 of the LSMHL	Dealt with under rights in the SAMHCA but not specifically addressed under the ZIMHA.	Not addressed under the TANMHA.	Not addressed.
V	Housing	The LSMHL in s. 52(4) protects the tenancy rights of mentally ill persons and prohibits eviction on the basis of mental illness.	Not specifically addressed under either the SAMHCA or the ZIMHA.	Not addressed under the TANMHA.	No information available
W	Employment	Covered under basic rights in the GMHA. Employment rights are specifically guaranteed under s. 58 of the LSMHL. The NLL is silent on this issue.	Not directly addressed under the SAMHCA or ZIMHA.	Not addressed under the TANMHA.	No information available
X	Social security	Not directly addressed under the GMHA or the LSMHL.	Not directly addressed under the SAMHCA or the ZIMHA.	Not addressed under the TANMHA.	No information available
Y	Civil issues	Not directly addressed under the GMHA or the LSMHL. However, s.	Not directly addressed under the SAMHCA or the ZIMHA.	Not addressed under the TANMHA.	No information available

		59(2) of the LSMHL states that men and women shall have equal social, cultural, economic, civil and political rights.			
Z	Protection of vulnerable groups	Under the GMHA and the LSMHL (sections 60–62), this covers children, women, aged persons and those with mental retardation. Provisions for protection of their rights are addressed in some detail.	Perhaps the capacity provisions in the SAMHCA may illustrate some protection for vulnerable groups such as those with severe/profound intellectual disability. Section 66(1)(h) further provides for the establishment of separate facilities for children/adolescents and elderly in mental health institutions.	Not addressed under the TANMHA.	No information available
AZ	Offenses	Only few specific offenses (neglect of mentally ill, discrimination or abuse of other rights) are outlined under the GMHA. The NLL shows high compliance in relation to outlined offenses and penalties. The LSMHL (s. 74) outlines specific offenses	Specific offenses mentioned under the SAMHCA include: misrepresentation of facts, obstruction of lawful duty, abuse/neglect/ill-treatment of mental health care user, inciting of absconding and false information to the police. Penalties are	Specific offenses mentioned in the TANMHA include: wrongful admission into a mental health facility, assisting absconding and acts of cruelty/neglect/abuse towards a mentally ill person. Penalties are clearly stated.	No information available

(*Continued*)

Table 11.2 (Continued)

Item	*Legislative Issue*	*West Africa*	*Southern Africa*	*East Africa*	*North Africa*
		such as misrepresentation of facts, obstruction of lawful duty, abuse/neglect/ill-treatment of mental health care user, inciting of absconding and false information to persons acting under powers granted by the Act. Penalties are clearly indicated.	clearly indicated. Under the ZIMHA, offenses outlined include: unlawful detention outside the provisions of the act, false statements, ill-treatment of patients, assisting absconding patients, obstruction and unlawful sexual intercourse with a patient. Penalties are clearly outlined as well.		

patients' autonomy, represented a threat to clinicians' judgment with its subtle paternalistic leanings (Loza & El Nawawi, 2012).

As part of considerations regarding self-determination, it is equally pertinent to note the inadequate treatment of social, cultural and economic rights specifically in many of the illustrative legislations within Africa. This trend had also been noted in mental health laws in non-African jurisdictions (e.g., England & Wales and Ireland) (Kelly, 2011). Arguments exist as to the reasonableness of leaving these aspects to be addressed by "general" or common law provisions as well as government policy. Evidence suggests, however, that the human rights of the mentally ill may be more efficiently protected by dedicated legislation (Kelly, 2011); although a combined approach of specific mental health legislation plus mental health–related elements in relevant laws appears most pragmatic (World Health Organization, 2005).

Definition of mental disorder

There are important ethical and human rights considerations in the definition of mental disorder within the context of mental health legislation (Pilgrim, 2005). Arguments have been made for both a broad and narrow interpretation (Fulford, 1998; Goldman & Grob, 2006; Regier, 2003). On the one hand, a broad definition of mental disorder is regarded as having little room for restrictive interpretation (Mason & Laurie, 2013) and is perceived as introducing uncertainty into mental health law (Glover-Thomas, 2011). Such wide definitions may also be prone to arbitrary use by the state especially in relation to providing limited exclusions under non-consensual treatment for mental disorders (Barber, Brown, & Martin, 2017). On the other hand, it has been advanced that a broad view of mental disorder accommodates dynamic changes in mental health diagnoses in an evolving field (*Winterwerp v Netherlands*, 1979; Leung, 2002) and does not necessarily violate human rights. It would appear that a balanced solution has been one of "broad definition and narrow use" (Fulford, 1998). It has equally been suggested that the focus of legislation should determine the form of definition. For instance, where the emphasis is on "care and treatment," definition should be narrow. Whereas if the focus is on protecting a broad range of "positive" rights, it should be broad and inclusive (World Health Organization, 2005).

Closely related to definitions is the legal context within which defined mental disorders may trigger the need for involuntary admission and treatment. Intellectual disability and substance-use disorders fall under this category and the basis for instituting care for these conditions under mental health law ought to be addressed frontally in their definition for legislative purposes (see Mental Health Act 1983 of the United Kingdom; see also Mental Health Act 2007 for further explanation of grounds upon which intellectual disability may be construed as mental disorder for the purposes of this bill.) This has been done in respect of intellectual disability but not substance use under some of the highlighted legislations (e.g., the Lagos State Mental Health law in its section 62). Such bases may be rendered in their definitions as: "evidence of misbehaviour or mental disorder …" (after the Lagos State Mental Health Law) or "abnormally aggressive or seriously irresponsible conduct" (after the Zimbabwean Mental Health Act, 2000 (ZIMHA)). This is vitally important since the mere presence of intellectual disability or substance use should not constitute grounds for involuntary treatment under the Act. A non-contextualized approach to these conditions under mental health law will not only impose a heavy care burden on the mental health system, it will likely lead to undue discrimination and possibly stigmatization of persons with intellectual disability or substance-use problems.

Personality disorders and/or psychopathy occupy a slightly different sphere because there are still arguments as to whether they can be diagnosed or defined as mental disorders (Kendell, 2002). Notwithstanding this, the leading nosological classifications of mental disorders (World Health Organization, 1992; American Psychiatric Association, 2013) contain diagnostic criteria for different types of personality disorder thereby suggesting that in the clinical sense, these personality disorders are brought under the canopy of mental disorders. This inclusion of personality disorders under the rubric of mental disorder embraces a broad-based definition of mental disorder although some level of confusion arises when legislative attempt is made to limit personality disorders to those that portray social deviance that is, the so-called "psychopathic disorder" (such a specific mention of psychopathic disorder is observed in the ZIMHA). This confusion is based on two cardinal considerations. First, this limitation substantially negates the essence of regarding all personality disorders as mental disorders which is to incorporate them into the group of conditions that can be assessed and treated under mental health legislation. Second, the tendency of equating antisocial personality disorder with psychopathy engenders diagnostic confusion since there is emerging evidence that antisocial personality disorder may occur in the absence of psychopathy (De Brito, Viding, Kumari, Blackwood, & Hodgins, 2013; Gregory et al., 2012) even though psychopathy shows frequent comorbidity with the former (Blackburn, Logan, Donnelly, & Renwick, 2003). Nonetheless, it has been observed that personality or psychopathic disorders are not adopted wholesale under mental health law but usually put in the context of such disorders being associated with aggressive or irresponsible conduct. Indeed, a recent meta-analysis demonstrated that personality disorders significantly reduced the odds of involuntary hospitalization (Walker et al., 2019).

The legislative significance of the definition of key terms such as mental disorder, mental incapacity and associated expressions in mental health legislation is that it ensures consistency in the use of such terms throughout the document (World Health Organization, 2005). It will also undoubtedly reduce unnecessary ambiguity in the interpretations of the "interpretable terms" in the document. While definitions are provided for "incapacity," "mental retardation" and "personality disorder" in the GMHA, no definition is supplied for mental disorder per se. The Nigerian Lunacy Law (1916) (NLL) given its very archaic form, does not provide a definition for any form of mental disorder. However, the more recent LSMHL provides definitions for mental disorder-related terms such as "mental challenge," "mental disability" and "mental/psychological incapacity."

Similarly, the SAMHCA provides a broad-based definition for mental disorder simply as "mental illness" being a positive diagnosis of a mental health–related illnesses based on acceptable diagnostic criteria. The ZIMHA provides definitions for "mentally disordered or intellectually handicapped" as referring to a person suffering from "mental illness, arrested or incomplete development of mind, psychopathic disorder or any other disorder or disability of the mind." Psychopathic disorder lies defined in s. 2 as well. Uganda's Mental Health Act (UMHA) enacted in 1964 offers no definition for mental disorder and essentially uses derogatory terms such as "idiot," "lunatic" and "imbecile" as descriptors quite similar to the current framing of terms in the Nigerian Lunacy Law of 1916. The Tanzanian Mental Health Act (TANMHA) defines mental disorder under the term "medical disorder," which refers to a mental and behavioral disorder as classified under ICD. It also defines mentally disordered offender, although it fails to define mental incapacity.

Involuntary admission and treatment

One of the major mandates of mental health law is the setting of clear and objective criteria for involuntary admission as well as the establishment of specified procedures for the protection of the rights of those involuntarily committed due to mental disorder (World Health Organization, 2005). The existence and implementation of legislative provisions in respect of involuntary hospitalization involve complex socio-legal, political and resource-related considerations (Rains et al., 2019). More directly, in spite of the fact that the cornerstone of modern-day psychiatric practice is informed consent, hospitalization/treatment against a person's wish may be warranted under conditions of risks posed to self and others (Fistein et al., 2009). Involuntary hospitalization and treatment of individuals with mental disorders require society to strike a delicate balance between individual autonomy and right to liberty and public safety (Jones, 2014; Mason & Laurie, 2013). Yet, involuntary admission and treatment have been open to criticisms from the human rights perspective as being subversive of autonomy and supportive of degrading or cruel treatment (Jones, 2005).

As controversial as involuntary admission/treatment for mental disorder might seem, there are global benchmarks to be met (United Nations, 1991; World Health Organization, 2005) for invoking such legislative provisions and these include:

- The presence of a mental disorder.
- Serious likelihood of immediate danger.
- Serious likelihood of deterioration of mental health condition.
- Clear presence of a therapeutic purpose.
- Presence of formalized procedures for the admission and/or treatment including the designation of health facilities as well as application and appeal procedures.

In terms of illustrative legislations in Africa, involuntary admission is to be implemented by an application to the court under the GMHA suggesting a formalized procedure. This is similar to the NLL but the LSMHL provides for an application to the medical director of the designated treating hospital in keeping with more modern approaches as contained in s. 34 of the LSMHL and based upon the recommendation of two mental health professionals – "medical practitioner" and "medical social worker." The oversight of involuntary admissions is to be provided by the Mental Health Review Committee under the LSMHL. Applications for involuntary treatment are made to the head of the mental health institution in which care is sought under the SAMHCA section 33. It is based upon the recommendation of two "mental health practitioners," one of whom must be qualified to "conduct physical examinations." Appeals against involuntary treatment are to be directed to the Mental Health Review Board; where it fails, the decision of the Review Board must be statutorily reviewed by the High Court. In the North African sub-region, the Egyptian Mental Health Act (2009) (EMHA) distinguishes between compulsory admission and compulsory treatment. The legal process now includes notifying a judicial authority and a quasi-judicial body, called the Council of Mental Health, of the detention, to get an independent assessment within seven days of admission. The patient's condition should be reviewed 2 days, 7 days and 1 month after their compulsory admission, as well as every month thereafter. Mechanisms to oversee the involuntary treatment practices and involuntary hospitalization equally exist under the TUMHA.

It is to be noted that in the GMHA as well as the NLL and the LSMHL, there is no separation of admission and treatment in terms of involuntary hospitalization. Similarly, there is no separation of involuntary treatment from involuntary admission under the SAMHCA or the ZIMHA. However, the EMHA distinguishes between compulsory admission and compulsory treatment as stated in the foregoing and established different criteria and procedures for each situation.

The separation of involuntary admission from involuntary treatment is an attempt to ensure respect for individual autonomy and is an ethically sound posture. However, there are several important problems with this approach. First, it assumes that detention itself cannot be regarded as treatment. This is a narrow view of treatment. Case law from the UK seems to support the position that detention is not mere containment but provides benefits derivable from a ward environment (*MD v Nottinghamshire Healthcare NHS Trust*). Furthermore, in *Reid v Secretary of State for Scotland*, the court held that appropriate treatment could range from "cure" to "containment." Second, the separation of compulsory admission from involuntary treatment carries the risk of detention without treatment (Jones, 2014; Wessely, Gilbert, Hedley, & Neuberger, 2018; World Health Organization, 2005) thereby questioning the therapeutic purpose of such involuntary hospitalization. Such scenarios might easily project mental health services as mere agents of social control.

Emergency treatment

Emergency treatment is construed as situations in which there is high probability of immediate and imminent danger to self and/or others (World Health Organization, 2005). This aspect under mental health legislation focuses on the criteria, procedure and professional qualifications required for invoking the legal provisions as well as the time limit for such admissions. In addition, it seeks to prohibit certain treatments such as electroconvulsive therapy, use of depot neuroleptics, sterilization, psychosurgery as well as other irreversible treatments under emergency admission (World Health Organization, 2005). As shown in Table 11.2, the Ghanaian legislation documents a clear procedure and a time limit of 72 hours. The NLL provides for a "certificate of emergency" covering seven days while the more contemporary LSMHL allows for a "certificate of urgency" valid for 72 hours. South African legislation equally permits a 72-hour assessment period after which decisions as to further involuntary care (or conversion to voluntary care) must be taken within the oversight of the Mental Health Review Board. The Zimbabwean legislation is slightly different permitting the admission of patients as a matter of urgency based on an application accompanied by a medical certificate. An order is then made by a magistrate to this effect and may not exceed 14 days. A comparative study of legislation across the EU, the Americas, Australasia and Asia suggests a duration between 24 hours and 10 days (Zhang, Mellsop, Brink, & Wang, 2015). There are also clear instructions and procedures in emergency situations under Egyptian law, but the country suffers from a crucial shortage of mental health professionals, especially psychosocial workers. There is a total of human resource of 8 per 100,000 populations (Spagnolo et al., 2017).

Other forms of deprivation of liberty: Seclusion and restraints

Therapeutic strategies like seclusion and restraint invade the sphere of fundamental human rights and should be regulated in a bid to strike the delicate balance between autonomy and necessity with proportionality. Provisions regulating these specific forms of deprivation of liberty are covered under s. 58 of the GMHA and follow strict institutional guidelines and documentation. Specifically, they are not to be used for the punishment of patient or convenience of staff. Similarly, they are covered by s. 51 of the LSMHL with provisions on how to be deployed and the need for detailed documentation within the authorized facility. In a different approach, the two are brought under ministerial regulations within the SAMHCA. These issues are not addressed in the Ugandan or Tanzanian legislation.

Taking exemplars from more developed jurisdictions, Kelly (2011) noted that the Irish Mental Health legislation specifically regulates the use of seclusion. A more recent mental health law in India similarly regulates seclusion and restraint (Duffy & Kelly, 2017). In the UK Mental Health Act (1983) (as amended by the Mental Health Act 2007), these therapeutic procedures are regulated under its code of practice (Department of Health, 2015) although there have been recommendations to provide clear provisions regarding them in the act itself (Ogunwale, 2019). Akin to the UK approach, the South African MHCA's provision for ministerial regulation of seclusion and restraint leaves this in the purview of "practice regulations." Within the Egyptian experience, chemical restraints are considered by the majority of staff as necessary to cope with involuntarily admitted service users contesting their admission, refusing treatment, and/or labeled "dangerous." Data concerning the use of restraints were insufficiently systematic or comprehensive although it appears that a separate record of the use of mechanical restraints is maintained by nurses (Elnemais Fawzy, 2015).

Competence, capacity and guardianship

Some provisions for competence, capacity and guardianship exist under both Ghanaian and Nigerian legislations (see sections 68–70 and sections 63–66 of the LSMHL). Under Ghanaian law, guardians are appointed by the courts and they may be limited in their functions to the aspect of the patient's incapacity. Guardianship may be reviewed. These issues are similarly addressed in detail in the LSMHL with procedures outlined for the appointment of guardians as well as the scope and review of guardianship. Covered under sections 59–65 of the SAMHCA, the emphasis is on those with "mental illness or those with severe or profound intellectual disability." Evidently, this introduces a complexity of terms since intellectual disability is a variant of mental illness although with some emphasis on "nature" and "degree" in this case. Under the South African act, an "administrator" is court-appointed to manage the affairs of the affected patient.

Under the ZIMHA, issues of capacity and guardianship are addressed in sections 84–94. In the first instance, the spouse, children (>18 years) or other relatives of the incompetent patient may administer his/her property pending the appointment of a "curator" by a judge or a magistrate. The term "mental capacity" has been defined clearly under the EMHA. Under the TUMHA, competence, capacity and guardianship are not directly addressed. Thus, in Tunisia, issues regarding competency, capacity, and guardianship for the mentally ill are included in other common laws.

Clinical and experimental research

Apart from the Egyptian legislation that prohibits scientific research without the approvals from ethics committees (Elnemais Fawzy, 2015), clinical and experimental research in mental health settings are not frontally addressed by the GMHA, the NLL or the LSMHL. Similarly, the SAMHCA fails to provide clear provisions in this regard. Yet, clinical and experimental research constitute both ethical (World Medical Association, 2013) and human rights issues (United Nations, 1966). Specifically, article 7 of the International Covenant on Civil and Political Rights (ICCPR) prohibits medical or scientific experimentation without informed consent. Considerations relevant to clinical and experimental research apply to both voluntary and involuntary patients (Veer, Drachman, Ahad, Silvers, & Ramos, 2010). In practice, three cardinal elements are required for valid consent: (i) adequate information disclosure, (ii) capacity to consent and (iii) voluntariness (Appelbaum, Lidz, & Klitzman, 2009; Braude & Kimmelman, 2012; Grimes, McCullough, Kunik, Molinari, & Workman, 2000; Roberts, 2002; US Government Printing Office, 1949; Veer et al., 2010). For voluntary patients, the issues relevant to consent would be largely centered upon these three elements without a specific slant towards any of them. The matter is however more complex when the involuntary patient is involved since a more critical question arises around the extent of "voluntariness" that an "involuntary" patient would reasonably possess. Nevertheless, research seems to suggest that consent outcomes are not necessarily affected by admission status (Veer et al., 2010) and voluntariness could occur on a continuum (Appelbaum et al., 2009). Thus, a blanket prohibition of clinical and experimental research in involuntarily hospitalized patients potentially represents covert paternalism on the part of research ethics oversight bodies and could be unjust in denying that population of patients the benefits that may accrue from research (Veer et al., 2010).

Oversight and review mechanisms

These appear to be multi-layered in some countries and are presented in Table 11.2. For example, the Mental Health Authority, Mental Health Review Tribunal and Visiting committees are all recognized under the GMHA and have different remits of oversight. In Nigeria, visiting committees to the asylums reporting annually are equally recognized under the NLL while a Mental Health Commission and a Mental Health Review Committee are provided for under the LSMHL as oversight bodies. The SAMHCA provides for the establishment of Mental Health Review Boards to consider appeals against hospitals, involuntary admissions as well as transfers to high-security hospitals. In a similar vein, s. 68 of the ZIMHA provides for the establishment of mental health boards and special boards to oversee mental health institutions where patients are cared for. Under Tanzanian law, a regional human rights review body exists that has the authority to review involuntary admission, discharge procedures and review complaints investigation processes. The review body sends its reports to the Ministries of Health and Justice, which are the only ones to have the authority to impose the sanctions envisaged by law (including prison sentences).

"Forensic" mental health legislation: Treatment of mentally ill offenders under mental health law and relevant criminal legislations

The essence of legislative provisions for safeguarding the rights of mentally ill individuals who offend is justice as well as fairness (World Health Organization, 2005) and it is consistent with international law (United Nations, 1991). The assessment and treatment of mentally ill offenders under mental health legislation in different parts of the continent address eight broad areas of intervention, namely:

- Assessment and treatment at arrest.
- Rights of offenders undergoing treatment for mental disorders.
- Management of offenders found "unfit to plead."
- Sentencing of convicted mentally ill offenders.
- Transfer of mentally ill prisoners to hospital.
- Duration of hospitalization of mentally ill prisoners and considerations for term of imprisonment.
- The need role of psychiatric assessment in attempted suicide.
- Absconding offenders from mental health establishments.

It is important to note that the issue of attempted suicide is particularly crucial because it is criminalized in certain jurisdictions and would ordinarily be treated as a misdemeanor, attracting a fine or imprisonment term or both (e.g., section 327, Criminal Code Act, Laws of the Federation of Nigeria, 2004). To that extent, psychiatric assessment in cases of attempted suicide could serve a dual function in mental health legislation as well criminal procedure laws as follows:

- Signal the need for involuntary admission for the purpose of adequate observation and/or treatment under mental health law.
- Serve as a means of diversion from the criminal justice system.

Table 11.3 shows the current level of interventions provided under relevant mental health and criminal legislations in different African jurisdictions. In addition, the WHO has provided key recommendations regarding issues associated with mentally ill offenders that ought to be addressed in mental health legislation (shown in Box 11.1) and these serve a benchmarking function.

Mental health assessment at arrest

As shown in Table 11.3, within the West African sub-region, mental health assessment is to be conducted within 48 hours of arrest under the GMHA. Provisions of the 1960 Criminal and other offenses Procedure Act of Ghana equally apply to such offenders. Offenders suspected to have a mental disorder are to be sent to psychiatric facility for assessment and possible committal for treatment. In comparable terms, under s. 73(1) of the LSMHL, mental health assessment of an offender is required to be done within 48 hours if there is suspicion of mental disorder. There is allowance for transfer to a mental health facility for assessment and if necessary, treatment. This legislative approach is in keeping with diversion paradigms which not only reduce the disproportionately high rates of mental disorders in criminal justice systems but also lower re-offending rates (Adjorlolo, 2016; Munetz & Griffin, 2006).

Table 11.3 Comparing mental health law provisions for the treatment of mentally ill offenders within different African jurisdictions

Item	*Legislative issue*	*West Africa*	*Southern Africa*	*East Africa*
A	At arrest	Under the GMHA (s. 76; ss 1, 2 and 3), mental health assessment is to be done within 48 hours of arrest and police custody. Provisions of the 1960 Criminal and other offenses Procedure Act of Ghana apply to such offenders. Offender suspected to have mental disorder to be sent to psychiatric facility for assessment and possible committal for treatment (subsection 3). Under s. 73(1) of the LSMHL, mental health assessment of an offender to be done within 48 hours if there is suspicion of mental disorder. Subsection 2 of the said section allows for transfer to a mental health facility for	Under the SAMHCA, no provisions are stated with regard to the mental health assessment of offenders at arrest or in police custody. Similarly, under the ZAMHA, no such provisions are made. However, s. 29 of the ZAMHA provides for the designation of health facilities for the admission, care and treatment of the "forensic mental patient" defined as a person referred to a mental health facility for a court-ordered assessment of fitness to plead or clinical assessment for the purpose of determining criminal liability in the presence of mental disorder. Such patients are referred to as "state patients" under the SAMHCA (interpretation, s. 1) – in terms of sections 77(6)(a)(i) (unfit to plead) and 78(6)(i)(aa) (not guilty by reason of insanity) of the South African Criminal Procedure Act.	Mental health issues at arrest of offenders not addressed under the TANMHA. Similarly, these issues are not addressed by the Kenyan Mental Health Act(KMHA).

(*Continued*)

Table 11.3 (Continued)

Item	*Legislative issue*	*West Africa*	*Southern Africa*	*East Africa*
		assessment and if necessary, treatment.		
B	Offender undergoing treatment at a psychiatric facility	s. 76(4) of the GMHA and 73(3) of the LSMHL guarantee that offenders undergoing treatment at a mental health facility shall have similar rights to non-offenders, including right of judicial review by the court.	The rights of offenders undergoing treatment at a psychiatric facility are not specifically addressed by either the SAMHCA or the ZAMHA.	The TANMHA only defines a "mentally disorder offender" (sic) as a person confined for a crime suspected to have been due to mental disorder or a prisoner transferred to a mental health facility for proper treatment. No provisions regarding rights while in treatment. No definition of mentally disordered offender is provided by the KMHA.
C	Offenders found unfit to plead	Charges being faced by mentally ill offenders who are found unfit to plead are to be stayed while undergoing treatment under the terms of s.	Under the ZAMHA, forensic patients referred to mental health establishments are required to be assessed within 14 days of the court order. Under sections 42 and 43 of the SAMHCA, state patients found unfit to plead are to be	Not specifically addressed by the TANMHA or the KMHA.

(*Continued*)

Table 11.3 (Continued)

Item	*Legislative issue*	*West Africa*	*Southern Africa*	*East Africa*
		76(5) of the GMHA and s. 73(4) of the LSMHL.	admitted to designated health facilities for care and treatment pending further determination by a judge in chambers under the terms of s. 47 of the SAMHCA.	
D	Mentally ill offender at sentencing	Mentally ill offenders are not to be imprisoned but granted probation by way of hospital order (psychiatric hospital or security hospital depending on the seriousness of crime and risk to the public) (s. 76(6) of the GMHA and s 73(5) of the LSMHL). Under s. 73(6) of the LSMHL, offenders found "not guilty by reason of insanity" and reassessed to be free from mental disorder at a later date shall be discharged subject to further directives from the court.	Under sections 42 and 43 of the SAMHCA, state patients found "not guilty by reason of insanity" may be detained in a mental health establishment pending further determination by a judge in chambers under the terms of s. 47 of the SAMHCA.	Not specifically addressed by the TanMHA or the KMHA.
E	Convicted offender (prisoner)	Under s. 76(8) of the GMHA as well as s. 73(7)	The SAMHCA and the ZAMHA have robust provisions for the care	Not specifically addressed by the

(*Continued*)

Table 11.3 (Continued)

Item	*Legislative issue*	*West Africa*	*Southern Africa*	*East Africa*
	who becomes mentally ill	of the LSMHL, a prisoner who becomes mentally ill is to be transferred to a security hospital if his/ her condition sufficiently warrants it.	of mentally ill prisoners. s. 50 of the SAMHCA and s. 34 of the ZAMHA direct the head of prison or correctional service to ensure mental health assessment by requisite levels of professionals. s. 51 of the SAMHCA and s. 35 of the ZAMHA provide for mental health care in prison where the mental health status of the prisoner allows. s. 52 of the SAMHCA and s. 36 of the ZAMHA permit transfer of prisoners to a mental health facility outside the prison after due assessment; the SAMHCA requires a valid magisterial order for this. s. 54 of the SAMHCA and s. 37 of the ZAMHA apply to periodic review of the mental health of the prisoner while in hospital. s. 33 of the ZAMHA provides for such periodic reviews with regard to forensic mental patients. s. 56 of the SAMHCA as well as sections 33(2)(b) and 38 of the ZAMHA detail the procedure for the discharge report on the prisoner or forensic mental patient.	TANMHA or the KMHA.
F	Duration of hospital order in the case of a prisoner on	Prisoners in mental health facility shall not spend more time	s. 58 of the SAMHCA provides that mentally ill prisoners should be released from hospital at the expiry of the	Not specifically addressed by the TANMHA

(*Continued*)

Table 11.3 (Continued)

Item	*Legislative issue*	*West Africa*	*Southern Africa*	*East Africa*
	transfer direction	than required sentence unless she/he becomes civilly committed under the terms of s. 76(9) of the GMHA. Similar terms are detailed in s. 73(8) of the LSMHL.	term of imprisonment. Should the prisoner require further care, the head of the mental health establishment is expected to make an application for involuntary hospitalization/care at least 90 days before expiry of imprisonment term. These issues are not addressed by the ZAMHA. Section 47 of the SAMHCA details the procedure for the discharge of a state patient and indicates the possibility of "conditional discharge" under conditions specified by an order in terms of s. 47(6)(d) subject to periodic reviews under the oversight of the court.	or the KMHA.
G	Attempted suicide and the need for psychiatric assessment	Addressed by s. 76(10) of the GMHA. The court may authorize psychiatric assessment of suicide attempters. Section 73(9) of the LSMHL addresses the need for court-ordered psychiatric assessment of suicide attempters.	Not specifically addressed by the SAMHCA or the ZAMHA.	Not specifically addressed by the TANMHA or the KMHA.
H	Absconding offenders from mental health	Not directly addressed under the	The South African Mental Health Care Act provides for the transfer of absconders	Not specifically addressed by the TANMHA

(*Continued*)

Table 11.3 (Continued)

Item	*Legislative issue*	*West Africa*	*Southern Africa*	*East Africa*
	establish-ments	GMHA or the LSMHL.	(non-offenders) as well as those with high likelihood of inflicting harm on other patients in a mental health facility to high-security hospitals. s. 44 of the SAMHCA directs the head of mental health units housing state patients to inform the South African police service of any absconding. s. 32 of the ZAMHA directs the head of a forensic mental health facility to inform the police in the event of a forensic patient absconding from such facilities.	or the KMHA.

In examples drawn from Southern Africa, under the SAMHCA, no provisions are stated with regard to the mental health assessment of offenders at arrest or while in police custody. Similarly, under the ZAMHA, no such provisions are made. However, the Zambian mental health act (section 29) provides for the designation of health facilities for the admission, care and treatment of the "forensic mental patient." This is defined as a person referred to a mental health facility for a court-ordered assessment of fitness to plead or clinical assessment for the purpose of determining criminal liability in the presence of mental disorder. Comparably, such patients are referred to as "state patients" under the SAMHCA (interpretation, s. 1). The interpretation in the SAMHCA makes reference to sections 77(6)(a)(i) (unfit to plead) and 78(6)(i)(aa) (not guilty by reason of insanity) of the South African Criminal Procedure Act. In the Eastern African exemplars (Tanzania and Kenya), mental health issues at arrest of offenders are not addressed under the Tanzanian law or the Kenyan legislation.

Offender undergoing treatment at a psychiatric facility/ designation of health establishments for the treatment of the mentally ill offender

Legislation in Ghana and Nigeria clearly make provisions for the protection of the rights of mentally ill offenders undergoing psychiatric treatment. Relevant sections of the GMHA and the LSMHL (refer to Table 11.3) guarantee that

Box 11.1 Key recommendations on legislative provisions for the treatment of mentally ill offenders (Source: WHO checklist on mental health legislation (World Health Organization, 2005))

- Does the legislation allow for diverting an alleged offender with a mental disorder to the mental health system in lieu of prosecuting him/her, taking into account the gravity of the offense, the person's psychiatric history, mental health state at the time of the offense, the likelihood of detriment to the person's health and the community's interest in prosecution?
- Does the law make adequate provision for people who are not fit to stand trial to be assessed, and for charges to be dropped or stayed while they undergo treatment? Are people undergoing such treatment given the same rights in the law as other involuntarily admitted persons, including the right to judicial review by an independent body?
- Does the law allow for people who are found by the courts to be "not responsible due to mental disability" to be treated in a mental health facility and to be discharged once their mental disorder sufficiently improves?
- Does the law allow, at the sentencing stage, for persons with mental disorders to be given probation or hospital orders, rather than being sentenced to prison?
- Does the law allow for the transfer of a convicted prisoner to a mental health facility if he/she becomes mentally ill while serving a sentence? Does the law prohibit keeping a prisoner in the mental health facility for longer than the sentence, unless involuntary admission procedures are followed?
- Does the legislation provide for secure mental health facilities for mentally ill offenders?

offenders undergoing treatment at a mental health facility shall have similar rights to non-offenders including right of judicial review by the court. On the contrary, the rights of offenders undergoing mental health treatment are not specifically addressed by either the SAMHCA or the ZAMHA.

An evaluation of legislations from East Africa shows that while the TANMHA defines a "mentally disorder offender" (sic) as a person confined for a crime suspected to have been due to mental disorder or a prisoner transferred to a mental health facility for proper treatment, it makes no clear provisions regarding rights while in treatment. This picture is similar to that of the Kenyan mental act as well.

Offenders found unfit to plead

Under legislations in Ghana and Nigeria, charges being faced by mentally ill offenders who are found unfit to plead are to be stayed while undergoing treatment, state patients found unfit to plead are to be admitted to designated health facilities for care and treatment pending further determination by a judge in chambers under the terms of s. 47 of the SAMHCA. The treatment of offenders found unfit to plead are not specifically addressed by the TANMHA or the Kenyan Mental Health Act (KMHA).

Mentally ill offenders at sentencing

In the Ghanaian and Nigerian legislations, at sentencing, mentally ill offenders are not to be imprisoned but granted probation by way of hospital orders (psychiatric hospital or security hospital depending on the seriousness of crime and risk to the public). Furthermore, the LSMHL provides that offenders found "not guilty by reason of insanity" and reassessed to be free from mental disorder later are to be discharged subject to further directives from the court. Similarly, under the terms of the SAMHCA, state patients found "not guilty by reason of insanity" may be detained in a mental health establishment pending further determination by a judge in chambers (see Table 11.3). The sentencing direction for mentally ill offenders is not specifically addressed by the TANMHA or the KMHA.

Convicted offender (prisoner) who becomes mentally ill

Examples drawn from West Africa, as represented by both the Nigerian and Ghanaian laws, provide that a prisoner who becomes mentally ill is to be transferred to a security hospital if his/her condition sufficiently warrants it. With regard to this, the Southern African jurisdictions appear to have more robust provisions for the care of mentally ill prisoners. Both the SAMHCA and ZAMHA direct the head of prison or correctional service to ensure mental health assessment by requisite levels of professionals. Relevant sections of both laws (see Table 11.3) provide for mental health care in prison where the mental health status of the prisoner allows. However, while the SAMHCA and ZAMHA permit transfer of prisoners to a mental health facility outside the prison after due assessment, the SAMHCA requires a valid magisterial order for this. Furthermore, the two legislations provide for periodic review of the mental health of the prisoner while in hospital. The ZAMHA further provides for such periodic reviews regarding forensic mental patients. Both the SAMHCA and ZMHA detail the procedure for the discharge report on the prisoner or forensic mental patient. These issues are not specifically addressed by the East African jurisdictions as exemplified by the TANMHA or the KMHA.

Duration of hospital order in the case of a prisoner on transfer direction

In terms of length of incarceration based on a hospital order, prisoners in mental health facilities are not to spend more time than required by their prison sentence unless they become civilly committed under the terms of the GMHA as well as the LSMHL. Section 58 of the SAMHCA provides that mentally ill prisoners should be released from hospital at the expiry of the term of imprisonment. Should the prisoner require further care, the head of the mental health establishment is expected to make an application for involuntary hospitalization/care at least 90 days before expiry of imprisonment term. These issues are not addressed by the ZAMHA with regard to prisoners although it details the procedure for the discharge of the forensic mental patient under s. 38. Relevant sections of the SAMHCA details the procedure for the discharge of a state patient and indicates the possibility of "conditional discharge" under conditions specified by an order which is subject to periodic reviews under the oversight of the court. The TANMHA or the KMHA do not specifically address these issues.

Attempted suicide and the need for psychiatric assessment

The need for psychiatric assessment in attempted suicide is observed in legislation within West Africa. Under sections 76(10) of the GMHA and 73(9) of the LSMHL, the court may authorize psychiatric assessment of suicide attempters. None of the illustrative laws from Southern or East Africa address these issues.

Absconding offenders from mental health establishments

The South African Mental Health Care Act provides for the transfer of absconders (non-offenders) as well as those with high likelihood of inflicting harm on other patients in a mental health facility to high-security hospitals. In addition, the SAMHCA directs the head of mental health units housing state patients to inform the South African Police service of any absconding incidents. In analogous terms, the ZAMHA directs the head of a forensic mental health facility to inform the police in the event of a forensic patient absconding from such facilities. This important safety consideration is not specifically addressed by legislations in Tanzania, Kenya, Nigeria or Ghana.

Conclusion

Despite the critical function of mental health legislation in safeguarding patients' and society's well-being, only roughly half of African countries have mental health legislations. Where existent, there is a wide variation in their currency with a few countries having laws that were enacted in the 19th or early 20th century. There are also observable differences in legal frameworks and routine procedures which may be underpinned by subtle disparities in legal traditions across countries. In many instances, the laws are outmoded and fail to take cognizance of human rights since some of them pre-date the ascendancy of human rights considerations in mental health laws. Within the more specific context of "forensic" legislative provisions under the existing laws, some countries fall short of the global standards in protecting the rights of mentally ill offenders particularly in areas such as handling of mentally ill offenders at arrest, the treatment of offenders found unfit to plead, attempted suicide and the attendant need for psychiatric evaluation, duration of incarceration of mentally ill prisoners (deprivation of liberty) on hospital orders and sentencing direction of mentally ill offenders. Overall, mental health laws in a fair number of African countries require improvement in a broad sense as well as in particularities related to mentally ill offenders.

References

Adjorlolo, S. (2016). Diversion of individuals with mental illness in the criminal justice system in Ghana. *International Journal of Forensic Mental Health, 15*(4), 382–392. https://doi.org/10.1080/14999013.2016.1209597

American Academy of Psychiatry and the Law. (2005). *Ethics guidelines for the practice of forensic psychiatry*. https://aapl.org/guidelines-and-practice-resources

American Psychiatric Association (2013). Diagnostic and statistical manual of mental disorders (DSM-5) (5th ed.). Arlington, VA: American Psychiatric Association.

Appelbaum, P. S., Lidz, C. W., & Klitzman, R. (2009). Voluntariness of consent to research: A conceptual model. *Hastings Center Report, 39*(1), 30–39. https://doi.org/10.1353/hcr.0.0103

Barber, P., Brown, R., & Martin, D. (2017). *Mental health law in England & Wales: A guide for mental health professionals* (3rd ed.). Learning Matters, An imprint of SAGE Publications Ltd.

Blackburn, R., Logan, C., Donnelly, J., & Renwick, S. (2003). Personality disorders, psychopathy and other mental disorders: Co-morbidity among patients at English and Scottish high-security hospitals. *The Journal of Forensic Psychiatry & Psychology, 14*(1), 111–137. https://doi.org/10.1080/1478994031000077925

Braude, H., & Kimmelman, J. (2012). The ethics of managing affective and emotional states to improve informed consent: Autonomy, comprehension and voluntariness. *Bioethics, 26*(3), 149–156. https://doi.org/10.1111/j.1467-8519.2010.01838.x

Buchanan, A. (2012). Forensic Psychiatry By Nigel Eastman, Gwen Adshead, Simone Fox, Richard Latham, and Sean Whyte. Oxford: Oxford University Press. 691 pp. *The Journal of the American Academy of Psychiatry and the Law, 42*(2), 267–268.

De Brito, S. A., Viding, E., Kumari, V., Blackwood, N., & Hodgins, S. (2013). Cool and hot executive function impairments in violent offenders with antisocial personality disorder with and without psychopathy. *PLoS ONE, 8*(6), e65566. https://doi.org/10.1371/journal.pone.0065566

Department of Health (2015). Mental Health Act 1983: Code of practice. London: TSO.

Doku, V. C. K., Wusu-Takyi, A., & Awakame, J. (2012). Implementing the mental health act in Ghana: Any challenges ahead? *Ghana Medical Journal, 46*(4), 241–250.

Duffy, R. M., & Kelly, B. D. (2017). Concordance of the Indian Mental Healthcare Act 2017 with the World Health Organization's Checklist on Mental Health Legislation.

International Journal of Mental Health Systems, *11*(1), 48. https://doi.org/10.1186/s13033-017-0155-1

Eastman, N., Adshead, G., Fox, S., Latham, R., & Whyte, S. (2012). *Oxford specialist handbooks in psychiatry: Forensic psychiatry* (1st ed.). New York: Oxford University Press Inc.

Elnemais Fawzy, M. (2015). Quality of life and human rights conditions in a public psychiatric hospital in Cairo. *International Journal of Human Rights in Healthcare*, *8*(4), 199–217. doi: https://doi.org/10.1108/ijhrh-02-2015-0006

Fistein, E. C., Holland, A. J., Clare, I. C. H., & Gunn, M. J. (2009). A comparison of mental health legislation from diverse Commonwealth jurisdictions. *International Journal of Law and Psychiatry*, *32*(3), 147–155. https://doi.org/10.1016/j.ijlp.2009.02.006

Fulford, K. M. (1998). Invited commentaries on: Mental health legislation is now a harmful anachronism. Replacing the Mental Health Act 1983? How to change the game without losing the baby with the bath water or shooting ourselves in the foot. *Psychiatric Bulletin*, *22*, 666–670.

Glover-Thomas, N. (2011). The age of risk: Risk perception and determination following the Mental Health Act 2007. *Medical Law Review*, *19*(4), 581–605. https://doi.org/10.1093/medlaw/fwr023

Goldman, H. H., & Grob, G. N. (2006). Defining "mental illness" in mental health policy. *Health Affairs*, *25*(3), 737–749. https://doi.org/10.1377/hlthaff.25.3.737

Gregory, S., Ffytche, D., Simmons, A., Kumari, V., Howard, M., Hodgins, S., & Blackwood, N. (2012). The antisocial brain: Psychopathy matters: A structural MRI investigation of antisocial male violent offenders. *Archives of General Psychiatry*, *69*(9), 962. https://doi.org/10.1001/archgenpsychiatry.2012.222

Grimes, A. L., McCullough, L. B., Kunik, M. E., Molinari, V., & Workman, R. H. (2000). Informed consent and neuroanatomic correlates of intentionality and voluntariness among psychiatric patients. *Psychiatric Services*, *51*(12), 1561–1567. https://doi.org/10.1176/appi.ps.51.12.1561

Jones, M. (2005). Can international law improve mental health? Some thoughts on the proposed convention on the rights of people with disabilities. *International Journal of Law and Psychiatry*, *28*(2), 183–205. https://doi.org/10.1016/j.ijlp.2005.03.003

Jones, R. (2014). *Mental Health Act manual* (17th ed.). London: Thomson Reuters (Professional) UK Limited.

Kelly, B. D. (2011). Mental health legislation and human rights in England, Wales and the Republic of Ireland. *International Journal of Law and Psychiatry*, *34*, 439–454.

Kendell, R. E. (2002). The distinction between personality disorder and mental illness. *British Journal of Psychiatry*, *180*, 110–115.

Lagos State Mental Health Law (2018). Ikeja: Lagos State Government.

Laws of the Federation of Nigeria (2004). Criminal Code Act CAP C38. Federal Ministry of Justice.

Leung, W.-C. (2002). Human Rights Act 1998 and mental health legislation: Implications for the management of mentally ill patients. *Postgraduate Medical Journal*, *78*, 178–181. https://doi.org/10.1136/pmj.78.917.178

Loza, N., & El Nawawi, M. (2012). Mental health legislation in Egypt. International Psychiatry, 9, 64–66.

Mason, J., & Laurie, G. (2013). Law and medical ethics (9th ed.). Oxford: Oxford University Press.

Mental Health Care Act (2002). Act No. 17 (South Africa). Pretoria: Department of Health.

Mental Health Act (1983). London: HMSO.
Mental Health Act (2000). Chapter 15:12 (Zimbabwe).
Mental Health Act (2009). Law No. 71 (Egypt). Official Gazette Issue 20, 14 May 2009. Cairo: Government of Egypt.
Mental Health Act (2012). Act 846 of the Parliament of the Republic of Ghana. Accra: Government Printer Assembly Press Ltd.
Mental Health Act (2019). Act No. 6 of 2019. Government of Zambia.
Morakinyo, V. (1977). The law and psychiatry in Africa. African Journal of Psychiatry, *3*, 91–98.
Munetz, M. R., & Griffin, P. A. (2006). Use of the sequential intercept model as an approach to decriminalization of people with serious mental illness. *Psychiatric Services, 57*(4), 6.
Ogunlesi, A. O., Ogunwale, A., Roos, L., De Wet, P., & Kaliski, S. (2012). Forensic psychiatry in Africa: prospects and challenges. African Journal of Psychiatry, *15*, 3–7.
Ogunwale, A. (2019). Involuntary mental health treatment in England and Wales: A rights-based critique of current legal frameworks and recommendations for reform. International journal of law and psychiatry, *66*, 101451. doi: 10.1016/j.ijlp.2019.101451.
Organisation of African Unity (1986). *African charter on human and peoples rights.*
Pilgrim, D. (2005). Defining mental disorder: Tautology in the service of sanity in British mental health legislation. *Journal of Mental Health, 14*(5), 435–443. https://doi.org/10.1080/09638230500270750
Ramlall, S. (2012). The Mental Health Care Act No 17–South Africa. Trials and triumphs: 2002-2012. *African Journal of Psychiatry, 15*(6), 407–410.
Rains, L. S., Zenina, T., Dias, M. C., Jones, R., Jeffreys, S., Branthonne-Foster, S., & Johnson, S. (2019). Variations in patterns of involuntary hospitalisation and in legal frameworks: an international comparative study. The Lancet Psychiatry, 6, 403–417.
Regier, D. A. (2003). Mental disorder diagnostic theory and practical reality: An evolutionary perspective. *Health Affairs, 22*(5), 21–27. https://doi.org/10.1377/hlthaff.22.5.21
Roberts, L. W. (2002). Informed consent and the capacity for voluntarism. *The American Journal of Psychiatry, 159*, 705–712.
Spagnolo, J., Champagne, F., Leduc, N., Piat, M., Melki, W., Charfi, F., & Laporta, M. (2017). Building system capacity for the integration of mental health at the level of primary care in Tunisia: a study protocol in global mental health. BMC Health Services Research, *17*(1), 38. doi: 10.1186/s12913-017-1992-y.
United Nations (1948). *Universal Declaration of Human Rights.* United Nations.
United Nations (1966). *International covenant on civil and political rights. General Assemby resolution 2200A.* https://www.ohchr.org/Documents/ProfessionalInterest/ccpr.pdf
United Nations (1991). *Principles for the protection of persons with mental illness and the improvement of mental health care.* United Nations, Secretariat Centre For Human Rights.
United Nations (2006). *Convention on the rights of persons with disabilities.* United Nations.
US Government Printing Office (1949). *US Government Printing Office. Tribunals of war criminals before the Nuremberg Military Tribunals under Control Council Law No. 10.* Washington DC: US Government Printing Office.
Veer, N. L. V. D., Drachman, D., Ahad, S., Silvers, G., & Ramos, G. (2011). Voluntariness to consent to research in a voluntarily and involuntarily hospitalised psychiatric population. *Journal of Empirical Research on Human Research Ethics, 6*(1), 55–61.

Walker, S., Mackay, E., Barnett, P., Sheridan Rains, L., Leverton, M., Dalton-Locke, C., Trevillion, K., Lloyd-Evans, B., & Johnson, S. (2019). Clinical and social factors associated with increased risk for involuntary psychiatric hospitalisation: A systematic review, meta-analysis, and narrative synthesis. *The Lancet Psychiatry*, *6*(12), 1039–1053. https://doi.org/10.1016/S2215-0366(19)30406-7

Wessely, S., Gilbert, S., Hedley, M., & Neuberger, J. (2018). *The independent review of the Mental Health Act: Interim report* (pp. 1–60). Crown copyright.

World Health Organization (1992). The ICD-10 Classification of Mental and Behavioural Disorders. Geneva: World Health Organization.

World Health Organization (1996). *Mental health care law: Ten basic principles. Geneva: World Health Organization, Division of Mental Health and Prevention of Substance Abuse.* https://www.who.int/mental_health/media/en/75.pdf

World Health Organization (Ed.). (2005). *WHO resource book on mental health, human rights and legislation.* World Health Organization.

World Health Organization (Ed.). (2018). *Mental health atlas 2017.* World Health Organization.

World Health Organization (2020). *WHO|Mental health atlas-2017 country profiles.* WHO; World Health Organization. http://www.who.int/mental_health/evidence/atlas/profiles-2017/en/

World Medical Association (2013). *Declaration of Helsinki—Ethical principles for medical research involving human subjects.*

Zhang, S., Mellsop, G., Brink, J., & Wang, X. (2015). Involuntary admission and treatment of patients with mental disorder. *Neuroscience Bulletin*, *31*(1), 99–112. https://doi.org/10.1007/s12264-014-1493-5

Part III

Special forensic populations

12 Mental health of children and adolescents within the juvenile justice system in Africa

Olayinka Atilola and Gbonjubola Abiri

Introduction

Adolescence is a critical period of developmental transition from childhood to adulthood, and it is characterized by rapid biological and emotional changes. It is a dynamic phase shaped significantly by interaction with the social environment such that it supports the acquisition of emotional, psychosocial, and cognitive abilities that transforms the child into an adult. Adolescence is associated with risk-taking behavior arising from immature impulse control brought about by the rapid physiological (often hormonal) chances taking place in their bodies, inadequate planning skills and the desire to "feel among" and belong to a community of peers (Thompson et al., 2012). However, in the presence of neurodevelopmental disability, trauma experiences, adversity and/or mental health difficulties, the child's developmental trajectory can be significantly hampered leading to an increased risk of delinquency and subsequent contact with the juvenile justice system.

Adolescents' predisposition to risk taking often arises as a result of underestimating the consequences of the risks they take, and they go ahead to do things they know are prohibited or even dangerous such as rough driving, drug use, risky sexual practices, violence and general defiance. These patterns of behavior are not necessarily delinquent, but they provide an explanation for why individuals who are within the adolescence age bracket are more likely to break the law than during later life. These adolescents engage in these behaviors not because they do not understand the potential risks, but because they do not foresee the potential short- and long-term consequences of what they do, which may include arrest and prosecution. By going against laid-down rules and regulations, adolescents become more prone to getting apprehended by those who are saddled with the responsibility of keeping the law, getting prosecuted and potentially interfacing with the juvenile justice system.

Juvenile delinquency

Juvenile delinquency is a major social and public-health issue and has gathered increasing attention over the last decade due to several factors. The Second United Nations Congress on the Prevention of Crime and the Treatment of Offenders recommends that the meaning of the term *juvenile delinquency* should be restricted as far as possible to violations of the criminal law (Morris, 1960). Generally, the juvenile delinquent is an individual within the age of adolescence who engages in a behavior or action that has been defined by law as illegal and/or who is determined "delinquent" by an appropriate court (Igbinovia, 1988). The prevalence of delinquent behavior peaks during the adolescent phase on the "age-crime curve," especially between the ages of 15 and 19, and adolescent delinquency is a strong predictor of adult criminality (Thompson et al., 2012). Up until 2015, there had been an increasing trend in the proportion of crimes committed by adolescents; and at the moment, the total population of young people within the juvenile justice system is still very high (Penal Reform International, 2015). One factor associated with the increasing attention on juvenile delinquency is the increasing globalization and pervasiveness of social media that has increased public awareness of crimes committed by juveniles, as news now spread rapidly and easily (Stouthamer-Loeber and Loeber, 2002).

Definition of a child

The definition of who is considered a child with respect to the justice system is one that varies from country to country in Africa. Across many of these countries, the definition is hinged on the age of the individual and often restricted to those under the age of 21 years. In the Tanzanian court system, a juvenile is considered as a person under the age of 12 years, and is assumed not to be criminally responsible for any act or omission except it can be proven that he/she had the capacity to know what should or should not be done regarding the act or omission (Igbinovia, 1988). Similarly, in neighboring Kenya, a child between the age of 7 and 16 years is considered a juvenile and cannot be tried in an adult court.

Nigeria is another African country that has multiple definitions of who a child (or juvenile) is across its subnational demarcations. The Child's Rights Act and other laws enacted after it recognizes a child as an individual younger than the age of 18 years (Bamgbose, 2014). This is followed in a few states such as Lagos and Ogun. In the southern part of the country, Akwa Ibom state defines a child as one younger than 16 years while several states in the northern part contend that a child is no more a child once he/she reaches puberty. These northern states consider a female to be an adult once the first menstrual flow takes place (Abifarin, Abdulrasaq, & Olayemi, no date), a position that is considered child abuse by child activists.

Despite the lack of consensus on who should be considered a juvenile, it is a known fact that approximately half of the African population is below 25 years, and this has significant implications for the numbers of young people involved in crime and at risk of contact with the juvenile justice system (Economic Commission for Africa, 2016).

Mental health and juvenile delinquency

Researchers have over the years tried to draw links between mental health and juvenile delinquency. Studies have pointed at a significantly large number of children and adolescents within the juvenile justice system with mental-health difficulties. More specifically, evidence from the USA, UK, Europe and Australia demonstrates a high prevalence of mental health problems among incarcerated juveniles. According to researchers, 60–80% of adolescents within the juvenile justice system have mental health challenges as compared with estimates of 7–12% in adolescents in the general population (Golzari, Hunt, & Anoshiravani, 2006; Roberts, Attkisson, & Rosenblatt, 1998). Data from Africa is not very different, with rates of mental and behavioral disorders among incarcerated young offenders ranging between 44% and 63% (Atilola, 2012a; Atilola et al., 2017).

These studies suggest an association between mental health problems and juvenile delinquency even though this may not suggest a causal relationship. Against this background, this chapter examines research investigating the potential explanations for the link between mental ill health and delinquency. It provides an overview of the burden of psychiatric morbidity among adolescents within the juvenile justice system across the African continent using illustrative data. It also discusses policy regarding providing mental health services with such systems and the challenges inherent within existing services. It concludes with recommendations in terms of identifying and effectively responding to the health and developmental needs of those within and at risk of becoming involved with the juvenile justice system in the region.

The juvenile justice system in Africa: A description

The juvenile justice system globally is set up on a philosophy of concern, care and reformation as a way of protecting and subjecting young offenders to reformation and rehabilitation programs within relatively controlled settings (Igbinovia, 1988). It can be summarized as a government's formal responsive arrangement to handle a child that has gotten in conflict with the law in line with set laws and procedures while taking care to consider the child's rights and best interests (Okech, 1989). The United Nations in 1985 approved the Standard Minimum Rules for the Administration of Juvenile Justice as a way of protecting the interest of the child, which has also been imbibed and reiterated by the African Charter on the Rights and Welfare of the Child (Bamgbose, 2014). These guidelines have been adopted across many African countries with slight variations in its adoption and implementation. Many of these countries have adopted the concept of "reformatory rehabilitation" where adolescents who fit the criteria are sent to correctional facilities and passed through a process of remediation.

The juvenile justice system across Africa is an area in which not much research has been done, but widely agreed to be an important component to the development and enhancement of the rule of law, nationally and globally. Across the African continent, the basic elements of national judicial systems for juveniles are similar, consisting of, at the minimum, a juvenile penal law, sanctions for juvenile crimes ranging from warnings or cautions to incarceration in correctional facilities and special procedures for handling juveniles. For instance, the Kenyan juvenile justice system is based on a penal code (Children Act No. 8 of 2001) that describes specific procedures for handling juvenile delinquents and combines a welfare approach and the justice model driven by the principle of the best interests of the child; and in Cameroon, the 2005 Code of Criminal Procedure contains several procedural protections and processes for handling children who have come in conflict with the law (Dankoff, 2011; Okech, 1989). Some of the key differences across countries however include the definition of the age bracket of juvenile offenders, types of sanctions and procedural rules for handling juvenile offenders and the focus of criminal policies.

As an illustration, the Nigerian juvenile justice system is one of the most documented and described systems for criminal justice for the underaged in Africa. It is a typical illustration of juvenile justice systems in Africa in which the police as well as social service, welfare, educational and mental health agencies serve as initial contact points of children and adolescents with the justice system. It recognizes and emphasizes the importance of the well-being of the child and adolescent, and ensures that their rights to privacy, due process and fair hearing are protected. The system comprises all individuals, institutions and relevant agencies working toward this same goal. Understanding how the system works in Nigeria will not be possible without considering some of the acts and laws underpinning it. The Children and Young Persons Ordinance enacted in 1943 is the foundation on which the country's juvenile justice system is based. The Act made provisions for the establishment of juvenile courts in the country as well as the welfare of juvenile offenders. The Child's Rights Act of 2003 further ensured proper treatment of children with respect to care and rehabilitation.

Like in many other African countries, the Nigerian Police Force is often the first point of contact with the country's juvenile justice system, as the offender may be directly apprehended by the police or handed over to the police when found to have infringed a law. Under applicable laws, the police take necessary measures to prevent the juvenile offender from coming in contact with an adult charged with an offense while in custody and prior to handing over to the juvenile courts. However, this rarely happens as the police hardly consider the need to protect children. Akinseye–George indicates that juvenile offenders are unfairly ascribed adult ages by the police as a way of justifying their detention in adult settings (Akinseye, 2009). Where the police act in line with existing guidelines, they hand over young offenders to the juvenile court which then adjudicate. The juvenile courts do not only attend to issues of juvenile offending, they also cater for children appearing as victims of abuses or neglect and who require welfare and protection. In line with the Child Rights' Act, proceedings of the court are often kept from public glare and are often in the best interest of the child.

The final point of call of children in contact with the juvenile justice system in Nigeria is a correctional facility or prison in extreme cases. The Child's Rights Act and similar laws provide for imprisonment of the child in the case of grievous crimes; otherwise, children are kept in remand homes and approved schools that have been established across the country (Bamgbose, 2014). Children stay in these facilities until they respond to the training or they reach their 18th birthday. Similar measures of handling juvenile offenders exist in many other

African countries where borstals and approved schools of reformation and rehabilitation/re-education are widely used. These institutions are targeted at keeping juvenile offenders out of prisons and providing them with a safe space for constructive and reformative education targeted at getting them prepared for a civilized life outside (Igbinovia, 1988).

Kenya runs a juvenile justice system similar to Nigeria. There, young offenders are sent to remand homes, and thereafter to correctional or approved schools, when vacancies are available. The focus of these institutions is reformation rather than punishment. These schools emphasize the need to stay away from antisocial conduct and teach the children prosocial behavior. First offenders who are 17 years old or younger and/or those considered to have committed a serious crime are sent to borstal institutions for rehabilitation instead of being imprisoned. The approach is a little different in the Ivory Coast, where the options of sentencing for juvenile delinquents are more varied. Juveniles who are 13 years or less may be sentenced to (i) placement in the care of parents, guardians, tutors or some other trustworthy adult; (ii) placement in a licensed medico-pedagogic facility; (iii) placement in an approved private or public educational institution, or vocational training facility; (iv) placement in an approved boarding school for young offenders of school age or (v) placement in the care of a Children's Aid Service (Igbinovia, 1988). Juvenile delinquents above the age of 13 years may be sentenced to any of the above or placed in a public correctional facility for supervised reformation/rehabilitation (Igbinovia, 1988).

In Uganda, there are four categories of correctional facilities for young offenders. These are prisons for young offenders, reformatory schools, approved educational facilities and remand homes, in order of decreasing gravity (United Nations Social Defence Research Institute, 1971). The first two are managed by the country's prisons service while the other two are administered by the Department of Community Development and Social Welfare. The young persons' prisons cater to adolescent males between 17 and 21 years and focus on getting them to participate in vocational training. These adolescents are required to participate in classes as well as sporting activities and compete with those from neighboring facilities. The reformatory schools, on the other hand, only admit males between the ages of 14 and 17 years who have been convicted of a criminal offense. The boys in these reformatory facilities are provided with remedial education that emphasizes vocational training and formal education. Upon discharge from the facility, the boys are supervised by the Probation Service for a period as determined by the court.

Approved schools and remand homes in Uganda are for adolescents with less serious offenses or requiring social protection. The schools provide character training, care, and guidance with the intent of stopping criminality and providing adjustment to those with behavioral and personality issues. The Ugandan remand homes serve four purposes: as temporary detention for adolescents with planned court hearings, observation facility for social welfare officers and those dealing with juvenile offenders to observe the behavior of juveniles within a secure environment, temporary probational facility (not longer than six months) for very young juveniles waiting to be matched to a foster home, and a temporary place of safety/protection (not longer than 12 months) for those suffering neglect and/or abuse.

While the justice system for young offenders across Africa have been set out in line with the United Nations' and the regional African Charter with respect to the administration of juvenile justice and protecting the interest of the child, available evidence indicates that many African countries have not been performing up to par in caring for young offenders adequately (Igbinovia, 1988). Juvenile justice systems on the continent are still rudimentary often tilting towards detaining both juvenile offenders (for reformation and rehabilitation) and victims of neglect/maltreatment (for protection) together in the same institution. In Nigeria, for instance, the inadequacy of correctional facilities has led to the detention of juvenile offenders in prisons even when what they have done does not deserve that. Furthermore, part of protecting the interest of the child is to ensure that the mental health of the juvenile is optimized and necessary provisions made to detect and respond quickly to mental health issues when they occur in children and adolescents. Sadly, the mental health needs of these juveniles in many African countries have not been properly served, often perpetuating adolescent's functional impairment and increasing recidivism, leading to a reduction in public safety.

Epidemiology of mental disorders among adolescents in Africa's juvenile justice system

Empirical evidence has indicated a rise in the prevalence rates of mental health challenges among young people in the general population over the last few decades (Atilola, Abiri, & Ola, 2019). This has been attributed in part to changes in the social context of growing children and adolescents (Fombonne, 1998). Globally, the average prevalence of mental health disorders in this population is about 20%, suggesting that one in every five young persons will have at least one mental health problem (Patel et al., 2007). The evidence shows an increase in the prevalence of mental disorders among youth within the JJS in high-income countries (Bronsard, Alessandrini, & Fond, 2016; Fazel, Doll, & Långström, 2008; Grisso, 2004). A similar picture appears to be emerging in Africa.

For instance, studies from Kenya have documented prevalence rates of current mental and behavioral morbidity of as high as 44.4% among juvenile offenders in correctional institutions (Maru, Kathuku, & Ndetei, 2003). In Nigeria, the psychiatric morbidity amongst incarcerated youths is as high as 67.6% (Atilola, 2012b). Atilola et al. (2019) particularly described youth correctional facilities in Nigeria as *"warehouses"* for youth mental and behavioral disorders because of the wide discrepancies in the prevalence rates of mental health conditions found in these facilities as compared with the rest of the general population of adolescents (Atilola et al., 2019). These results point to a huge unchecked mental health crisis in the juvenile justice system across the African continent. The common mental health problems that have been identified areas follows.

Mood and anxiety disorders

Mood disorders are some of the most commonly found mental health disorders among juvenile offenders in more developed countries with rates of about 33.3% for anxiety, 11% for depression and 40–50% for PTSD among young offenders as opposed to 0.2–3% prevalence rates among the general population who have not been in contact with the justice system (Ruchkin et al., 2002; Shufelt & Cocozza, 2006). Similar findings have also been documented amongst African juvenile populations. A Nigerian study investigating psychopathology and the psychosocial needs of children within the juvenile justice system found out that as much as 20.3–33% of the juvenile population had depressive symptoms and/or anxious preoccupations (Bella, Atilola, & Omigbodun, 2010). This is much higher than the prevalence rates of between 0.2% and 4.4% reported among the general population. In the same manner, the prevalence rates of PTSD among a cohort of Nigerian juvenile justice inmates was found to be as high as 5.8% for current PTSD and 9.7% for lifetime PTSD as opposed to 1.4% and 2.8% for current and lifetime PTSD, respectively, among similar aged controls in the general population (Atilola, Omigbodun, & Bella-Awusah, 2014a). This is not surprising as the lifetime exposure to traumatic events among the incarcerated youths were significantly more likely, with as much as 75% of them reporting exposure to at least one traumatic event.

Behavioral disorders

Attention-deficit hyperactivity disorder (ADHD), oppositional defiant disorder (ODD) and conduct disorder (CD) are a cluster of diagnostic categories characterized by distinctive features such as impulsivity and/or hyperactivity, inattention in ADHD; oppositional, hostile and negative behaviors in ODD and violation of the basic rights of other people in CD. Fazel, Doll, and Långström (2008) reported pooled prevalence rates of 18.5% to 52.8% for ADHD and CD, respectively, among adolescents in correctional facilities. Children and adolescents with these behavioral disorders often exhibit a higher frequency of physically aggressive behavior as compared with other individuals within the same age range. Unsurprisingly, the prevalence of ADHD and CD appears to be a lot higher in juvenile delinquents than comparable general populations. In fact, studies have pointed out CD to be the most prevalent mental health diagnosis in young offenders, with prevalence rates as high as 90% (Maniadaki & Kakouros, 2008).

In Africa, the figures are between 15% and 64%. A study assessing prevalence of disruptive behavioral disorders among youths at a Nigerian borstal institution reported that as much as 15.1% had ADHD, 64.2% had CD and 60.4% had ODD (Adegunloye et al., 2010). Similarly, another cross-sectional study reported prevalence rates of 56.5% of conduct disorders among another sample of incarcerated young offenders in Nigeria (Olashore, Ogunwale, & Adebowale, 2016). These figures are much higher than what is obtainable among the general population of adolescents. For instance, the prevalence of CD in a population of 885 secondary school children was found to be 15.8%, as opposed to the 64.2% and 56.5% documented among incarcerated adolescents (Frank-Briggs & Alikor, 2011).

Alcohol/substance-use disorder

Substance abuse is a major mental health problem affecting young people and has received increasing attention in recent time. In the United States and many other developed countries, at least one-third to one-half of the adolescent population have experimented with an illicit drug, with marijuana being the most commonly abused drug (Office of Applied Studies Substance Abuse and Mental Health Services Administration, 2002; Robertson, Dill, & Husain, 2004). McClelland et al. (2004) reported that approximately 50% of the 1829 randomly sampled young offenders at a temporary detention center abused two or more illicit substances, indicating a close relationship between substance-use disorder and juvenile delinquency.

Beyond studies conducted among Western populations, a recent study reported the lifetime prevalence rate of substance (including alcohol) abuse among adolescent in youth correctional facilities in Nigeria to be 22.5% (Atilola, Ola, & Abiri, 2016). This figure is similar to those reported by other Nigerian studies using similar study approaches: 28% prevalence rate among institutionalized adolescents in Ibadan (Atilola, 2012a) and 26.4% prevalence among adolescents in an Ilorin borstal home (Ajiboye et al., 2009). When compared with the 21% prevalence rate among school-going adolescents, the difference between incarcerated adolescents and those outside the juvenile justice system with respect to substance abuse is not so much. It is also important to note that the 22.5% lifetime prevalence rates of substance abuse among young offenders in Nigeria is much lower than the average prevalence rate of 50% reported among similar youths outside Nigeria. This may be due to potential recall bias in the Nigerian cohort as studies were conducted after about 12 months of incarceration, as opposed to other studies where data was collected shortly after the adolescents were incarcerated.

Neurodevelopmental disorders

Neurodevelopmental disorders become apparent early in an individual's life and characterized by different combination of functional impairments. Studies over the years have highlighted the link between neurodevelopmental disorders and criminality, especially with reports that more than 50% of juvenile offenders have difficulties with reading (Svensson, Lundberg, & Jacobson, 2001). Researchers estimate that 27–32% of young offenders had features indicative of learning or intellectual disability as opposed to a prevalence rate of 2–4% among the general adolescent population (Kroll et al., 2002; Rayner, Kelly, & Graham, 2005; Hughes et al., 2020).

In Nigeria, Atilola, Omigbodun, and Bella-Awusah (2014b) reported significantly lower average intellectual quotient (IQ) scores for remand home participants relative to controls (77±11 vs. 99±14; $p = 0.001$) indicating that adolescents in correctional facilities are more likely than their counterparts outside the juvenile justice system to have intellectual disabilities; which suggests a higher risk of neurodevelopmental disorders. In the same study, up to 22.4% of the institutionalized adolescents qualified for intellectual disability in contrast with an average of 2–4% in general populations.

Overall, studies examining the prevalence of mental health disorders among African juvenile offenders are scarce. However, the few available studies conducted on African juveniles suggest that there is indeed a higher prevalence of mental health challenges that require closer attention. As part of an ongoing systematic review of research on the mental health of adolescents within the juvenile justice system in Africa (Atilola, 2020), Table 12.1 shows the range of the prevalence rates of psychiatric disorders that have been reported.

Relationship between mental health and juvenile delinquency

The high prevalence rates of mental health disorders among juvenile delinquents suggests a relationship between the two concepts. However, there is as yet no firm understanding of this relationship. One major problem with trying to explain the relationship in question is the lack of consensus on the operational definition of some of the mental health and juvenile criminality concepts that determine how countries and their justice systems perceive and respond to problems of mental health in juveniles. Terms such as *"juvenile delinquency," "conduct disorder"* and *"antisocial behavior"* have been observed to be used interchangeably in a way that causes confusion (Tremblay, 2003). These terms represent distinct concepts that should not be mixed up. Conduct disorder is recognized by both the American Psychiatric Association (APA) and the World Health Organization (WHO) as a pattern of severe aggressive and anti-social behavior, and should be diagnosed only when a child or adolescent exhibits at least three of a set of 15 behaviors relating to theft, destruction of property, aggression or serious violations of existing rules (American Psychiatric Association, 2000). On the other hand, delinquency is a legal terminology that describes actions and behaviors relating to breaking the law and may include some of the behaviors that constitute conduct disorder, while anti-social behavior is a more generic term that summarizes aggression, delinquency, substance abuse, vandalism, noncompliance with existing rules, etc. (Maniadaki, Kakouros, & Karaba, 2009).

Following the distinction in the above terms, this chapter looks at the two most prevalent models that have tried to explain the relationship between mental health of adolescents and juvenile delinquency, with a focus on two causal hypotheses: (1) pre-existing social, demographic, and environmental risk factors for both juvenile delinquency and childhood neuro-psychiatric disorders intersects

Table 12.1 Range of psychiatric disorders that has been reported among adolescents within the juvenile justice system in Sub-Saharan Africa

	Lifetime prevalence rate (range)	*Number of studies*	*Current prevalence rate (range)*	*Number of studies*
Any psychiatric disorder	59.7–63.0%	3	22.0%	1
Any disruptive behavior disorders	40.8–63.1%	2	---	------
Conduct disorder	36.5–87.1%	6	----	-------
Oppositional defiant disorder	60.4%	1	------	--------
ADHD	15.1%	1	------	------
Any mood disorders	5.0–40.0%	2	------	----
Depression	11.3–35.8%	4	11.8–17.0%	2
Dysthymia	------	-----	7.5%	1
Suicidality	6.3–20.8%	2	------	------
Bipolar disorder	8.4%	1		
Any anxiety disorders	-----	----	14.2–27%	2
Generalized anxiety disorder	11.3–31.2%	2	4.7%	1
PTSD	9.7–11.6%	3	4.7%	1
Separation anxiety disorder	10.4%	1	-----	-----
Phobic anxiety disorder	------	-----	------	------
OCD	-------	-----	------	------
Panic disorders	8.3%	1	------	-----
Agoraphobia	10.4%	1	------	-----
Any alcohol/substance-use disorders	13.0–43.3%	4		
Any alcohol/substance use	88.0%	1	----	-----
Alcohol use	66.7%	1	-----	-------
Alcohol abuse/dependence	11.3–26.4%	3	------	------
Substance abuse/dependence	4.2–48.1%	6	-----	------
Neurodevelopmental disorders				
Intellectual development disorders	46.7%	1	-----	------
Specific learning disorders	----	-----	-----	------
Language/communication disorders	----	-----	-------	------
Autistic spectrum disorders	------	------	-------	------
Nocturnal enuresis	17.1%	1	------	----
Psychotic disorders	6.7–8.0%	3	---------	----

ADHD: Attention Deficit/Hyperactivity Disorder; PTSD: Posttraumatic Stress Disorder; OCD: Obsessive-Compulsive Disorder

and overlap, such that they co-produce the two phenomena (that is; juvenile delinquency and psychiatric disorders) in the same individual and (2) mental health disorders experienced by children and adolescents lead to juvenile delinquency and subsequent involvement with the juvenile justice system.

One can summarize the relationship between mental health disorders and juvenile delinquency as being one where the disorders arise as a consequence of involvement with the juvenile justice system. One evidence that supports this is the increased feeling of alienation, reduced self-esteem, anxiety and/or depression that adolescents placed in family-deprived, unfamiliar and restrictive settings commonly experience (Bohnstedt, 1978). It is not unsurprising to find adolescents in remand homes and other correctional facilities anxious and/or depressed at some point during their stay. In fact, researchers have documented significantly high prevalence rates of suicidal ideations and attempts among incarcerated juveniles (Junger-Tas, 1992). This goes further to corroborate the idea that placing children and adolescents in correctional facilities is a risk in itself for depression and potentially suicidal behavior.

Conversely, there are researchers who believe that incarceration only serves to unearth already existing symptoms of depression and other mental health disorders in adolescents. Anger and irritability that leads to subsequent delinquency have been identified as closely associated with adolescent depressive disorders (Knox et al., 2000). In the same vein, anger has been described as a motivator for aggressive and deviant behavior. In 1994, the APA made a provision to substitute "irritable mood" for "depressed mood" in response to the pervasiveness of irritability amongst adolescents with dysthymia and major depression (American Psychiatric Association, 1994). The expression of anger and irritability, which are motivators of aggressive behaviors, suggests that symptoms of depression may have been present even before the action that precipitates contact with the juvenile justice system have taken place. This makes it easy to surmise that placing a young person in a restrictive correctional environment may trigger the symptoms of depression (and potentially other mental health disorders) or precipitate a major episode of depression in an already vulnerable adolescent. Regardless of the side one chooses, there is evidence suggesting that factors within the juvenile justice system as well as vulnerability of some adolescents interact to precipitate mental health disorders in those incarcerated in juvenile justice facilities.

The second hypothesis describes the relationship as one where the symptoms of previously existing mental health disorders precipitate juvenile delinquency and contact with the justice system. Evidence that supports this hypothesis is the discovery that childhood traumatic brain injury increases the risk of involvement in crime when controlled for other factors (McKinlay et al., 2014). More specifically, a Swedish study reported that siblings who had experienced traumatic brain injury during childhood were two times more likely to be involved in a violent crime than their other siblings unaffected by the condition (Fazel et al., 2011). This study corrected for the effects of genetics and socio-economic factors that may confound the effects of traumatic brain injury, providing a strong evidence for the link with juvenile delinquency. Already, childhood traumatic brain injuries have been previously associated with functional deficits in behavior, social communication, cognition, empathy, impulse control and emotional response – all of which have been identified as harbingers of juvenile delinquency.

These two hypotheses underscore the significant overlap (co-variance) between the risk for mental and behavioral disorders among children and adolescents, and those for involvement with the juvenile justice system. For instance, family problems (instability, disruption, insufficiency, transitions, etc.), disruptive life changes (e.g., trauma and childhood adversity) and deprivation and want are risk factors for both juvenile justice contact and mental health disorders. The overlap will be better appreciated by examining each of the various categories of mental health disorders and how their psychopathologies relate closely with the risk factors of contact with the juvenile justice system.

Neurodevelopmental disorders

There are two considerations in understanding the link between neurodevelopmental disorders and adolescent offending. The first is that delinquency and neuro-developmental disorders share common risk factors (Maniadaki et al., 2009). For instance, children who grew up in an environment of rife psychosocial adversity are more likely to have poorer neuro-cognitive development; and they are also more likely to have poorer social adjustment and with a higher tendency towards delinquency (Svensson et al., 2001). The second consideration is the manifestations of neuro-developmental disorders being criminalized. Neuro-developmental disorders are associated with poor learning, truancy, poor school engagement and eventual dropout. Poor school engagement can make children and adolescents to divert their time and energy into something else, often in the context of antisocial behavior. Truancy can be categorized as a status offense, while children who are out of school are more likely to be in circumstances that puts them in conflict with the law. Retrospective studies of young offenders have pointed at a previous history of academic failure, truancy and high dropout levels (Maniadaki & Kakouros, 2008). On another note, the cognitive deficits and behavioral dysregulation that is sometimes associated with neuro-developmental disorders may increase the risk of engaging in violent behaviors due to poor judgment (Hammill, 1990). It is also thought that adolescents with poor neuro-cognitive abilities are more susceptible to negative peer influence and that they are easier to apprehend when involved in crime (Svensson et al., 2001).

Behavioral disorders

Youths with any of the behavioral disorders (attention deficit/hyperactivity disorder; ADHD, conduct disorder; CD, and oppositional defiant disorder; ODD) often exhibit physically aggressive behaviors at a more frequent rate than other youth populations. These behavioral manifestations can result in unlawful behavior, giving rise to delinquency and contact with the juvenile justice system. Longitudinal studies on disruptive behavioral disorders such as ADHD and CD have provided more evidence showing that the presence of ADHD and/or any other behavioral disorder is a predictor of later anti-social behavior (Moffitt, 1993). On the other hand, young offenders already in the system have been documented to suffer from these behavioral disorders at a more frequent rate than non-delinquents (Maniadaki & Kakouros, 2008). Some of the data presented previously indicates that CD is the most prevalent diagnosis for young offenders, with between 40% and 90% of them suffering from the disorder (Robertson et al., 2004). As explained earlier, this is not unexpected, as some of the criteria for diagnosing CD overlaps with features of juvenile delinquency. This is not to say however that CD is the only psychopathology that juvenile delinquents have as many have suggested (Maniadaki et al., 2009). Available evidence indicates that even after correcting for the presence of CD, up to 60% of juvenile delinquents still meet the criteria for a mental health disorder different from CD (Shufelt & Cocozza, 2006).

ADHD is another behavioral disorder common among juvenile delinquents. Longitudinal studies following children with ADHD into adolescence show that these children are more likely to become delinquents compared to those without ADHD (Sourander, Elonheimo, & Niemela, 2006). The co-existence of ADHD with CD or any other behavioral disorder has even been associated with an increased risk of arrest, conviction and incarceration of adolescents at a much early age than those with a single diagnosis of either CD or ADHD (Maniadaki et al., 2009). Also, the cognitive deficits that belie ADHD have been shown to not only slow learning of academic concepts but also impede the learning of prosocial rules and behaviors (Loeber, 1990).

This is of utmost importance in resource-poor African settings within which ADHD may not be diagnosed early enough. The combination of the underlying neurocognitive deficits of this disorder with the adverse psychosocial and economic environment in which the child is forced to grow up may place the child at a risk of repeated failures in school. With time, the child learns to hate school, avoid anything academic and drop out of school, all of which worsen learning difficulties. Other risk factors that increases the risk of juvenile delinquency include the drive for excitement, impulsivity, difficulty in understanding consequences of risky behavior, low threshold for frustration, inability to delay gratification and manage emotions, etc. (Sonuga, 2003).

Mood and anxiety disorders

When adolescents are removed from social environments they are used to (such as families and communities) and put in an unfamiliar and restrictive environment, it is easy to understand why they may become withdrawn and depressed (Robertson et al., 2004). However, it is also possible that the occurrence of mood disorders may precede incarceration. Research in developmental psychopathology suggests that there is a relationship between mood disorders and behavior problems. According to Bleiberg (1991), male juveniles are more likely to manifest their depression through aggressive behaviors, which supports previous propositions that depression may exacerbate or contribute to delinquency in some ways (Bleiberg, 1991). This is in line with data presented by Loeber that suggests that depression in children and adolescents may be a predictor of subsequent delinquency through the externalization of the symptoms of depression (Loeber, 1990). Symptoms of conduct disorder have been reported to occur much earlier in the life of depressed adolescents (Riggs et al., 1995). In addition, when a young person suffers from depression, his/her social functioning can be impaired in such a way that makes the adolescent more likely to engage in delinquent behavior.

Anxiety disorders, especially posttraumatic stress disorder (PTSD), are also common among justice-involved adolescents. This is linked to the fact that exposure to trauma, which is a fact of life for most children and adolescents within the juvenile justice system (Abram et al., 2007), is associated with anxiety disorders. Most of the children who end up within the juvenile justice system often come from family and environmental settings fraught with violence and adversities. A significant proportion are also exposed to various forms of violence in the course of their offending life or during incarceration. Studies have found higher prevalence rates, compared with a matched normative sample or national average among normative samples, among adolescents within the juvenile justice system (Atilola et al., 2014b).

Alcohol/substance-use disorder

As previously pointed out, the abuse of alcohol and other illicit substances is more prevalent amongst juvenile offenders. It is not clear how substance abuse leads to juvenile delinquency or vice versa. One way to look at this is to consider the risk factors of each. Psychosocial and economic challenges in the environment an adolescent grows up are known to increase the risk of juvenile delinquency. In the same way, these challenges also increased the risks of adolescents engaging in substance abuse (Siegel & Welsh, 2008). Adolescence is associated with a greater propensity for risky behaviors, one of which is substance abuse. But in the same way adolescents are more likely to engage in substance abuse, which is a deviant behavior, they are also more likely to engage in other deviant behavior that may bring them at crossroads with the law.

Neighbors, Kempton, and Forehand (1992) view substance abuse as deviant behavior that is more likely to be exhibited alongside other deviant behaviors, including those that constitute the criteria for disruptive behavioral disorders (Neighbors et al., 1992). The relationship between conduct disorders and substance abuse, especially among young offenders, has been described as strong (Shufelt & Cocozza, 2006); even though this relationship may be sequential instead of being causal. The existence of other mental health disorders increases the chance of substance abuse while substance abuse increases the risk of other mental health disorders. It is one coming up after the other rather than one being a cause of the other. Furthermore, both substance abuse and behavioral disorders have been associated with aggressiveness, impulsivity and thrill/novelty seeking, suggesting common genetic backgrounds (Kreek et al., 2005). The overlapping risk factors of both substance abuse and juvenile delinquency is in line with interrelationships between risk factors of other mental health disorders and juvenile delinquency.

Challenges with responding to the mental health crisis in Africa's juvenile justice system

While it is obvious that there is a huge mental health crisis in Africa's juvenile justice system, especially with the disproportionately high prevalence rates of mental health illnesses among incarcerated adolescents, addressing this problem is not so straightforward as there are a number of existential issues that countries still need to deal with. These challenges include the high prevalence of social and family problems that drive mental health problems and juvenile justice, insufficiency of community youth mental health resources and diversion programs and the lack of mental health services in many African juvenile facilities in spite of the fact that mental health problems are very common.

Firstly, all the myriads of environmental, social and family problems that co-produce mental disorders and juvenile justice contact are still alive and well in Africa. The combination of an extraordinarily large population of young people, together with chronic poverty and social inequality, is the right mix for youth crime, delinquency and criminalization. For instance, Nigeria is one of the countries with the lowest human development index (HDI) globally. Even though the country is currently recognized as having the largest economy on the continent following South Africa's fall into recession, recent reports indicate that between 60% and 90% of the country's population live below the poverty line (depending on the benchmark used: USD $1.25 to $2 per day) (Ogwumike & Ozughalu, 2018). Youth unemployment is still at an all-time high, estimated conservatively at 24% (according to official government data) (National Bureau of Statistics, 2010). Social inequality is also another major problem as the bulk of the country's financial resources is concentrated in the hands of the richest 10% of the population.

Ghana is another West African country that still battles problems with poverty and illiteracy. Recent data from the World Bank shows that the country has about 23% of its population living below the poverty line and a net human capacity index of 0.44 on a scale of 1 to 4. Even though youth literacy in Ghana is one of the highest on the continent, with 91.3% and 89.9% of males and females classified as being literate, youth unemployment is still a big issue (Adeniran, Ishaku, & Yusuf, 2020). Estimates from the country's statistical service indicates that only 53.7% of eligible youths are engaged in the labor force (World Bank, 2018). Several other Sub-Saharan countries have similar poor human development indices. In Uganda, about one-quarter of the population lives in poverty, and the Uganda Bureau of Statistics has pointed out that youth unemployment increased from 23% in 2002 to approximately 32% in 2012. Other countries such as Kenya, Tanzania and South Africa have reported similar figures pointing at adverse socioeconomic and environmental conditions in which many African children are brought up, and which continue to perpetuate the cycle of mental health disorders and juvenile delinquencies on the continent.

Secondly, the lack of community youth mental health resources and lack of diversion programs are contributing to the dumping of disadvantaged youth with mental health problems into the juvenile system. One would expect that with the recognition of the disproportionate prevalence of mental health disorders among youths in the juvenile justice system, countries will put necessary measures in place to optimize the mental health of young people before and after they get into the system. The reverse is often the case in many African settings. Researchers have repeatedly highlighted the lack of community-based diversion programs for young people in Nigeria and many other countries. The result of this is that youths arrested for status offenses (such as loitering around when they should be in school or staying out during a night curfew) and minor offenses (such as street hawking, non-aggressive stealing or trespassing) are incarcerated in correctional facilities with youths who have committed more serious offences. The appropriate thing to do is to divert such youths into non-incarcerating community programs like is being done in the United States and other better developed settings (Atilola et al., 2019).

Also, when children who do not meet the relevant criteria for incarceration continue to pile into correctional facilities, the end result is a severe stretch of an already strained juvenile justice system. For instance, the three available federal correctional facilities for young people in Nigeria are often overfilled and spill over into state-run remand homes and other rehabilitation centers. The continued mix of children who require protection with gross offenders in an overstretched system creates an environment in which mental health issues can be precipitated and perpetuated.

Closely related to the lack of community diversion programs in African juvenile justice systems is the rarity of mental health services within juvenile facilities. Even though mental health problems are common, effective, and efficient mental health services are hard to come by in many of the correctional facilities across Africa. One of the reasons for this is the dearth of youth mental health professionals on the continent. The few that are available are often overburdened and do not have the capacity to manage the burgeoning mental health crises within the system (Robertson et al., 2004).

Future directions

This chapter has provided evidence supporting the strong association between mental health disorders and juvenile delinquency. African youths with mental health disorders are at a high risk of coming in contact with the juvenile justice system in their respective countries. On the other hand, youths incarcerated in correctional facilities and other relevant institutions are more likely to have a mental health disorder precipitated and, in many cases, perpetuated. These facts point to the need to find ways to reduce the increasing prevalence of juvenile delinquency and associated mental health illnesses.

1. Addressing socio-economic disadvantage

Considering the significant overlaps in the risk factors of both mental health disorders and juvenile delinquency, one important solution is to address all relevant social and developmental risk factors that places children and young adults at increased risk of both mental health challenges and juvenile delinquency. Countries on the African continent need to address issues of poverty and illiteracy that appear to be fundamental problems across many African countries. With increasing evidence showing that socio-economic advantage confers some protection against mental health disorders, there is a need to fix issues such as community deprivation, youth unemployment, educational disengagement and family poverty.

2. Developing a framework for mental health services in the juvenile justice system

Beyond the underlying predisposing socio-economic factors, earlier intervention in suspected cases of mental health difficulties is another way to ensure that adolescents do not become involved in delinquency and subsequent contact with the justice system. In many African settings, there is a poor understanding and response to early warning signs of behaviors suggestive of a mental health disorder (Hughes et al., 2020). These behaviors are also more often than not warning signs of potential future delinquency, which if picked up on early enough, allows for measures to be put in place to address potential delinquent actions. A mental health service framework will be useful in this regard, and an optimal and robust framework will involve assessment, diagnosis, early intervention and follow-up.

Earlier identification of potential mental health challenges in incarcerated juveniles can be achieved through routine assessments of children at various points during their journey through the juvenile justice system, including when a child is first apprehended. Juveniles need to be monitored for potential mental health problems at set intervals and information shared between mental health services, health system, family support services and other key stakeholders involved in the process. With the introduction of routine assessments, diagnoses of mental health disorders are made earlier and faster, which in turn enables early intervention.

Early identification of potential behavioral challenges, and prompt response and provision for the health and developmental needs of children and adolescents significantly increases the chance of reducing the risk of contact with the criminal justice system. However, this will require an efficient and well-coordinated system where parents, caregivers and teachers are aware and sensitive to potential behavioral problems of their children and wards; and information sharing and referrals take place seamlessly between educational institutions, mental health services, health systems and families/family support services.

3. Making a case for diversion programs

The peculiarities of the juvenile justice system across Africa, which has a problem of poor distinction between children with mental health problems and overstretched juvenile incarceration facilities, indicates the need for community-based diversion programs. Diversion programs run by non-governmental organizations and community-based organizations across Africa have been shown to be cost-effective options of reducing the risk of recidivism and getting young people the help they need to be weaned off delinquent behavior and adapt seamlessly to proper adult life (Atilola, 2013). The involvement of communities in this model has been demonstrated to be even more beneficial. For instance, Uganda's Village Resistance Committee Courts managed by elders in the community have been found to provide a familiar environment for a child under "trial" as well as give the community a sense of responsibility in the training of "their own child" (Andersson & Stavrou, 2010). An ideal model of a diversion program is one in which the state and community collaborate to provide a rehabilitation platform that takes into consideration the local context and meets the peculiar needs of children and adolescents at all levels – local, regional and/or national.

As pointed out earlier, many of the children and adolescents who find themselves in the juvenile justice system have significant health and developmental difficulties. This means that the juvenile justice is directly or indirectly the primary service provider for the mental health needs of these children. Unfortunately, these needs are often not being met across many African settings. There is a need for countries to address these needs in a systematic way by providing routine screening for mental health challenges to all children and adolescents prior to entering the system and within the system. One option to consider is to set up mental health services/posts manned by well-trained staff within juvenile correctional facilities. Such outposts serve as a primary point to address all mental health challenges experienced by the wards of the system. However, this option will be feasible in a situation where there are enough mental health professionals trained to manage children and adolescents. Available evidence suggests these types of professionals are few and far between (Robertson et al., 2004).

Conclusion

There is no one-size-fits-all approach to solving the problems of the burgeoning mental health crises in Africa's juvenile justice system. Each country needs to conduct in-depth situational analysis to understand what is driving the problem and develop contextualized solutions. This chapter presents an important bird's eye view of the problem, provides potential considerations for solving the problem, and serves as a guide for African nations to use in reforming their criminal justice systems, especially for children and adolescents. Countries need to set up diversion programs to address specific problems of juveniles and separate actual offenders from victims, support capacity building interventions and trainings for mental health professionals and incorporate mental health services into the juvenile justice system. These are crucial to addressing health and developmental needs of children and adolescents and, in the long run, reducing criminalization among young people.

References

Abifarin, O., Abdulrasaq, F. F., & Olayemi, S. (no date). *Reflections on marriageable age, child marriage, Child Rights Act and the health of the child in Nigeria.* Retrieved from https://unilorin.edu.ng/publications/abdulrasaqff/Reflections_on_marriageable_age_Child_Rights_Act.pdf.

Abram, K. M. et al. (2007). Posttraumatic stress disorder and psychiatric comorbidity among detained youths. *Psychiatric Services, 58,* 1311–1316.

Adegunloye, O. A. et al. (2010). Prevalence and correlates of disruptive behavior disorders in youths in a juvenile Borstal Institution. *Nigerian Journal of Psychiatry, 8*(3), 12–17.

Adeniran, A., Ishaku, J., & Yusuf, A. (2020). Youth employment and labor market vulnerability in Ghana: Aggregate trends and determinants. In M., McLean (Ed.) *West african youth challenges and opportunity pathways. Gender and cultural studies in Africa and the diaspora.* Cham: Palgrave Macmillan.

Ajiboye, P. O. et al. (2009). Current and lifetime prevalence of mental disorders in a juvenile Borstal Institution in Nigeria., *Research Journal Medical Science, 3*(1), 26–30.

Akinseye, Y. (2009). *Juvenile justice system in Nigeria.* Abuja, Nigeria: Center for Socio-Legal Studies.

American Psychiatric Association (1994). *Diagnostic and statistical manual of mental disorders* (4th ed.). Washington, DC: American Psychiatric Association.

American Psychiatric Association (2000). *Diagnostic and statistical manual of mental disorders* (4th ed.). Washington, DC: American Psychiatric Press Inc.

Andersson, C., & Stavrou, A. (2010). *Youth* delinquency and the criminal justice sys*tem in Dar Es Salaam, Tanzania: A* snap shot sur*vey*. Nairobi: Safer Cities Programme.

Atilola, O. (2012a). Different points on a continuum? Cross sectional comparison of the current and Pre-contact Psychosocial problems among the different categories of adolescence in institutional care in Nigeria. *BMC Public Health, 12,* 554.

Atilola, O. (2012b). Prevalence and correlates of psychiatric disorders among residents of a juvenile remand home in Nigeria: Implications for mental health service planning. *Nigerian Journal of Medicine, 21*(4), 416–426.

Atilola, O. (2013). Juvenile/youth justice management in Nigeria: Making a case for diversion programmes. *Youth Justice, 13*(1), 3–16.

Atilola, O. et al. (2017). Status of mental-health services for adolescents with psychiatric morbidity in youth correctional institutions in Lagos. *Journal of Child and Adolescent Mental Health, 29*(1), 63–83.

Atilola, O. (2020). Psychiatric morbidity among adolescents and youth involved with the juvenile justice system in sub-Saharan Africa: Systematic scoping review of current studies and research gaps. *Journal of Law and Psychiatry, 73,* https://doi.org/10.1016/j.ijlp.2020.101633.

Atilola, O., Abiri, G., & Ola, B. (2019). The Nigerian juvenile justice system: From warehouse to uncertain quest for appropriate youth mental-health service model. *British Journal of Psychiatry, 16*(1), 63–83.

Atilola, O., Ola, B., & Abiri, G. (2016). Service and policy implication of substance use disorders among adolescents in juvenile correctional facilities in Lagos, Nigeria. *Global Mental Health, 3,* e30. doi: https://doi.org/10.1017/gmh.2016.25.

Atilola, O., Omigbodun, O., & Bella-Awusah, T. (2014a). Post-traumatic stress symptoms among juvenile offenders in Nigeria: Implications for holistic service provisioning in juvenile justice administration. *Journal of Health Care for the Poor and Underserved, 25,* 991–1004.

Atilola, O., Omigbodun, O., & Bella-Awusah, T. (2014b). Neurological and intellectual disabilities among adolescents within a custodial institution in South-West Nigeria. *Journal of Psychiatric and Mental Health Nursing*, *21*(1), 31–38.

Bamgbose, O. (2014). *Re-evaluating the juvenile/child justice system in Nigeria, Nigerian Institute of Advanced Legal Studies (NIALS)*. Abuja: Nigerian Institute of Advanced Legal Studies.

Bella, T., Atilola, O., & Omigbodun, O. (2010). Children within the juvenile justice system in Nigeria: Psychopathology and psychosocial needs. *Annals of Ibadan Postgraduate Medicine*, *8*(1 SRC-GoogleScholar FG-0), 34–39.

Bleiberg, E. (1991). Mood disorders in children and adolescents. *Bulletin of the Menninger Clinic*, *55*(2), 182–204.

Bohnstedt, M. (1978). Answers to three questions about juvenile diversion. *The Journal of Research in Crime and Delinquency*, *15*(1), 109–123.

Bronsard, G., Alessandrini, M., & Fond, G. (2016). The prevalence of mental disorders among children and adolescents in the child welfare system: A systematic review and meta-analysis. *Medicine*, *95*(7), e2622.

Dankoff, J. (2011). An assessment of Cameroon's justice system for children: Formal and Traditional responses to children in conflict with the law and child victims. Retrieved from http://www.youthmetro.org/uploads/4/7/6/5/47654969/cameroon_final_assessment_17.1.11.pdf.

Economic Commission for Africa. (2016). *The demographic profile of African countries*. Addis Ababa, Ethiopia: United Nations Economic Commission for Africa.

Fazel, S. et al. (2011). Risk of violent crime in individuals with epilepsy and traumatic brain injury: A 35-year Swedish population study. *PLoS Med*, *8*(12), e1001–e1150.

Fazel, S., Doll, H., & Långström, N. (2008). Mental disorders among adolescents in juvenile detention and correctional facilities: A systematic review and metaregression analysis of 25 surveys. *Journal of the American Academy of Child Adolescent Psychiatry*, *47*(9), 1010–1019.

Fombonne, E. (1998). Increased rates of psychosocial disorders in youth. *European Archives of Psychiatry and Clinical Neuroscience*, *248*, 14–21.

Frank-Briggs, A. I., & Alikor, E. A. D. (2011). Sociocultural issues and causes of cerebral palsy in Port Harcourt, Nigeria. *Nigerian Journal of Paediatrics*, 38, 115–119.

Golzari, M., Hunt, S. J., & Anoshiravani, A. (2006). The health status of youth in juvenile detention facilities. *Journal of Adolescent Health*, *38*, 776–782.

Grisso, T. (2004). *Double jeopardy: Adolescent offenders with mental disorders*. University of Chicago Press.

Hammill, D. D. (1990). On defining learning disabilities: An emerging consensus. *Journal of Learning Disabilities*. Sage Publications Sage UK: London, England, *23*(2), 74–84.

Hughes, N. et al. (2020). Health determinants of adolescent criminalisation. *The Lancet Child & Adolescent Health*, *4*(2), 1–12.

Igbinovia, P. (1988). Perspectives on juvenile delinquency in Africa. *International Journal of Adolescence and Youth*, *1*(2), 131–156.

Junger-Tas, J. (1992). An empirical test of social control theory. *Journal of Quantitative Criminology*, 8, 9–28.

Knox, M. et al. (2000). Aggressive behavior in clinically depressed adolescents. *Journal of the American Academy of Child and Adolescent Psychiatry*, *39*, 611–618.

Kreek, M. J. et al. (2005). Genetic influences on impulsivity, risk taking, stress responsivity and vulnerability to drug abuse and addiction. *Nature Neuroscience*, *8*(11), 1450–1457.

Kroll, L. et al. (2002). Mental health needs of boys in secure care for serious or persistent offending: a prospective, longitudinal study. *The Lancet, 359*, 1975–1979.

Loeber, R. (1990). Development and risk factors of juvenile antisocial behavior and delinquency. *Clinical Psychology Review, 10*, 1–41.

Maniadaki, K., & Kakouros, E. (2008). Social and mental health profiles of young male offenders in detention in Greece. *Criminal Behaviour and Mental Health*, 18, 207–215.

Maniadaki, K., Kakouros, E., & Karaba, R. (2009). Juvenile delinquency and mental health. In A. Kakanowski & M. Narusevich (Eds.) *Handbook of social justice* (pp. 1–44). New York, USA: Nova Science Publishers, Inc.

Maru, H. M., Kathuku, D. M., & Ndetei, D. M. (2003). Psychiatry morbidity among children and young persons appearing in the Nairobi juvenile court Kenya. *East African Medical Journal, 80*(6), 281.

McClelland, G. M. et al. (2004). Multiple substance use disorders in juvenile detainees. *Journal of the American Academy of Child Adolescent Psychiatry, 43*, 1215–1224.

McKinlay, A. et al. (2014). Substance abuse and criminal activities following traumatic brain injury in childhood, adolescence, and early adulthood. *The Journal of Head Trauma Rehabilition, 29*, 498–506.

Moffitt, T. E. (1993). Adolescence-limited and life-course-persistent antisocial behavior: A developmental taxonomy. *Psychological Review, 100*(4), 674–701.

Morris, T. P. (1960). Second United Nations congress on prevention of crime and the treatment of offenders. *The British Journal of Criminology*, HeinOnline, *1*, 261.

National Bureau of Statistics. (2010). *Statistical news: Labor force statistics.* Abuja: The NBS Publication.

Neighbors, B., Kempton, T., & Forehand, R. (1992). Co-occurrence of substance abuse with conduct, anxiety, and depression disorders in juvenile delinquents. *Addictive Behaviors, 17*(4), 379–386.

Office of Applied Studies Substance Abuse and Mental Health Services Administration. (2002). *National survey on drug use and health.* Washington, DC: Office of Applied Studies, Substance Abuse and Mental Health Services Administration.

Ogwumike, F., & Ozughalu, U. (2018). Empirical evidence of child poverty and deprivation in Nigeria. *African Development Review, 77*(1), 12–22.

Okech, C. (1989). *The juvenile justice in Kenya: Growth, system, and structures.* Nairobi: United Nations Asia and Far East Institute.

Olashore, A. A., Ogunwale, A., & Adebowale, T. O. (2016). Correlates of conduct disorder among inmates of a Nigerian Borstal Institution. *Child and Adolescent Psychiatry and Mental Health, 10*, 13.

Patel, V. et al. (2007). Mental health of young people: A global public-health challenge. *The Lancet, 369*, 1302–1313.

Penal Reform International. (2015). Global prison trends. Penal Reform International. Retrieved from https://www.penalreform.org/resource/global-prison-trends-2015/.

Prichard, J., & Payne, J. (2005). *Alcohol, drugs and crime: A study of juveniles in detention.* Canberra: Australian Institute of Criminology.

Rayner, J., Kelly, T. P., & Graham, F. (2005). Mental health, personality and cognitive problems in persistent adolescent offenders require long-term solutions: A pilot study. *The Journal of Forensic Psychiatry & Psychology*, 16, 248–262.

Riggs, P. D. et al. (1995). Depression is substance-dependent delinquents. *Journal of the American Academy of Child and Adolescent Psychiatry, 34*, 764–771.

Roberts, R. E., Attkisson, C. C., & Rosenblatt, A. (1998). Prevalence of psychopathology among children and adolescents. *The American Journal of Psychiatry*, *155*, 715–725.

Robertson, A., Dill, P., & Husain, J. (2004). Prevalence of mental illness and substance abuse disorders among incarcerated juvenile offenders in Mississippi. *Child Psychiatry and Human Development*, *35*(1), 55–74.

Ruchkin, V. V. et al. (2002). Violence exposure, posttraumatic stress, and personality in juvenile delinquents. *Journal of the American Academy of Child & Adolescent Psychiatry*. Elsevier, *41*(3), 322–329.

Shufelt, J., & Cocozza, J. (2006). *Youth with mental health disorders in the juvenile justice system: Results from a multi-state prevalence study*. New York, USA: National Center for Mental Health and Juvenile Justice.

Siegel, L. J., & Welsh, B. C. (2008). *Juvenile delinquency: The core* (3rd ed.). Belmont, CA: Wadsworth Cengage Learning.

Sonuga, B. E. (2003). The dual pathway model of AD/HD: an elaboration of neuro-developmental characteristics. *Neuroscience & Biobehavioral Reviews*, 27(7), 593–604.

Sourander, A., Elonheimo, H., & Niemela, S. (2006). Childhood predictors of male criminality: A prospective population-based follow-up study from age 8 to late adolescence. *Journal of the American Academy of Child and Adolescent Psychiatry*, *45*(5), 578–586.

Stouthamer-Loeber, M., & Loeber, R. (2002). Lost opportunities for intervention: Undetected markers for the development of serious juvenile delinquency. *Criminal Behaviour and Mental Health*, *12*, 69–82.

Svensson, I., Lundberg, I., & Jacobson, C. (2001). The prevalence of reading and spelling difficulties among inmates of institutions for compulsory care of juvenile delinquents. *Dyslexia*, *7*, 62–76.

Thompson, M. E. et al. (2012). *Child and adolescent mental health: Theory and practice*. London, UK: Hodder Arnold.

Tremblay, R. E. (2003). Why socialization fails: The case of chronic physical aggression. In B. B. Lahey, T. E. Moffitt, & A. Caspi (Eds.), *Causes of conduct disorder and juvenile delinquency* (pp. 182–226). New York: The Guilford Press.

United Nations Social Defence Research Institute. (1971). *Social defence in Uganda: A survey for research*. Rome.

World Bank. (2018). *World development indicators*. Retrieved from http://datatopics.worldbank.org/world-development-indicators/ (Accessed 20 March 2020).

13 Forensic mental health care services for the elderly in Africa

Emmanuel Oluyinka Majekodunmi and Aishatu Yusha'u Armiya'u

Introduction

Prison remains a harsh environment for anyone, significantly so for those who are aging (Fazel, Hope, O'Donnell, & Jacoby 2001; Chiu, 2010). Elderly prisoners constitute a group of vulnerable individuals in correctional institutions with more propensities for the negative effect of incarceration with its attendant public health problems. In Sub-Saharan Africa, the number of older persons has doubled since 1990 and is projected to more than triple between 2015 and 2050 (United Nations, Department of Economic and Social Affairs, Population Division, 2015). Studies on the other hand have reported an increase in the number of elderly prisoners across the globe and could be a reflection of the growth of ageing populations outside prison (Fazel, Hayes, Bartellas, Clerici, & Trestman, 2016; Pro & Marzell, 2017). This increase in the number of elderly prisoners has also been noted in African countries (Obioha, 2011; Omale, 2011; Ojo & Okunola, 2014), although the data supporting this observation is not readily available. Changes in legal systems such as modifications in sentencing practices have been reported to be among the causes of such a rise (Vogel, Languillon, & Graf, 2013). These modifications have manifested as the hardening of sentencing practices, the increased use of imprisonment and reduced mechanisms for early release in some countries. They may also be demonstrated by longer prison terms being handed down by the courts under mandatory sentencing laws. In a recent report, the observation about the rise in the number of aging prisoners was made as follows: "*The increasing warehousing of aging prisoners for low-level crimes and longer sentences is a nefarious outgrowth of the 'tough on crime' and 'war on drugs' policies of the 1980s and 1990s*" (ACLU, "The Mass Incarceration of the Elderly," 2012, 2).

In some societies, it is reported that the gradual breakdown of traditional family and community ties has led to older persons turning to crime due to poverty and isolation (Onishi, 2007). Even though there is a dearth of empirical studies on factors responsible for the growing rate of elderly prisoners in Africa, worsening socio-economic conditions and social neglect of the aged have been reported to account for the increasing numbers of elderly offenders in the criminal justice system (Kumolu, 2012). Unfortunately, these factors that are currently unrelenting may contribute to a continued growth in the older prison population in many countries worldwide, including those in Africa.

According to Loeb and Abudagga (2006), prisoners who are 50 years and older have accounted for the most rapidly increasing age group among prisoners. In more developed economies, the number of prisoners aged 55 and above increased by 400% from 26,300 in 1993 to 131,500 in 2013 (Bureau of Justice Statistics, 2016). On the other hand, prisoners aged 65 and above recorded 94 times the rate of growth in overall prison population between 2007 and 2010 (Fellner, 2012). Among incarcerated prisoners, older prisoners with mental illness are not just the fastest-growing sub-population, but also the ones with the worst health outcomes (Chodos, Ahalt, Cenzer, Myers, Goldenson, & Williams, 2013; Pro & Marzell, 2017).

Elderly prisoners are more prone to health-related conditions and thus incure higher costs of care. One of the leading costs specific to them is that related to the provision of mental health services for dementia, anxiety disorders and schizophrenia (Maschi, Kwak, Ko, & Morrissey, 2012; Maschi & Aday, 2014). Recent literature on the cost of care for elderly prisoners with such diagnoses shows that it is about three times the cost of caring for an average healthy elderly inmate (Maschi, Viola, & Sun, 2013; Swanson, Frisman, Robertson, & Lin, 2013). Other costs include indirect costs related to prison conditions, such as lack of ventilation and poor temperature regulation that often worsen medical problems for elderly inmates (Reimer, 2008). In line with the factors highlighted by Reimer (2008), attention was also drawn by Maschi and Aday (2014) in arguing that poor confinement conditions for older persons could represent a type of elder abuse and neglect.

The majority of elderly prisoners are likely to have lost touch with their families and friends, who have either died or are no longer strong enough to visit while others could have moved on with their lives. For this population, health concerns are rampant and feeling isolated in that situation is possible. In the prison, the opportunity to enjoy the small things in life, as inmates grow older, is gradually lost. It instead becomes an unceasing grind in which one is forced to endure unstimulating, routinized and frequently unsanitary custodial environments.

Managing elderly prisoners is one of the most significant and unplanned crises in the correctional system (Williams, 2012). The Human Rights Watch puts it this way:

> *Life in prison can challenge anyone but it can be particularly hard for people whose bodies and minds are being whittled away by age. Prison around the world contain an ever growing number of aging men and women who cannot readily climb stairs, haul themselves to the top bunk, or walk distances to meals or the pill line; whose old bones suffer from thin mattresses and winters cold; who need wheelchairs, walkers, canes, portable oxygen, and hearing aids; who cannot get dressed, go to the bathroom, or bath without help; and who are incontinent, forgetful, suffering chronic illness, extremely ill and dying.*
>
> (Human Rights Watch, Old Behind Bars, 2012, p. 4)

Though the aging population in prison had been more of a problem in developed countries where life expectancy has steadily and significantly increased, it is also becoming a problem in developing countries, such as those in Africa, largely due to the increasing use of custodial sentences (Williams, 2012).

The concept of elderly inmates

Defining elderly inmates is a challenging exercise. There is currently no consensus on what constitutes the lower age limit for "older," or "elderly," inmates. Different studies and correctional facilities have used different ages, varying from as low as 40 to as high as 65. Some authors placed the lower limit at 50 years (Aday, 2003; Luallen & Kling, 2014). Some chose 55 years and over, while others, mostly from Europe, used the higher age limit of 60 years (Fazel, Hope, O'Donnell, & Jacoby, 2001; Fazel & Danesh, 2002; Fazel & Grann, 2002; Chodos, Ahalt, Cenzer, Myers, Goldenson, & Williams, 2014). In some other cases, the age of 65 is considered the basal limit (Tomar, Treasaden, & Shah, 2005). Setting the age threshold for defining the elderly inmate is therefore almost an arbitrary determination (Fazel & Grann, 2002; Loeb & Abudagga, 2006). Evidently, this makes comparison across studies difficult. However, in most literature, particularly in North America from where most studies on elderly offenders emanate, the age threshold of 50 years is commonly used. For Africa, the 50-year lower limit might be more plausible when consideration is made of the average life expectancy of most countries on the continent.

What types of crimes do elderly offenders commit?

A study conducted at Kakamega Main Prison, Kenya in 2015 reported that 58% of the elderly prisoners had committed the crime of rape, 16% had committed capital offenses and 10% were charged with theft. Others included assault, burglary and drug trafficking. In a recent Nigerian study by Majekodunmi, Obadeji, Oluwole, and Oyelami (2017), 64.7% of the inmates had committed or were charged with violent crimes. Murder/manslaughter and armed robbery accounted for 56.3% and 27.3% of the offenses, respectively. In South Africa, the majority of elderly offenders were sentenced for aggressive crimes (assault, culpable homicide, murder, attempted murder, robbery), followed by sexual crimes (sexual assault, intercourse with a minor, rape, attempted rape), economic crimes (car theft, breaking and entering, fraud and forgery, livestock theft) and narcotic-related crimes (possession, distribution and manufacturing of illegal substances). It appears that common offences committed by elderly prisoners in African settings include rape, theft and assault.

This pattern is comparable with that reported in a study in England and Wales where the majority of elderly prisoners aged 50 and above were serving prison sentences for sexual offences compared to all prisoners serving the same prison sentence (Omolade, 2014).

Demographic information

Demographic information on elderly prisoners in Africa is scarce due to paucity of research in the area. In 2010, however, a total number of 722 inmates (sentenced offenders *and* remand detainees) older than 61 years were incarcerated in South Africa; this number increased to 744 in 2011, 778 in 2012, 862 in 2013, 996 in 2014 and 2015, the total number of incarcerated elderly offenders (sentenced offenders and remand detainees) was 1065. Though there are no official statistics to support their claims, recent studies in Nigeria affirm the growing rate of elders in Nigeria prisons (Obioha, 2011; Omale, 2011; Ojo & Okunola, 2014). The findings are similar to those of a longitudinal study conducted in England and Wales in 2004–2014. Prisoners aged 60 years and above were observed to be the fastest-growing age group, followed by those aged 50–59 years (104% increase) (Omolade, 2014). In the United States, there were 14 times as many incarcerated individuals who were at least 55 years old in 2011 as were found in 1981, and it has been estimated that by 2030, more than one-third of the entire prison population will be individuals aged 55 years or older according to Skarupski, Gross, and Schrack (2018).

The few studies in African countries commenting on the socio-demographic characteristics of prisoners showed an overwhelming majority of elderly offenders in prison being males. Most were relatively elderly before incarceration. About 60% of elderly prisoners (above 50 years) reported never being sentenced to prison previously, compared to younger prisoners (Omolade, 2014; Langat et al., 2015; Aborisade et al., 2016). Mostly they were within the age group of 55–60 years, and were frequently married (Omolade, 2014; Aborisade et al., 2016). In terms of prison status, most of them were awaiting trial. In a study conducted within five federal prisons in Nigeria, Majekodunmi et al. (2017) equally observed that the average age of elderly prisoners was about 59 years, with 62% of them being between 50 and 59 years old. All of them were male and most were married (85%) within a monogamous context (62.4%). The majority were employed prior to incarceration (91%) but had little or no education (61.2%). A slim majority of the study participants were awaiting trial (54%).

A similar age distribution was found in a Kenyan study but 34% of the elderly prisoners were reported to be either divorced or separated (Langat et al., 2015). This finding with regard to marital difficulties among elderly prisoners appears to be supported by Njeru (2009) who observed that crime was relatively caused associated family breakdown. One elderly offender reported that *"my wife left me when i was arrested and taken to prison. My neighbors burned my houses because of the crime i had committed by killing my brother over a land dispute."* The same study found that four out of ten elderly prisoners did not know how to read or write (Langat et al., 2015). This is an indicator that quite a number of the elderly offenders had little or no education. This was in contrast to a study in England and Wales where older offenders were more likely to report higher levels of education and were about four times more likely to have completed apprenticeship than young offenders (Omolade, 2014). They were also less likely to require help to complete their education or work-related skills.

A study from Kenya by Sereria reported that the statistics of elderly offenders from Kenyan prisons indicated that over 5000 offenders were either under life imprisonment or facing the death penalty, and the number might increase significantly. Over half of those convicted, in the Majekodunmi et al. (2017) study, were also facing the death penalty. These findings appear to be corroborated by a study from England and Wales in which older offenders were found to be serving long terms in prison (Omolade, 2014).

Overall morbidity among elderly prisoners

Elderly inmates are more likely to have health-related problems such as hypertension, pneumonia, diabetes, gastritis, arthritis, cancer, kidney and heart problems and bladder and prostate problems. It has also been found that elderly offenders may suffer from an average of three chronic illnesses while incarcerated (Aging Inmate Committee, 2012; Stal, 2012; Maschi, Viola, & Sun, 2013). The most prevalent reported medical problems among prisoners aged 45 years and older were arthritis (30.5%), hypertension (29.5%), heart problems (13.1%), tuberculosis (13.0%), diabetes (12.1%) and hepatitis (9.8%) (Bureau of Justice Statistics, US Department of Justice, 2008). According to Aborisade et al. (2016), most elderly prisoners have hypertension, diabetes mellitus, tuberculosis and heart disease at the time of entry to the prison. However, not all of them reported their ailment to the prison authorities upon admission. Omolade (2014) similarly reported that older prisoners were significantly more likely to experience medical problems prior to incarceration. The study by Majekodunmi et al. (2017) observed that 43.5% of the inmates were currently receiving medical care in prison at the time of the study. The most common ailments were eye and skin diseases, hypertension, hernia and diabetes. Close to 70% (69.4%) of the inmates admitted a change in their medical condition while in prison. Of these, 56.5% expressed worsening of their medical condition, while the remaining 11 (18.6%) claimed improvement in their physical health. Nearly 5% (4.7%) required some form of physical support, while only 3.5% used some form of dental devices. About a third (74.1%) of the inmates visited their various prison clinics within the preceding 30 days. About 1.2% of the inmates were receiving mental health care.

This pattern appears consistent with the observation that the most commonly prescribed medications for the older offender population are those for cardiovascular-, musculoskeletal- and gastrointestinal-related illnesses (Fazel et al., 2004). Apart from the chronic health problems already highlighted, older offenders are also more likely to require the use of reading glasses, hearing aids, wheelchairs, walkers and canes (Human Rights Watch, 2012). Consistent with this observation, the Bureau of Justice Statistics, US Department of Justice (2008) noted that 37.5% of prisoners aged 45 years and above reported having a chronic impairment or condition, such as vision (17.4%), learning (13.3%), hearing (11.4%), mobility (6.1%), mental (5.0%) and/or speech (3.5%).

Psychiatric morbidity of elderly prisoners

Mental health problems are the most significant cause of morbidity in prisons (Birmingham, 2003) and prisoners with mental disorders create a major challenge for the correctional service. Over 90% of prisoners have a mental disorder, with a study reporting diagnosable mental disorders in 50% of older prisoners (Kingston, Mesurier, & Yorston, 2011). The prison environment as well as the rules and regimes governing daily life inside prison can be seriously detrimental to mental health (Birmingham, 2003). Mental health issues affecting older offenders comprise, among others, substance use, anxiety disorders, psychotic disorders, mood disorders, neurodevelopmental disorders and personality disorders with an onset that often starts at a younger age, but the additional disease burden of old age includes age-related neuropsychiatric disorders like dementia or depression (Fazel & Grann, 2002; Hayes, Burns, Turnbull, & Shaw 2012; Davoren, Fitzpatrick, & Caddow, 2015). Generally, prisoners with mental disorders also suffer from the additional burden imposed by comorbid physical illnesses.

Substance-use disorder in elderly prisoners

No statistics have been found on substance-use disorder (SUD) in elderly prisoners in Africa. However, studies on elderly prisoner across the world reported similar rates for SUD among both older and younger prisoners. While older prisoners were more likely to misuse alcohol, younger prisoners misused illicit drugs (cited in Haesen et al., 2019). Older prisoners are also less likely to need assistance for drug-related problems compared to younger prisoners (Omolade, 2014). Among elderly prisoners, those aged 50–54 years have been found to suffer more from SUD compared to those who were between 65 and 69 years (Hayes et al., 2012).

Depression in elderly prisoners

Among elderly offenders, depression has been found to be three times higher than in younger inmates or elderly in the community (Yorston & Taylor, 2006; Collins & Bird, 2007; Dawes, 2009; Williams, 2012; Maschi et al., 2013). A Nigerian study found a prevalence rate of 24.7% for depression in elderly prisoners and it was observed to be associated current medical care and perception of the prison environmental conditions. It also reported that physical comorbidity and perception of prison conditions were major predictors of depression in older prisoners (Majekodunmi et al., 2017).

Human rights of elderly prisoners

The human rights of elderly prisoners appear to have been neglected for a long time. As noted earlier on, an "ageing crisis" within correctional systems is brewing and many of such systems are poorly equipped to meet the complex needs of elderly prisoners (Williams, Stern, Mellow, Safer, & Greifinger, 2012). This failure to meet these needs could potentially result in violation of their rights.

In a survey cited in Maschi (2013), many incarcerated older adults reported some of the harsh realities of incarceration, ranging from being a victim of and/or witnessing minor to severe trauma, abuse, violence and exploitation. Some older prisoners also described "being picked on for petty things by guards," having "constant shakedowns" or "canceled recreation" and "being denied medical/medical help and phone privileges for no reason at all." Others reported "being punished for other people's actions" and "being accused of things you didn't do" and their jobs taken away. Elderly prisoners also described experiences of isolation or being victims of and/or witnesses to forms of torture or cruel and unusual punishment. Mental health can be affected by feelings of isolation in the correctional setting. When compared to younger prisoners, elderly prisoners generally have fewer regular visitors and fewer connections within the prison to social networks (Williams, Baillargeon, Lindquist, & Walter, 2010) thus making them feel isolated. Their comments included: "prison officers confine them in two cages 15–20 minutes 25 at times…"; "I've been locked up in a room for 23 hours a day for the past four months without an explanation from administration." This relative social isolation can lead to diminished functional capacity or may be exacerbated by it, putting older adult prisoners at a heightened risk for subsequent worsening of loneliness and physical disability (Perissinotto, Cenzer, & Covinsky, 2012). Overall, these scenarios represent some violation of their human rights when viewed in line with the United Nations standard minimum rules for the treatment of prisoners (the "Nelson Mandela Rules," see Table 13.1), which guarantee respect for human dignity and the prohibition of degrading treatments while in prison (United Nations, 2015).

Many elderly prisoners equally reported poor nutrition and inadequate healthcare within the prison. Some of their statements included: "food nutrition – poor, variety – poor, balance – none, lack of use of utilities, water – no water to drink for 2 days, food, meat not cooked, not getting out to yard enough" (Maschi, 2013). Rule 22 of the Nelson Mandela Rules states that "Every prisoner shall be provided by the prison administration at the usual hours with food of nutritional value adequate for health and strength, of wholesome quality and well prepared and served. Drinking water shall be available to every prisoner whenever he or she needs it." Thus, it is a violation of the basic rights of prisoners not to have proper food and clean water. Most correctional facilities were designed to restrict the liberty of young people, not to provide optimal care for the aged in incarceration. As a result, correctional facilities are often ill-equipped to meet the needs of elderly prisoners with complex medical conditions and physical disabilities. These facilities often require residents to contend with challenging environmental features such as poor lighting, steep staircases, dimly lit walkways, poor ventilation, high bunk beds and low toilet seats. However, with the rise in the population of older prisoners, some correctional facilities have introduced environmental modifications for

Table 13.1 "The Nelson Mandela Rules" and its impact on service planning for elderly prisoners

S/N	*the Nelson Mandela Rules*	*Impact on service planning*
1	**Rule 1** All prisoners shall be treated with the respect due to their inherent dignity and value as human beings. No prisoner shall be subjected to, and all prisoners shall be protected from, torture and other cruel, inhuman or degrading treatment or punishment, for which no circumstances whatsoever may be invoked as a justification. The safety and security of prisoners, staff, service providers and visitors shall be ensured at all times.	The principle of human dignity implies that the prison administration also has a special duty to care for prisoners. In view of the strong dependence of prisoners on the authorities for meeting their needs and enjoying their rights, authorities have an obligation to take concrete positive measures to protect and promote human dignity. Therefore, in a broader sense that may also be interpreted as extending of duty of care vis-à-vis prison staff (i.e., for shaping their conditions of service in a way that enables them to discharge their duties in a professional manner). When implemented properly there will be a positive impact on service planning.
2	**Rule 2 no 2** In order for the principle of non-discrimination to be put into practice, prison administrations shall take account of the individual needs of prisoners, in particular the most vulnerable categories in prison settings. Measures to protect and promote the rights of prisoners with special needs are required and shall not be regarded as discriminatory.	Protecting the rights of prisoners without discrimination especially with the basis of age in this case elderly prisoners will enhance quality of life of these already fragile population of inmates.
3	**Rule 5 no 2** Prison administrations shall make all reasonable accommodation and adjustments to ensure that prisoners with physical, mental or other disabilities have full and effective access to prison life on an equitable basis.	Loss of muscle mass, pain due to arthritis, impaired balance due to loss of nerve sensation and hearing or visual impairment are examples of the many drivers of high fall risk among older adults including those in prisons. In the correctional setting, many factors can heighten the risk of falls, such as dimly lit or crowded walkways. Therefore, environmental manipulations need to be made to accommodate the needs of elderly prisoners.
4	**Rule 11** The different categories of prisoners shall be kept in separate institutions or parts of institutions, taking account of their sex, age, criminal record, the legal reason for their detention and the necessities of their treatment (though no older prisoners included).	Elderly prisoners have unique problems, and they require special care. The physical impairment they might have need not lead to disability if the environment can be modified to meet their individual's needs; installation of grab bars and seats in the shower and the placement of special doorknobs to accommodate poor dexterity due to arthritis are examples of environmental modifications that can improve independent living in their own area.
5	**Rule 12 no 2** Where dormitories are used, they shall be occupied by prisoners carefully selected as being suitable to associate with one another in those	To mitigate elderly abuse, some facilities developed age-segregated housing to overcome the common mismatch between correctional housing units and

(*Continued*)

Table 13.1 (Continued)

S/N	*the Nelson Mandela Rules*	*Impact on service planning*
	conditions. There shall be regular supervision by night, in keeping with the nature of the prison.	the needs of older adults. Such units can be constructed and staffed to mitigate environmental hazards and facilitate access to clinical health care staff and can sometimes minimize fear of elder abuse.
6	**Rule 13** All accommodation provided for the use of prisoners and in particular all sleeping accommodation shall meet all requirements of health, due regard being paid to climatic conditions and particularly to cubic content of air, minimum floor space, lighting, heating and ventilation.	Making age-sensitive adjustments to prison accommodation will go a long way in ensuring an enhanced milieu for elderly inmates. This implies the need to take appropriate measures of care for prisoners with special needs in this case elderly prisoners, including, for example, reasonable adjustments for their disabilities.
7	**Rule 22** 1. Every prisoner shall be provided by the prison administration at the usual hours with food of nutritional value adequate for health and strength, of wholesome quality and well prepared and served. 2. Drinking water shall be available to every prisoner whenever he or she needs it.	The elderly prisoners are already frail and require balance diet for strength and clean water to avoid infections due to low immunity.
8	**Rule 24 no 1** The provision of health care for prisoners is a state responsibility. Prisoners should enjoy the same standards of health care that are available in the community and should have access to necessary health care services free of charge without discrimination on the grounds of their legal status.	The provision of health care in prisons is a crucial element of prison management for various reasons. First, the right to the highest attainable standard of physical and mental health provision for elderly prisoners is important. Thus, assessing and optimizing functional ability in older adults is critical to maximizing their health, safety and well-being, which is a critical component in service planning. When implemented the impact will be felt significantly.
9	**Rule 25** 1. Every prison shall have in place a health care service tasked with evaluating, promoting, protecting and improving the physical and mental health of prisoners, paying particular attention to prisoners with special health care needs or with health issues that hamper their rehabilitation. 2. The health care service shall consist of an interdisciplinary team with sufficient qualified personnel acting in full clinical independence and shall encompass sufficient expertise in psychology and psychiatry. The services of a qualified dentist shall be available to every prisoner.	Elderly prisoners as a vulnerable group have greater health care needs based on both physical and psychiatric morbidity. Given dental problems that tend to arise with age, dental health care needs must be given special attention among this population. Multi-disciplinary teams which have some level of training in geriatric practice should be deployed in prison health care services that cater for the health of elderly offenders.
10	**Rule 27** 1. All prisons shall ensure prompt access to medical attention in urgent cases. Prisoners who require specialized	Serious, life-limiting illnesses are often debilitating for a long period of time before death among the elderly in prison

(*Continued*)

Table 13.1 (Continued)

S/N	*the Nelson Mandela Rules*	*Impact on service planning*
	treatment or surgery shall be transferred to specialized institutions or to civil hospitals. Where a prison service has its own hospital facilities, they shall be adequately staffed and equipped to provide prisoners referred to them with appropriate treatment and care. 2. Clinical decisions may only be taken by the responsible health care professionals and may not be overruled or ignored by non-medical prison staff.	and require enhanced medical attention. This can create challenges for correctional staff and strain health system resources. Clinicians with advanced training in the management of symptomatic distress in advanced illness are needed so that incarcerated patients do not experience severe pain or distressing symptoms that unnecessarily cause a loss of their functional capacity. End-of-life care arrangements are also important for elderly prisoners who may eventually die from terminal diseases during incarceration.

residents with physical disabilities thus enhancing management of complex health needs although with additional correctional cost (Maschi et al., 2013). The Nelson Mandela Rule 13 had also provided that "All accommodation provided for the use of prisoners and in particular all sleeping accommodation shall meet all requirements of health, due regard being paid to climatic conditions and particularly to cubic content of air, minimum floor space, lighting, heating and ventilation" so as to respect the human rights of prisoners.

In spite of the highlighted human rights concerns, the existing UN documents protecting prisoner rights such as the Standard Minimum Rules for the Treatment of Prisoners and the Handbook on Prisoners with Special Needs are not directly enforceable at the national level. This could limit the expectation of older prisoners with regard to access to prison rehabilitation, physical and mental health care, geriatric-specific care and family programming and linkages to community services. The community reintegration or resettlement of older prisoners with their families is a critical issue that requires attention from corrections officials and others involved in reentry.

Service implication

A monumental consequence of the aging prison population is the increase in health-related cost (Maschi & Aday, 2014). In addition, many older prisoners may require treatment and/or counseling for depression and fear of dying (Maschi et al., 2012; Maschi & Aday, 2014). Thus, the health care of older prisoners necessitates the engagement of a multidisciplinary team of specialist staff, including a medical specialist, a nurse and psychologist as a minimum. Prison authorities need to establish close cooperation with community health services to ensure that specialist care is provided by outside medical services, as necessary, and that prisoners whose needs cannot be met in prison are transferred to hospitals without delay.

Older prisoners do need to have access to special programs addressing these needs. These could include: instruction on health care for older persons, counseling related to growing old, fear of death, isolation and substance abuse and special education courses that meet the needs of this age group. Specialized counseling may also include those designed for prisoners with terminal illness and those who have received a life sentence without parole. All of these requirements place a heavy burden on prison authorities and prison health care staff, impossible to cope with in most prison systems of the world. It is therefore highly recommended that older prisoners suffering from health conditions, which cannot be adequately treated in prison, are considered for compassionate release at the earliest possible time while still taking account of public safety requirements.

Generally, safe guarding life and property of all categories of inmates including secure environment is the responsibility of the correctional services of the country as well as the establishment of an environment aimed at correcting offending behavior (Annual Report of the Department of Correctional Services, 2014/2015). However, due to the frail nature of most elderly prisoners', victimization may result due to prison overcrowding and custodial staff shortages.

The vulnerability of elderly inmates is also compromised by the physical structure and conditions inside the prison. Most or all African prisons were designed and built to accommodate young offenders. As such elderly inmates are forced to learn to adapt and cope with the physical environment, such as climbing stairs to have access to various parts of the facility such as communal or single cells, kitchen or recreational area, slippery tiled shower cubicles without grab rails or antislip mats for those with this facilities, squatting to use the toilet facility. There are no wheelchair ramps in most cases as well. Older inmates may not always have lower bunk beds and may have to sleep on mats or untiled cold floors. An older prisoner in one study of well-being in prison had been reported to have observe as follows: "*…since I have been here, I am no longer as strong as before. I don't take my bath regularly because I am too weak to carry kegs of water and there is no one to assist me. They (younger inmates) won't offer to help you except you are ready to pay them…*" (Aborisade et al., 2016).

Additionally, the elderly offender population is diverse in terms of their socio-economic background, health, crime history, motivations for committing crime, adjusting to prison life and coping with reintegration and release. As a result of this diversity, correctional services in Africa must focus on the individualized assessment, rehabilitation and monitoring of this unique inmate population. Such an approach to offender treatment is the Risk-Need-Responsivity (RNR) model of rehabilitation. Relapse prevention is one of the major goals for correctional settings. The RNR model contends that high-risk offenders benefit more from intervention programs than low-risk offenders (risk principle), and interventions are more effective if they target criminogenic needs (need principle) and engage offenders (Basanta, Farina, & Arce, 2018). To summarize, RNR refers to identifying offender risk and matching the level of services to the offender's level of risk for reoffending (greater risk requiring greater and more intensive intervention; Risk Principle), identifying and treating changeable (dynamic) risk factors directly linked to criminal behavior (criminogenic needs; Need Principle) and finally, providing cognitive–behavioral treatments tailored to the specific needs of the offender such as the offender's learning style, motivation, personality functioning or cognitive functioning (Responsivity principle). It has been considered the best model that exists for determining offender treatment, and some of the best risk-assessment tools used on offenders are based on it (Andrews, Bonta, & Wormith 2011).

Furthermore, the engagement of community services and non-governmental organizations (NGOs) working with older persons in the community is of great value in designing and delivering programs and activities for older prisoners especially in resource-constrained correctional services as those found in many parts of Africa. Enabling contact with civil society is also beneficial to the elderly prisoners in order to reduce their prevalent sense of isolation particularly when they have lost family contacts.

In terms of service planning, correctional services across Africa should consider alternative polices such as creating separate facilities to accommodate elderly inmates thereby segregating them from the younger general prison population. This may involve providing a unit for them within the larger prison setting. Providing separate unit for older inmates will protect them against victimization by younger inmates. Additionally, programs which are more age-sensitive can be developed and delivered by specialized staff. In theory, separation may encourage identification with peers and stimulate social interaction thus reducing emotional distress among elderly prisoners. The downside to this segregation approach must equally be examined. Mental health of elderly prisoners can be further affected by feelings of isolation which could result from being separated from the larger prison population. Compared to incarcerated younger prisoners, older prisoners generally have fewer regular visitors and fewer connections within the prison to social networks and self-help groups (Williams et al., 2010). This relative social isolation can lead to diminished functional capacity or may be exacerbated by it, putting older prisoners at a heightened risk for subsequent worsening loneliness (Perissinotto et al., 2012). Another problem with separating elderly prisoners from the main prison is their exclusion from serving as role models to younger inmates through their calming effects, and vocational training which some find fulfilling (Kerbs & Jolley, 2007). Furthermore, elderly offenders are not necessarily a homogenous group with entirely similar needs. While segregation may be good for the sick and frail elderly inmates, others could prefer having a "senior" status among younger inmates. Within this context, they could remain in the same prison but in separate units such that they can enjoy the desired protection while fulfilling the need for generativity be serving as pro-social role models for younger prisoners.

With regard to the cost of planning new services or upscaling existing ones, there is need for correctional services to pursue innovative strategies in dealing with the increasing number of elderly prisoners. Geriatric or nursing home types of programs which have been designed in developed countries can be replicated in Africa, ranging from specially designed facilities for aged or special unit within a larger prison setting. In these models, prisoners with similar health care needs are grouped together which is more cost effective, allows for a design for more age-sensitive, as well as healthier and safer environment for elderly prisoners. This can help the inmates to avoid further deterioration in their health while encouraging preventive self-care (access to appropriate medication, special diet, low-impact sport and geriatric walking programs). These services will be provided by multidisciplinary geriatric teams and trained correctional care staff. Geriatrics training programs for health care providers should be adapted to correctional health care settings and more training programs for custody staff should be developed and implemented. In particular, custodial staff (correctional, parole and probation officer) training programs should focus on helping officers to become familiar with the following:

1. Common normative age-associated conditions (e.g., vision loss and hearing deficits).
2. Common pathological age-associated physical conditions (e.g., falls and incontinence).
3. Common age-related clinically diagnosed cognitive conditions (e.g., dementia and delirium).
4. The challenges that all such conditions can pose in the custodial setting.
5. Ways to identify patients who need rapid assessment by a health care provider.

For instance, such training could help correctional officers recognize that an elderly prisoner who seems to be disobeying orders may actually have a hearing impairment and prompt officers to seek a medical evaluation for the prisoner.

Conclusion

Elderly prisoners, as a heterogeneous group, are a separate category from other prison inmates and have special mental and physical health needs. This places an additional burden of care on prison systems. A multi-disciplinary and innovative approach to healthcare for elderly prisoners in resource-constrained correctional systems within Africa is crucial in meeting these health care needs in a way that improves inmates' quality of life and prevents abuse of their basic rights. As a result of the diversity in offending patterns among elderly prisoners, correctional services in Africa must focus on individualized assessment, treatment and rehabilitation of this unique inmate population by adopting effective offender treatment approaches such as the RNR model. Given the psychosocial circumstances of elderly prisoners upon release, it is expedient for correctional services to work with relevant non-governmental actors to ensure the sustainable re-integration of elderly offenders into their social milieu which could have been remarkably altered during their long incarcerations or the realities of individual aging during imprisonment.

References

Aborisade, R. A., Omotayo, T. O., & Oshileye, T. A. (2016). Elders in prison: Their health status, well-being and health promoting behaviours. *Nigerian Journal of Social Studies, XIX*(2), 86–104.

Aday, R. H. (2003). Aging prisoners: Crisis in American corrections. Westport, CT: Praeger Publishers.

Aging Inmate Committee. (2012). Aging inmates: Correctional issues and initiatives. *Corrections Today, 74*, 84–87.

Andrews, D. A., Bonta, J., & Wormith, J. S. (2011). The risk-need-responsivity (RNR) model: Does adding the good lives model contribute to effective crime prevention?. *Criminal Justice and Behavior, 38*(7), 735–755. doi: 10.1177/0093854811406356.

Annual Report of the Department of Correctional Services for the period 1 April 2014 to 31 (March 2015). Pretoria: Department of Correctional Services.

Annual Report of the Department of Correctional Services for the period 1 April 2015 to 31 (March 2016). Pretoria: Department of Correctional Services.

Basanta, J. L., Farina, F., & Arce, R. (2018). Risk need responsivity model: Contrasting criminogenic and non criminogenic needs in high and low risk juvenile offenders. *Children and Youth Services Review, 85*, 137–142.

Bezuidenhout, C., & Booyens, K. (2018). The elderly offender and the elderly victim of crime: A South African overview. In P. C.,Kratcoski & M. Edelhacher (Eds), *Perspectives in elderly crime and victimization* (pp. 79–97). Springer. ISBN: 978-3-319-72681-6 ISBN 978-3-319-72682-3 (eBook) https://doi.org/10.1007/978-3-319-72682-3

Birmingham, L. (2003). The mental health of prisoners. *Advances in Psychiatric Treatment, 9*(3), 191–199.

Bureau of Justice Statistics, US Department of Justice. (2008). Medical problems of prisoners. Washington, DC: Bureau of Justice Statistics. https://www.bjs.gov/index.cfm?ty=pbdetail&iid=1097 (Accessed June, 2nd 2020).

Bureau of Justice Statistics (2016). Prisoners in 2016. Retrieved from: http://www.bjs.gov/index.cfm?ty=pdbdetail&id=6187

Chiu, T. (2010). Aging prisoners, increasing costs, and geriatric release. Center on Sentencing and Correction. Retrieved from https://www.ojp.gov/library/abstracts/its-about-time-aging-prisoners-increasing-costs-and-geriatric-release

Chodos, A. H., Ahalt, C., Cenzer, I. S., & Goldenson, J. (2013). Characteristics of older adults who use the emergency room prior to jail detainment. *Conference: 36th Annual Meeting of the Society of General Internal Medicine, SGIM 2013. Denver, CO United States. Conference Start: 20130424. Conference End: 20130427. Conference Publication: (var.pagings)* (p. 28).

Chodos, A. H., Ahalt, C., Cenzer, I. S., Myers,J., Goldenson,J., & Williams, B. A. (2014). Older jail inmates and community acute care use. *American Journal of Public Health, 104*(9), 1728–1733.

Collins, D. R., & Bird, R. (2007). The penitentiary visit—A new role for geriatricians? *Age and Ageing, 26*, 11–13.

Davoren, M., Fitzpatrick, M., Caddow, F., et al. (2015). Older men and older women remand prisoners: Mental illness, physical Illness: offending patterns and needs. *International Psychogeriatrics, 27*(5), 747–755.

Dawes, J. (2009). Ageing prisoners: Issues for social work. *Australian Social Work, 62*(2), 258–271.

Fazel, S., & Danesh, J. (2002). Serious mental disorder in 23,000 prisoners: A systematic review of 62 surveys. *The Lancet, 359*, 545–550.

Fazel, S., & Grann, M. (2002 Oct). Older criminals: A descriptive study of psychiatrically examined offenders in Sweden. *International Journal of Geriatric Psychiatry, 17*(10), 907–991

Fazel, S., Hayes, A. J., Bartellas, K., Clcrici, M., & Trestman, R. (2016). Mental health of prisoners: Prevalence, adverse outcomes, and interventions. *Lancet Psychiatry, 3*(9), 871–881. https://doi.org/10.1016/S2215-0366(16)30142-0

Fazel, S., Hope, T., O'Donnell, I., & Jacoby, R. (2001). Hidden psychiatric morbidity in elderly prisoners. *British Journal of Psychiatry, 179*, 535–539.

Fazel, S., Hope, T., O'Donnell, I., & Jacoby, R. (2004). Unmet treatment needs of older prisoners: A primary care survey. Age and Ageing, 33, 396–398.

Fellner, J. (2012). Old behind bars: The ageing prison population in the United States. Human Rights Watch. Retrieved from:http://www.hrw.org/sites/default/files/reports/usprisons0112_brochure_web.pdf

Haesen, S., Merkt, H., Imber, A., Elger, B. , et al.(2019). Substance use disorder and other mental health disorders among older prisoners. International Journal of Law and Psychiatry, *62*, 20–31. doi:10.1016/ijlp.2018.10.004

Hayes, A. J., Burns, A., Turnbull, P., & Shaw, J. J. (2012 Nov). The health and social needs of older male prisoners. *International Journal of Geriatric Psychiatry, 27*(11), 1155–1162. https://doi.org/10.1002/gps.376

Human Rights Watch. (2012). *Old behind bars: The aging prison population in the United States.* New York: Human Rights Watch.

Kerbs, J. J., & Jolley, J. M. (2007). Inmate-on-inmate victimization among older male prisoners. *Crime & Delinquency, 53*(2), 187–218.

Kingston, P., Mesurier, N. L., Yorston, G., et al. (2011). Psychiatric morbidity in older prisoners: Unrecognized and untreated. *International Psychogeriatric Association, 23*(8), 1354–1360.

Kumolu, C. (2012). Nigeria's Problem is Poverty. Vanguard Online News. Retrieved from http://www.vanguarrdngr.com/2012/06 (Accessed 27 May 2020).

Langat, K., Kabaji, E., & Poipoi, M. (2015). Efficacy of rehabilitation programmes on psychosocial adjustment of elderly male offenders in Kakamega main prison Kenya. *The International Journal of Humanities & Social Studies, 3*(11), 70–80.

Loeb, S. J., & Abudagga, A. (2006 Dec). Health-related research on older inmates: An integrative review. *Research in Nursing & Health, 29*(6), 556–565.

Luallen, J., & Kling, R. A. (2014). Method for analyzing changing populations explaining the growth of the elderly in the prison. *Evaluation Review, 38*(6), 459–486.

Majekodunmi, O. E., Obadeji, A., Oluwole, L. O., & Oyelami, O. (2017). Depression and associated physical co-morbidity in elderly prison inmates. *International Journal of Mental Health, 46*(4), 269–283.

Maschi, T. (2013). Elderly abuse in prisons: The call for elderly justice and human rights protections behind bars. Prison Legal News, 52. Retrieved from https://www.prisonlegalnews.org/news/2013/dec/15/elder-abuse-in-prisons-the-call-for-elder-justice-and-human-rights-protections-behind-bars/ (Accessed 17 July 2020).

Maschi, T., & Aday, R. R. H. (2014). The social determinants of health and justice and the aging in prison crisis: A call for human rights action. *International Journal of Social Work, 1*(1), 15–33.

Maschi, T., Kwak, J., Ko, E., & Morrissey, M. B. (2012). Forget me not: Dementia in prison. *The Gerontologist, 52*(4), 441–451.

Maschi, T., Viola, D., & Sun, F. (2013). The high cost of the international aging prisoner crisis: well-being as the common denominator for action. *The Gerontologist, 53*(4), 543–554.
Njeru, M. (2009). Factors responsible for violent crimes among prisoners in Kamiti and Langat prisons in Kenya. Master's Thesis of University of Nairobi.
Obioha, E. (2011). Challenges and reforms in the Nigerian prison system. *Journal of the Social Sciences, 27*(2), 95–109.
Ojo, M., & Okunola, R. (2014). The plights of the aged inmates in Nigerian prison system: A survey of two prisons in Ogun State, Nigeria. *Bangladesh e-Journal of Sociology, 11*(1), 54–73.
Omale, M. (2011). *Prison reformation, rehabilitation and reintegration programmes in Nigeria: A study of selected prisons in Nigeria.* Nigeria Correctional Reports.
Omolade, S. (2014). The needs and characteristics of older prisoners: Results from the Surveying Prisoner Crime Reduction (SPCR) survey. Analytical Summary. London: Ministry of Justice. https://assets.publishing.service.gov.uk/government/uploads/system/uploads/attachment_data/file/368177/needs-older-prisoners-spcr-survey.pdf
Onishi, N. (2007). Elderly inmates find amenities in Japan's prisons. https://www.nytimes.com/2007/11/02/world/asia/02iht-japan.1.8161091.html
Perissinotto, C. M., Cenzer, I. S., & Covinsky, K. E. (2012). Loneliness in older persons: A predictor of functional decline and death. *JAMA Internal Medicine, 172*(14), 1078–1083.
Pro, G., & Marzell, M. (2017 Apr). Medical parole and aging prisoners: A qualitative study. *Journal of Correctional Health Care, 23*(2), 162–172. https://doi.org/10.1177/1078345817699608.
Reimer, G. (2008). The graying of the U.S. prisoner population. *Journal of Correctional Health Care, 14*(3), 202–208.
Skarupski, K. A., Gross, A., Schrack, J. A., et al. (2018). The health of America's aging prison population. *Epidemiologic Reviews, 40*, 157–165.
Stal, M. (2012). Treatment of older and elderly inmates within prisons. *Journal of Correctional Health Care, 19*(1), 69–73.
Swanson, J. W., Frisman, L. K., Robertson, A. G., Lin, H. J., et al. (2013). Costs of criminal justice involvement among persons with serious mental illness in Connecticut. *Psychiatric Services, 64*(7), 630–637. doi: 10.1176/appi.ps.002212012
Tomar, R., Treasaden, I. H., and Shah, A. K. (2005). Is there a case for a specialist forensic psychiatry service for the elderly? *International Journal of Geriatric Psychiatry, 20*(1), 51–56.
United Nations (2015). United Nations standard minimum rules for the treatment of prisoners. A/Res/70/175.
United Nations, Department of Economic and Social Affairs, Population Division (2015). *World Population Ageing 2015.*
Vogel, T., Languillon, S., & Graf, M. (2013). When and why should mentally ill prisoners be transferred to secure hospitals: A proposed algorithm. *International Journal of Law and Psychiatry, 36*(3-4), 281–286. https://doi.org/10.1016/j.ijlp.2013.04.021Epub
Wan He, D. G., & Paul K. (2016). An Aging World: 2015, US Census Bureau, International Population Reports, P95/16-1, US Government Publishing Office, Washington, DC, 2016.
Williams, J. (2012). Social care and older prisoners. *Journal of Social Work, 13*(5), 471–491.
Williams, B., Stern, M., Mellow, J., Safer, M., & Greifinger, R. (2012). Aging in correctional custody: Setting a policy agenda for older prisoner health care. *American Journal Public Health, 102*(8), 1475–1481.

Williams, B. A., Baillargeon, J., Lindquist, K., Walter, L. C., et al. (2010).Medication prescribing practices for older prisoners in the Texas prison System. *American Journal of Public Health, 100*(4), 756–761.

Yorston, G., & Taylor, P. (2006). Commentary: older offenders – No place to go? *The Journal of the American Academy of Psychiatry and the Law Online, 34*(3), 333–337.

14 Occupational therapy in forensic mental health: An occupational justice perspective

Theoca Moodley, Nafisa Abdulla, Zerina Hajwani, Madri Engelbrecht, and Gail Whiteford

Introduction

Occupational therapists view humans as occupational beings whose participation in meaningful occupations are essential to their health and well-being. Occupations, in this sense, are not just work or vocations that people participate in, but all things that people do on a day-to-day basis and that occupy their time. Within the forensic context specifically, a patient's access to meaningful occupations is limited by legislative, systemic and environmental structures that are unique to different custodial practices. These limitations represent a form of *occupational injustice*, a concept discussed in this chapter alongside the means by which occupational therapists in forensic settings can mitigate the negative impacts of such an injustice through the provision of occupational opportunities. We expand this discussion through a description of what an overt commitment to occupational justice looks like within occupational therapy service design and delivery.

Forensic occupational therapy practice in the African context

Trained occupational therapists and occupational therapy services are still scarce in African countries, although a greater number of services are found in the southern regions of the continent. Occupational therapists work in a variety of settings across countries; for example, non-governmental organizations, government hospitals, schools and private practices (Sherry, 2010) with foci in different occupational therapy fields such as pediatrics, physical rehabilitation and mental health. Clients of forensic mental health services are legally referred to as forensic *patients* to distinguish their status as being *in treatment within health facilities* as opposed to being incarcerated *as prisoners in the criminal justice system.* (Whiteford et al., 2019). Forensic patient populations in Africa comprise of male and female children and adolescents from 10 to 18 years old, as well as adult men and women older than 18 years, who are diagnosed with severe psychiatric conditions such as schizophrenia, bipolar affective disorder, comorbid substance abuse and intellectual impairment. These patients do not always have access to occupational therapy in services, for example, where prisoners with mental health issues are not transferred to psychiatric hospitals or are not given access to occupational therapy in general hospitals due to security concerns and a lack of human resources.

The majority of this population comes from low socio-economic circumstances where social contexts are dominated by gangsterism, substance abuse, low or no education, unemployment and a lack of affordable and adequate mental health care (Kaliski, 2013; Wegner, 2016). Single-income households are prevalent in these communities, with members living below the breadline rendering them dependent upon social assistance from the state, albeit a minimal contribution to household incomes in overpopulated homes (Duncan, 2009; Duncan, Swartz, & Kathard, 2011; Dubihlela & Dubihlela, 2014).

The influence of the social contexts extends beyond the attainment of education to employment for forensic patients. Many forensic patients are unskilled work seekers with limited education and work experience, who may have been subjected to violence and abuse, contributing to offending behaviors in adulthood. Such predispositions created by challenging life circumstances present more frequently among non-white forensic patient populations and draw significant influence from historical a socio-economic and political events. Examples of events are the previous apartheid regime in South Africa, colonization of the continent as well as genocide and dictatorship in African countries resulting in prevailing systemic racial and ethnic segregation.

The apartheid regime in South Africa brought with it the pursuit of systemic racial segregation including political and economic discrimination against non-white people. Similarly, colonialization, genocide and dictatorship in other African countries have affected the range, choice and accessibility of occupations available for people to engage in due to the adverse effects of these historical events on economic growth in these countries. An informal survey conducted by the authors in December 2019 noted that extreme political and economic challenges in Zimbabwe have resulted in overall reduced health care service provisions due to poor resources, inadequate funding and a general incapacitation of health care workers according to the surveyed occupational therapists from the country.

In keeping with many low- and middle-income countries, many African countries have mental health and social services that are not fully developed and often underfinanced (Burns, 2011), especially in comparison to their South African counterparts. In Nigeria, for example, there are occupational therapy services in most psychiatric hospitals, but these services are not available to mentally ill prisoners. Even when these prisoners are transferred to non-secure hospitals, they are unable to participate in occupational therapy services because of security concerns.

As much as attempts have been made to readdress historical damage and its impact on the patterns of occupational engagement of whole populations of people, the aftermath of this is still evident in the chronic poverty in which people live, their low education status, limited employment opportunities, poor access to medical services and other inequalities that are prevalent across African societies. Accordingly, an understanding of these political, economic, religious, ethnic and cultural influences on occupational participation and engagement of forensic patients is essential in a client-centered approach to occupational therapy assessment and intervention.

Forensic patients or state patients are offenders with mental health conditions who have been found "not guilty" by reason of insanity or "unfit to plead" due to their psychiatric illness or disability. These patients undergo court-ordered rehabilitation while being detained in institutions for indefinite periods of time. They are commonly incarcerated within one of two main types of correctional facilities, namely jails or secure units within a mental health facility. Incarceration continues until patients are eligible for periods of leave, reclassification or conditional or unconditional discharge. These correctional environments can impact negatively on the mental health and well-being of forensic patients as opportunities for occupational engagement within them are severely restricted for a number of reasons (Molineux & Whiteford, 1999).

Occupational rights and occupational justice in health promotion and risk management

While the laws that govern incarceration and treatment of forensic patients differ across African countries, this population's plight for community reintegration is similar (Bone & Roberts, 2019; Chichaya, Joubert, & McColl, 2019; Herbig & Hesselink, 2012; Kaliski, 2012; Krüger & Lewis, 2011). Court-mandated institutionalization legislatively and practically restricts opportunities for the forensic patient to rejoin society and reintegrate into their communities. Forensic patients tend to experience greater levels of social stigma. Therefore, to ensure good clinical governance and the advocacy of patients' rights, risk assessments are conducted to balance clinical decisions regarding a forensic patient's detention versus his or her freedom (Roffey & Kaliski, 2012). Risk assessment is the appraisal of an individual's risk for future propensities to commit a violent offense. Assessment may comprise of the identification of potential harm, ascertaining risk factors that are present and determining the likelihood the person will act violently and harm themselves or others (Kaliski, 2006; Nilsson et al., 2009). The assessment and management of risk is considered prior to and during leave periods for participation in community life. Risk assessment involves assessing the ability of the forensic patient to function and participate in occupations that can contribute to improved mental health and lowered recidivism (Kaliski, 2013).

The profession of occupational therapy promotes the occupational rights of individuals, groups and populations to engage in occupations that have positive outcomes for their health and well-being. Occupations are always meaningful and some, understood as socially sanctioned occupations, promote good health, quality of life and community well-being (Mace et al., 2018). Some do not, however, contributing instead to ill health, poverty and marginalization and are often referred to as non-sanctioned occupations because of their negative social impact (Kiepek, Beagan, Laliberte Rudman, & Phelan, 2018) Living in an incarcerated environment can create either an opportunity or impossibility for the forensic patient to enjoy occupational rights that leads to engagement in socially sanctioned occupations with positive outcomes – for example, skills development. The context is instrumental in determining both *what* is participated in over time, as well as *how* the individual participates and experiences specific occupations (Pierce, 2001; Stadnyk, Townsend, & Wilcock, 2010). When the forensic patient's occupational rights are infringed upon over a prolonged period of time, an occupationally unjust situation is created. Occupational injustice is therefore a problem that occurs in a variety of restricted environments, especially when the individual does not find themselves in that situation by choice (Stadnyk et al., 2010). Occupational injustice stems from a denial of access to resources and opportunities that promote participation in occupations, with restrictions imposed by policies, structural and systemic barriers outside of the control of the individual (Durocher, Gibson, & Rappolt, 2013; Chichaya et al., 2019). The impacts of such a denial are serious and pervasive. It should be noted that restricted access to certain forms of participation can result in disease or even death (Christiansen, 1999).

In forensic settings, risk monitoring and management is reliant on the assessment of the patient's behavior in everyday activities, their ability to engage with community resources, adequate functioning as assessed in occupational therapy programs, stable mental state as well as good social support (Kaliski, 2013). If they lack access to opportunities for occupational participation, however, the assessment of risk could be unfairly compromised. For this reason, the occupational therapist's approach to treatment and rehabilitation in the forensic context is vital as it combats occupational injustice(s) through actively creating opportunities for participation in occupations.

Types of occupational injustices in forensic contexts

Individuals or groups in forensic mental health settings may experience a range of negative occupational outcomes due to the limitations imposed on their occupational participation and engagement. These occupational outcomes, namely occupational deprivation, occupational imbalance, occupational alienation and occupational marginalization (Wilcock, 1998; Stadnyk et al., 2010), contribute to and enforce occupational injustices arising from conditions found in forensic mental health settings and can hinder the forensic patient's recovery.

Occupational deprivation

Forensic patients experience occupational deprivation when restrictions are placed on opportunities and resources for occupational participation (Wilcock, 2003). These restrictions can prevent a patient from acquiring, using or enjoying occupations over a period of time (Whiteford, 1997) and culminate in difficulties experienced by patients to structure their time in ways that promote their health and variation in occupations to meet personal goals. How and what they do with their time is influenced by what resources and occupations are available to them. In forensic contexts, patients spend most of their time engaged in unstructured leisure and passive activities. See Box 14.1.

Box 14.1 Typical time use of forensic patients

Typical forensic time use activities include:

Sleeping, sitting around and performing passive and solitary activities and substance use.

Humans have the right to develop themselves through participating in health building occupations and those that promote social inclusion (Townsend & Wilcock, 2004). Occupational deprivation works against this as people are excluded from engaging in occupations that are necessary for survival and are meaningful due to factors that are outside of their control (Whiteford, 1997). Examples of these may include discriminatory policies and practices, cultural aspects, politics and economic systems (Whiteford, 2000). Injustices persist for these vulnerable groups of men and women who find themselves oppressed due to their disability, forensic status, skin color, substance-use behavior, prolonged incarceration or even in some cases, their refugee status. See Box 14.2.

Box 14.2 Example of discriminatory practices toward foreign nationals

Example of discriminatory practices toward foreign nationals:

South Africa has seen an influx of foreign nationals seeking refuge after fleeing their countries due to intolerable living conditions. Some of these foreign nationals have been admitted within forensic psychiatric hospitals and face further isolation and marginalization in the community reintegration process as viable opportunities for this population are minimal. Additional difficulties, such as attaining documentation or xenophobia in communities, contribute to limited occupational participation and engagement in meaningful occupations such as formal work and learning programs.

Occupational deprivation is proposed to be the ultimate form of punishment for its isolating effects on individuals and their deprivation from occupational involvement (Townsend & Wilcock, 2004). The prolonged occupational deprivation from engaging in productive roles such as work, education/learning, skills development and socialization may result in gross estrangement to community life for forensic patients. The lack of opportunities to have productive life roles impacts risk management, resulting in negative outcomes in patient preparation for community reintegration (Farnworth & Muñoz, 2009; Whiteford et al., 2019, p. 2).

Adequate opportunities to engage in occupations of choice are required for development, health and well-being (Wilcock, 2003). When patients are prevented from exerting choice in their occupations, their capacity to function adequately and independently in everyday life can become diminished. Long periods of confinement in restrictive, institutional environments limit opportunities for forensic patients to participate in self-selected, meaningful occupations (Townsend & Wilcock, 2004). When these opportunities to assert choice, autonomy and decision making in daily routines are absent and high instances of boredom are present, occupational deprivation is exacerbated (Molineux & Whiteford, 1999).

Personal choice is one of the bases for individual development and without allowing for this frequently in life, one's motivation, sense of ownership and hope begins to diminish. This furthermore affects a patient's future occupational choices, performance and recovery (Bassman, 1997). In a forensic setting, the regulation of shower times, meal options and the enforcement of uniform dress codes are examples of how autonomy and choice are removed and the effects of institutionalization are intensified.

Occupational imbalance

Occupational imbalance results from the imposition of certain occupations to the detriment of participation in other occupations. This imposition is brought on by structures or forces outside of the individual's control and can be a direct result of occupational deprivation (Stadnyk et al., 2010). When people are over-occupied, unoccupied or under-occupied, their health and well-being are negatively impacted. Within the forensic context, occupational imbalance occurs when there is a disjuncture between what a patient wants to do and what he or she is expected to do and when available opportunities for engagement as well as restrictions to participation are determined by the forensic environment (Wagman, Håkansson, & Björklund, 2011).

Promoting change and creating opportunities for occupational participation

Occupational therapists in forensics have a dynamic role in counteracting occupational injustices by creating opportunities for participation in pro-social and health-building occupations, and in effect, to contribute to a reduction in recidivism. Occupational therapy promotes the occupational rights of forensic patients through advocating and providing access to resources and opportunities for meaningful engagement. Participation opportunities may be extensive and can take the form of health- and fitness-related programs, psychoeducation on diseases of lifestyle and understanding one's mental illness, managing side effects of medication and medication compliance. Dual diagnosis programs are also run to improve patients' knowledge on how best to manage their illness and minimize the harmful effects of substance abuse. See Box 14.3.

Box 14.3 Forensic OT services offered within a psychiatric hospital in South Africa (Valkenberg Hospital)

Examples of OT services offered in forensic contexts that promote occupational justice

OT services include a range of exploration and engagement in:

- Self-care and hygiene activities
- Psychoeducation and life-skills groups
- Dual diagnosis interventions
- Health and fitness activities
- Leisure and recreational activities
- Community-based social events
- Adult-based education and literacy programs that include apprenticeships and learnerships.
- Work preparation and supported employment programs

(*Moore, 2005*)

Community reintegration is integral to forensic occupational therapy programs as it provides opportunities for practical implementation of learned skills and assists the patient in navigating the challenges associated with community reentry. Occupational therapy intervention may, therefore, incorporate opportunities for social participation such as outings into the community. While risk management strategies are important to consider when working in a forensic setting, adopting an entirely risk-averse approach is not encouraged when weighed against the benefit of graded community participation. Despite the time limit associated with granting town paroles, hospitals that provide these opportunities promote the practice of life skills necessary for community reentry and increase independence while decreasing institutionalization and occupational imbalance and deprivation.

Specific occupational therapy interventions in forensic settings

Learning and skills development programs

Occupational therapy interventions focused on learning and skills development promote personal development and upskill patients to become more employable.

Skills development may include facilitating participation in adult-based education and literacy programs, apprenticeships and learnerships, but can also be related to practical community skills such as learning to drive a car or electrical or plumbing work. Learning is often seen to be a huge challenge for this population due to poor literacy levels, learning difficulties, language barriers as well as prolonged time periods since a patient may have participated in a structured program.

Learning and apprenticeship opportunities in forensic mental health settings are limited across the African context. When these opportunities are available, they often have strict exclusion criteria such as limited age ranges, secondary education levels and documentary proof. Even when patients fulfill the educational requirements, patients often struggle to access educational documents due to administrative challenges within education facilities, with a subsequent impact on their ability to participate in available learning opportunities. Occupational therapists play an important advocacy role in obtaining access to learning opportunities for forensic patients, despite the challenges. Unfortunately, learnership and apprenticeship training often do not translate into employment. Some patients choose to participate in additional learnerships for monetary benefits from the associated stipends received from program funders funding the participation of people with disabilities in these opportunities. The continued movement through learning programs that may be personally less relevant or beneficial to patients poses a challenge for forensic patients in establishing a career path.

Work programs

Occupational injustices often manifest within the employment domain for forensic patients in the form of stigma, discrimination and inadequate support or opportunities for career development (Engelbrecht, Van Niekerk, Coetzee, & Hajwani, 2017). Forensic patients are often unskilled with limited opportunities for employment in the context of high unemployment rates in low- and middle-income countries. While prolonged periods of unemployment adversely impacts people's health and well-being, the restrictive contexts of forensic patients with poor social support compounds the effects of unemployment for this population. Forensic occupational therapy services attend to the life sphere of work, to influence the lowering of recidivism rates and the increase of self-efficacy and capacity in forensic patients (Molineux & Whiteford, 1999; Brooke, 2015). This is promoted through engaging patients in productive occupations to counteract unhealthy and passive occupations such as substance misuse. Therefore, one of the cornerstones of an occupational therapy service in forensic mental health is the incorporation of a work program.

An integral element of an occupational therapy work program is a graded process to cater to a variety of skills and abilities of patients, with the end goal of acquiring gainful and meaningful employment within the community setting. It should integrate elements of vocational rehabilitation, prevocational training and work hardening that simulate natural work settings. These programs may include practical work tasks such as packaging, assembling, beading, sorting and woodwork. Thereafter, patients should have the opportunity to participate in skills development programs that target résumé development, job application, interview preparation and education on disclosure and consent. Additionally, the running of work-related personal and interpersonal skills development sessions on life skills such as stress management, conflict management and communication skills could be included.

Case example

The case example in Table 14.1 demonstrates how an occupational justice perspective is used to promote occupational rights for a forensic patient within a work setting. The screening guideline has been inspired from the occupational justice framework by Wolf, Ripat, Davis, Becker, and MacSwiggan (2010) and incorporates human rights considerations.

Challenges and recommendations

Recommendations that can strengthen and support forensic occupational therapy services that promote occupational justice across Africa, to better rehabilitate forensic patients, with the intention to improve community re-integration and reduce recidivism.

1 Guidelines and assessment tools

While no clear guidelines exist for the assessment of occupational injustices, an occupational justice framework can be utilized to identify and address human right infringements from an occupational perspective within a forensic context. This framework could inform the development of guidelines and assessment tools for forensic occupational therapy services around issues of injustice and assist multi-disciplinary teams with formulating a plan of action to combat injustices identified. Tools should consider enablers and barriers within forensic settings that impact occupational participation and engagement (*see* Table 14.2 *in addendum A*).

2 Client-centered approaches to recovery

A patient-centered approach is vital to promoting patient autonomy, decision making and choice, and in doing so, promotes occupational justice. A contextual, historical view that informs occupational therapists' awareness and sensitivity is needed to understand a forensic patient's occupational profile and to plan for interventions that will promote meaningful occupational participation and engagement that could be more equitable to comparison to other citizens. Intervention can include empowerment and enablement strategies so that

Table 14.1 Occupational injustice screening guideline

- **Identify the key problem**

Mr C. is a 40-year-old male from the Democratic Republic of Congo. He is married with one child and lives in a low-income area in the Western Cape Province. As a foreign national he does not have access to governmental grants despite having a disability. He has a diagnosis of bipolar mood disorder and has been a forensic patient in South Africa since 2013, following a charge of assault. He has a diploma in automotive mechanics and repairs which he attained in the DRC with five years working experience as a mechanic. He managed to acquire informal employment as a mechanic's assistant in the community while on a long leave from the forensic unit.

Subsequent to defaulting on his medication and struggling to cope with life stressors, he had relapsed and was readmitted to the maximum-security forensic ward after six months of employment. He stayed away from work and his home environment for an extended period of time while in recovery. His employer was not aware that he had a psychiatric illness and absence from work put him at risk of losing his job.

Mr C's condition stabilized quickly but he faced the challenge of being placed on a long waiting list for transfer to a less secure ward, which would allow him to go out on leave and fulfill his usual life roles. According to the forensic unit policy, this process of transfer usually takes four to six months due to minimal available beds. Shortage of beds is ultimately the result of limited movement of patients that are successfully integrated into the community. This further increased Mr C's risk of being dismissed from work. Additionally, he was separated from his wife for a long period of time, which negatively impacted their relationship.

- **Define the occupational injustice and provide an explanation**

Occupational Deprivation

Mr C. is not able to participate in work as a meaningful occupation, and has become deprived from fulfilling important life roles due to systemic barriers created by hospital policies.

Occupational Imbalance

Mr C. experiences restrictions in his ability to participate in activities of his choice that are meaningful to him (e.g., participation in work as well as caring and supporting his family) (*Wilcock & Townsend, 2000).*

- **Use the "but why?" technique to identify the reasons for the occupational injustice** *(Federal, Provincial and Territorial Advisory Committee on Population Health, 1999)*

But why is this a human rights infringement for Mr C.?

A ***The right to have freedom of movement and residence*** *The hospital policy is preventing Mr C. (who is psychiatrically stable) from re-integrating into community and work due to strict policies around the transfer of patients to less secure wards. This is compounded by the ward's difficulties in managing bed pressure and could take months for him to engage in important and meaningful occupations.*

B ***To have rights without discrimination, seek and enjoy asylum from persecution in other countries, access to social security and to have citizenship*** *Mr C. has the right to seek asylum in South Africa but has difficulty in applying for refugee status and benefitting from privileges associated with citizenship, such as disability- and child grants. He is a foreign national but has a family and children that need financial assistance from the government. He may have experienced additional stressors in relation to his mental illness, forensic patient status as well as having inadequate support structures as most of his family live in the DRC.*

C ***The right to work; the right to protection against unemployment and to just and favorable remuneration as well as the right to equality and dignity*** *Mr C's qualification is not recognized in South Africa, which limits his access to work opportunities within*

(*Continued*)

Table 14.1 (Continued)

his field. He was therefore only able to acquire a job that was below his skill level, with earnings commensurate to a lower level of qualification. While he retains the right not to disclosure information about his diagnosis, his decision not to disclose for fear of stigmatization could result in him losing his job. The impact of the possible job loss could have dire effects on his family and personal life as he would not be able to contribute financially to his household.

(The Universal Declaration of Human Rights, 1948)

- **Identify measures that can be put into place to combat these issues from a micro, meso and macro level** *(Restall & Ripat, 2008)*

The occupational therapist who worked with Mr C. did the following:

- **Micro (patient–clinician relationship)**
  - Conducted individual patient sessions focused on stress management, relapse prevention and medication compliance, disclosure and consent.
  - Coached Mr C. on mental health care-user rights as well as worker rights and assisted in the development of advocacy skills.
- **Meso (practice environment)**
  - Liaised with Forensic Business Unit clinical manager regarding adapting leave and/or transfer policy.
  - Liaised with MDT regarding leave to attend work from maximum security or to prioritize Mr C. for transfer.
  - Provided work support for Mr C. in relation to disclosure and liaised with employer regarding reintegration into work.
  - Sessions with the employer focused on psychoeducation and stigma following patient's choice to disclose his psychiatric diagnosis.
  - Engaged with MDT about review of hospital policies to allow for conjugal spaces for couples.
- **Macro (structure and organization of health/social/education/political)**

  This could not be acted upon due to poor access for occupational therapy to interact with macro-level structures. The following recommendations would have been made:
  - Advocate and encourage Mr C. to join Cape Consumer Advocacy Body, which could have advocated for his rights as a person with mental illness.
  - Advocate and encourage Mr C. to access the Commission for Conciliation, Mediation and Arbitration (CCMA) regarding his rights as a worker in line with the employment equity act.
  - It was noticed that there is a lack of support services for forensic patients in the community. Advocating for foreign nationals who are forensic patients to get assistance with obtaining refugee status and accessing government financial support is a need.

Summary:

For foreign nationals, participation in occupations of choice are often so restricted that some patients request assistance to return to their home countries, despite their initial reasons for immigration related to better living, working conditions and other opportunities. Those who stay often live in fear and in oppressive conditions and are generally exploited by the community. These circumstances negatively impact their health and well-being and their ability to successfully integrate and participate in society.

(Continued)

Table 14.1 (Continued)

In Mr C's case, occupational therapy provided extensive intervention aimed at all aspects of community integration and work engagement. The occupational therapist also assisted with personal needs and advocated for systemic changes at the FBU level which allowed for the patient to successfully reintegrate into his work. Continuous support and skills development allowed for Mr C. to fulfil his life roles as a father, husband and worker. This particular patient experienced many injustices in relation to his status as a foreign national coupled with being a forensic patient. He was also separated from his wife and this may have contributed to relationship difficulties and stress. Although the facility could not offer to meet these needs, there was at least an attempt made to address this by the occupational therapist. This highlights some of the challenges that our forensic population face in trying to reintegrate into general life following their incarceration.

patients can self-advocate in addressing their occupational and human rights needs. Patient feedback on rehabilitation programmes should be prioritized as it can be used to measure effectiveness and can promote program development and modification. Beyond the multi-disciplinary teams' assessment, opportunities should be created where patients and staff can communicate about perceived injustices and thereby promote patients' sense of agency and self-advocacy. Staff should encourage patients in accessing advocacy bodies for support in advocating for their rights.

3 Research needs

Forensic occupational therapy practice in Africa includes the use of a variety of occupation-based models and tools to guide assessment and intervention. Although these models assist in describing a person's occupational profile, they do not all consider culturally diverse needs of the forensic population. Occupational therapists therefore rely on clinical observations, collateral information from various sources and basic activity engagement to assess patients for intervention and risk. There is a need for more research that validates tools and assessments of occupations that are appropriate for the African context and target populations. These assessments should be sensitive to change and should be able to predict community functioning as well as establish the effectiveness of rehabilitation programs (Durocher et al., 2013). A further need exists for the development of suitable occupational therapy intervention methods that are outcomes-based and measurable.

4 The development of occupational therapy services in Africa

Forensic patients from the continent often reside in underdeveloped and resource-constrained settings. Individuals within a forensic system are treated by a multi-disciplinary team generally consisting of psychiatrists, psychologists, social workers, occupational therapists and nursing personnel. In African countries with limited resources, forensic patients may not have access to a multidisciplinary team that can impact their risk assessment and community participation (Monteiro, 2015). In addition to these challenges facing forensic patients in Africa, manpower shortages in occupational therapy services seem to compound the problem. Occupational therapy services, in particular, need to be established and/or further developed in some African countries as promoted by affiliations of occupational therapists from various regions to the Occupational Therapy Africa Regional group ("otarg.org.za," n.d.). There is a need for appropriate policies, programs and service developments to allow for the bridging of significant treatment gaps that exist, especially in the field of forensic mental health services. Alongside poor access to physical resources, limited opportunities for occupational participation persist for patients in these settings. Occupational therapy interventions thus have to take innovative approaches including low-cost programs which can, for example, utilize recyclable materials. Additionally, entrepreneurial skills development can be a core aspect of therapeutic programs, to promote income generation and to acquire physical resources. Low-cost and innovative approaches to occupational engagement in under-resourced countries within Africa may improve time use for patients as well as increase mental health knowledge and solidify group identity and purpose.

5 Facilitating community reentry

Occupational therapy strategies can focus on providing opportunities for community reintegration where community mapping, utilization of public transport and other life skills can be practiced. Advocating for patients to have graded town paroles into the community can contribute to the reentry process. Additional costs associated with patients accessing health care services need to be considered, as this can impact community mobilization. Occupational therapists can continue to network and create partnerships with key community role players to facilitate reintegration. This risk-tolerant approach may contribute to lower recidivism and reoffending rates and decrease the effect of institutionalization.

6 Accessing learning and work opportunities

To promote learning and work opportunities for forensic patients, occupational therapy interventions can include the psychoeducation of learning institutions, employers and patients to minimize stigma, provide ongoing support and advocate for reasonable accommodation. Although there is a drive for skills development for youth, along with new developments in legislation that promote the employment of people with disabilities in workplaces, there is much resistance towards the inclusion of people with psychiatric illnesses. Occupational therapists should build their knowledge of relevant legislation related to people with disabilities within the workplace to best support the patient and advocate for the psychiatric patient's right to be included and to participate in these opportunities.

7 Advocacy for legislative and policy-related recommendations that promote occupational justice

Occupational therapists could influence policies and legislation that govern forensic patients and the community reintegration process. Some recommendations that can be reflected upon forensic facilities to consider are:

- Advocating for more community supportive structures such as halfway houses or residential care facilities to promote community living. This includes advocating for the aging forensic population who would benefit from living in retirement homes that can offer psychiatric and medical support. Low-cost options are vital to this population as patients' sole form of income may be governmental grants that do not cover residential and living expenses.
- Having clinical staff and institutions advocate for patients to access public transport at lower costs in order to travel home and to health care service providers.
- Providing safe conjugal spaces for long-term forensic patients who reside within correctional facilities.
- Addressing the increasing substance-use problem. Ease of access to substances and unclear legislation regarding the legalization of cannabis in some African countries, for example, can add to the uncertainty of rights for patients who have comorbid diagnoses.
- Providing more opportunities and access for patients, including foreign nationals, to participate in occupations of citizenship such as voting, applying for grants and acquiring of identity documentation. Patients who are psychiatrically stable should be afforded the opportunity to participate in these roles.

Conclusion

Considerable structural, economic and socio-political factors continue to put forensic patients at risk of experiencing occupational injustices. Occupational risk factors, such as occupational deprivation and imbalance, hamper the impact of mental health care and impede the recovery of forensic patients. Occupational therapists strive towards occupational justice in forensic mental health settings and use occupation as a means to promote health and well-being and the participation of forensic patients as equal citizens in their community and the country in which they reside.

The struggle for justice will not end easily by simply rewriting policies and changing legislation, as much as this is important to address as well. Greater effort needs to be put into reforming existing legislation and policies so that it becomes clear where accountabilities lie and so that the relevant role players at various levels can be held responsible to work towards ensuring that the practical realities are met for the forensic patient. This, we hope, will allow for forensic patients to benefit from more relevant and supportive legislation over time.

Despite facing numerous challenges, occupational therapists need to constantly work towards the promotion and enablement of occupational justice, for forensic patients to experience enriching, meaningful lives regardless of their forensic status and the context within which they live. All people who access forensic services as forensic patients should have the right to freely choose and engage in meaningful occupations that are often limited during confinement. This calls for a proactive multi-disciplinary team approach to curtail injustices and instill hope for an otherwise marginalized and incarcerated population.

References

Bassman, L. (1997). Holistic mental health care: Alternatives and adjuncts to psychotherapy and medication. *The Humanistic Psychologist, 25(2)*, 138. doi: 10.1080/08873267.1997.9986877

Bone, T. A., & Roberts, M. (2019). An investigation into the routes to inpatient care at the Pantang Hospital in Ghana via the criminal justice system. *Ghana Medical Journal, 53(2)*, 100–108.

Brooke, C. (2015). Selected psychometric properties of the activity participation outcome measure to describe trends in a forensic population of mental health care users. Dissertation submitted to the Faculty of Health Sciences, University of the Witwatersrand, Johannesburg, in fulfilment of the requirements for the degree of Master of Science in Occupational Therapy. http://hdl.handle.net/10539/18684

Burns, J. K. (2011). The mental health gap in South Africa: A human rights issue. *The Equal Rights Review, 6(99)*, 99–113.

Chichaya, T. F., Joubert, R., & McColl, M. A. (2019). Applying the occupational justice framework in disability policy analysis in Namibia. *South African Journal of Occupational Therapy, 49(1)*, 19–25.

Christiansen, C. H. (1999). Defining lives: Occupation as identity: An essay on competence, coherence, and the creation of meaning. *The American Journal of Occupational Therapy, 53(6)*, 547–557.

Dubihlela, J., & Dubihlela, D. (2014). Social grants impact on poverty among the female-headed households in South Africa: A case analysis. *Mediterranean Journal of Social Sciences, 5(8)*, 160–166. doi: 10.5901/mjss.2014.v5n8p160

Duncan, M. (2009). Human occupation in the context of chronic poverty and psychiatric disability. Dissertation submitted to the Faculty of Psychology, Stellenbosch University, Cape Town, in fulfilment of the requirements for a doctoral degree. *91*, 34–48. http://scholar.sun.ac.za/handle/10019.1/1120

Duncan, M., Swartz, L., & Kathard, H. (2011). The burden of psychiatric disability on chronically poor households: Part 1 (costs). *South African Journal of Occupational Therapy, 41*, 55–63.

Durocher, E., Gibson, B. E., & Rappolt, S. (2013) Occupational Justice: A conceptual review. *Journal of Occupational Science, 21(4)*, 418–430. doi: 10.1080/14427591.2013.775692

Engelbrecht, M., Van Niekerk, L., Coetzee, Z., & Hajwani, Z. (2017). Supported employment for people with mental disabilities in South Africa: Cost calculation of service utilization. *South African Journal of Occupational Therapy, 47(2)*, 11–16.

Farnworth, L., & Muñoz, J. (2009). An occupational and rehabilitative perspective for institutional practice. *Psychiatric Rehabilitation Journal, 32(3)*, 192–198.

Federal, Provincial and Territorial Advisory Committee on Population Health. (1999). Toward a healthy future: Second report on the health of Canadians. Public Health Agency of Canada. Retrieved from http://www.phacaspc.gc.ca/phsp/reportrapport/toward/pdf/toward_a_healthy_english.PDF

Herbig, F. J. W., & Hesselink, A. E. (2012). Seeing the person, not just the number: Needs-based rehabilitation of the offenders in South African prisons. *SA Crime Quarterly, 41,* 29–37. doi: 10.17159/2413-3108/2012/v0i41a838

Kaliski, S. Z. (2006). The dangerous offender and risk assessment. In S. Z. Kaliski (Ed.) Psycholegal assessment in South Africa (pp. 113–125). Cape Town: Oxford University Press.

Kaliski, S. Z. (2012). Does the insanity defence lead to an abuse of human rights? *African Journal of Psychiatry, 15,* 83–87. doi: 10.4314/ajpsy.v15i2.11

Kaliski, S. Z. (2013). Reinstitutionalization by stealth: The Forensic Mental Health Service is the new chronic system. *African Journal of Psychiatry, 16*(*1*), 13–17. doi: 10. 4314/ajpsy.v16i1.2

Kiepek, N., Beagan, B., Laliberte Rudman, D., & Phelan, S. (2018). Silences around occupations framed as unhealthy, illegal, and deviant. *Journal of Occupational Science.* doi: 10.1080/14427591.2018.1499123

Krüger, C., & Lewis, C. (2011). Patient and social work factors related to successful placement of long-term psychiatric in-patients from a specialist psychiatric hospital in South Africa. *African Journal of Psychiatry, 14,* 120–129. doi: 10.4314/ajpsy.v14i2.3

Mace, J., Hocking, C., Waring, M., Townsend, L., Whalley Hammell, K., Galheigo, S., Aldrich, B., Bailliard, A., Adams, F. & Whiteford, G. (2018). Occupational Justice as the Freedom to Do & Be: A conceptual tool for advocating for human rights. WFOT Congress, Cape Town South Africa, May 2018.

Molineux, M. L., & Whiteford, G. E. (1999). Prisons: From occupational deprivation to occupational enrichment. *Journal of Occupational Science, 6*(*3*), 124–130. doi: 10.1080/14427591.1999.9686457

Monteiro, N. (2015). Addressing mental illness in Africa: Global health challenges and local opportunities. Clinical *and Counselling Psychology, 1,* 78–95. doi: 10.1285/i24212113v1i2p78

Moore, M. (2005). Forensic psychiatry and occupational therapy. In R. Crouch & V. Alers (Eds.), *Occupational Therapy in Psychiatry and Mental Health* (4th ed., pp. 256–260). England: Whurr Publishers Ltd.

Nilsson, T., Munthe, C., Gustavson, C., Forsman, A., & Anckarsäter, H. (2009). The precarious practice of forensic psychiatric risk assessments. *International Journal of Law and Psychiatry, 32*(*6*), 400–407. doi: 10.1016/j.ijlp.2009.09.010

Occupational Therapy Africa Regional Group Membership. (n.d). Retrieved from https://www.otarg.org.za/membership/member-countries-of-otarg.html

Pierce, D. (2001). Untangling occupation and activity. *American Journal of Occupational Therapy, 55*(*3*), 138–146. doi: 10.5014/ajot.55.2.138

Restall, G., & Ripat, J. (2008). Applicability and clinical utility of the client-centred strategies framework. *Canadian Journal of Occupational Therapy, 75,* 288–300.

Roffey, M., & Kaliski, S. Z. (2012). "To predict or not to predict - that is the question." An exploration of risk assessment in the context of South African forensic psychiatry. *African Journal of Psychiatry, 15*(*4*), 227–233. doi: 10.4314/ajpsy.v15i4.29

Royal College of Occupational Therapists. (2012). Occupational Therapists' Use of Occupation-Focused Practice in Secure Hospitals: Practice Guidelines. London: Royal

College of Occupational Therapists Ltd. 12–45. Retrieved from https://www.rcot.co.uk/practice-resources/rcot-practice-guidelines/secure-hospitals

Sherry, K. (2010). Voices of occupational therapists in Africa. In V. Alers & R. Crouch (Eds.) Occupational Therapy: An African Perspective (pp. 26–47). Johannesburg: Sarah Shorten Publishers.

Stadnyk, R., Townsend, E., & Wilcock, A. (2010). Occupational justice. In C. H. Christiansen & E. A. Townsend (Eds.), *Introduction to occupation: The art and science of living.* (Vol. 2, pp. 329–358).Upper Saddle River, NJ: Pearson Education.

Townsend, E. A., & Wilcock, A. (2004). Occupational justice and client-centred practice: A dialogue in progress. *Canadian Journal of Occupational Therapy, 71(2)*, 75–85.

United Nations. (1948). Universal declaration of human rights. Retrieved from https://www.ohchr.org/EN/UDHR/Documents/UDHR_Translations/eng.pdf

Wagman, P., Håkansson, C., & Björklund, A. (2011). Occupational balance as used in occupational therapy: A concept analysis. *Scandinavian Journal of Occupational Therapy, 19*, 322–327. doi: 10.3109/11038128.2011.596219

Wegner, L. (2016). Meaning and purpose in the occupations of gang-involved young men in Cape Town. *South African Journal of Occupational Therapy, 46(1)*, 53–58. doi: 10.17159/2310-3833/2016/v46n1a11

Whiteford, G. (1997). Occupational deprivation and incarceration. *Journal of Occupational Science, 4(3)*, 126–130. doi: 10.1080/14427591.1997.9686429

Whiteford, G. (2000). Occupational deprivation: Global challenge in the new millennium. *British Journal of Occupational Therapy, 63(5)*, 200–204.

Whiteford, G., Jones, K., Weekes, G., Ndlovu, N., Long, C., Perkes, D., & Brindle, S. (2019). Combatting occupational deprivation and advancing occupational justice in institutional settings: Using a practice-based enquiry approach for service transformation. *British Journal of Occupational Therapy*, *83*(1), 52–61.

Wilcock, A. A. (1998). Reflections on doing, being and becoming. *Canadian Journal of Occupational Therapy, 65(5)*, 248–256.

Wilcock, A. A., & Townsend, E. (2000). Occupational terminology interactive dialogue. *Journal of Occupational Science, 7(2)*, 84–86.

Wilcock, A. (2003). Occupational science: The study of humans as occupational beings. In P. Kramer, J. Hinojosa, & C. B. Royeen (Eds.), *Perspectives in human occupation: Participation in life* (pp. 156–180). Philadelphia: Lippincott Williams & Wilkins.

Wolf, L., Ripat, J., Davis, E., Becker, P., & MacSwiggan, J. (2010). Applying an occupational justice framework. *Occupational Therapy Now, 12(1)*, 15–18.

Addendum A.

Table 14.2 Assessment of occupational injustices in a forensic context

Assessment areas		
Assessment of basic needs	**YES**	**NO**
Does the patient have access to means that satisfy physiological needs such as showers, toilets, toiletries, food, shelter and clothing?		
Comment:		
Assessment of individuality and autonomy	**YES**	**NO**
Is patient individuality supported?		
Are patients able to participate in religious and spiritual activities?		
Are their rights as citizens being violated in any way?		
Are patients allowed to keep personal/electronic items with them for use (i.e., a cellphone/laptop)?		
Are patients given an opportunity to make decisions and choices in relation to their recovery (management of illness, activity participation, daily routine and engagement as well as input into their use of medication)		
Do patients have choices around participating in the available groups/interventions?		
Are patient requests accommodated within reason?		
Comment:		
Assessment of the environment and living conditions	**YES**	**NO**
Does the physical environment satisfy principles of basic human rights?		
Is the environment spacious and comfortable?		
Is the environment safe?		
Does the environment allow for some level of privacy?		
Are allowances made for personalization of patients' living spaces?		
Does the environment promote interactive occupation and social engagement?		
Are patients able to independently access resources on-site that mimic community life such as		
• A television and video player		
• A radio/CD player		
• Use of a phone		
• Reading material/a library		
• A tuck-shop/coffee shop		
• A computer		
• TV games/computer games		
• A hairdresser/barber		
• A gym/sporting equipment		
• A kitchen and kitchen equipment		
• Outdoor resting area		

(*Continued*)

Table 14.2 (Continued)

Assessment areas		
Comment:		
Assessment of program development and maintenance	**YES**	**NO**
Is a person-centered model used in the recovery practice?		
Are cultural considerations included in program development?		
Are ward group programs adapted to patients' needs and interests?		
Are individual profiles and rehabilitation plans developed in collaboration with patients?		
Are therapies transparent in service delivery and managing patients' expectations?		
Do patients have a participatory role in forum discussions pertaining to their service needs?		
Are programs evaluated in relation to patients' evolving needs and input?		
Are programs adapted in relation to emerging patient needs?		
Is the program balanced in addressing needs in the various life areas – work, learning, socializing and living?		
Are programs tailored at the different levels of functioning of patients as well as their age and life stage?		
Do programs include skills development for income generation?		
Comment:		
Assessment of opportunities for community participation	**YES**	**NO**
Are patients allowed to leave the premises and access the community independently on a daily basis?		
Are patients allowed to go for short and long periods of leave?		
Are accommodations made for escorted parole if they are not allowed unsupervised leave?		
Are patients taken on community outings (to places of their choice)?		
Are patients allowed to travel independently with public transport?		
Are provisions made for those who are unable to travel independently?		
Are provisions made for patients who require financial assistance for traveling?		
Does the institution assist with grant applications for patients who are going on long periods of leave?		
Comment:		
Assessment of work and learning	**YES**	**NO**
Are there learning programs (learnerships, apprenticeships, adult-based education, tertiary education etc.) available to patients?		

(*Continued*)

Table 14.2 (Continued)

Assessment areas		
Are there on-site work programs available for patients to participate in?		
Are there voluntary work and learning programs available for skills development of patients?		
Do patients have a choice to participate in a work program?		
Are there restrictions on the type of work a patient is allowed to do?		
Do patients receive remuneration for on-site work?		
Do patients have full access to the income earned and can they choose how to use their income?		
Are patients allowed to enter the community to search, acquire and participate in employment?		
Is the employment and learning process facilitated and supported by the multi-disciplinary team (MDT)?		
Are patients assisted with traveling in their first month of participation in work/learning programs?		
Are patients fairly and equitably remunerated for work participation?		
Is ongoing support provided to the learner, worker or employer in the work or learning environment?		
Is disclosure around mental illness discussed with the patient and consent provided in preparation for work opportunities?		
Is confidentiality maintained when a patient chooses not to disclose their illness?		
Is confidentiality, at an institutional level, maintained around the patients' forensic status?		
Is stigma within the workplace proactively addressed by the MDT?		
Comments:		
Assessment of institutional policies and protocols	**YES**	**NO**
Do institutional policies and procedures empower and promote inclusion of patients?		
Do policies and procedures promote autonomy and support the rebalancing of power structures?		
Are privileges revoked/withheld if patients choose not to participate in the program?		
Do ward routines/protocols promote unconstructive use of time and participation in passive occupations?		
Comments:		
SUMMARY		
ASSESSMENT AREA	**ENABLERS**	**BARRIERS**
Basic needs		
Individuality and autonomy		
Environment and living conditions		
Program development and maintenance		
Community participation		
Work and learning		
Institutional policies and protocols		

(Royal College of occupational therapists, 2012, p. 12; Whiteford et al., 2019)

15 Best practices with female patients in African forensic mental health care

Aishatu Yusha'u Armiya'u and Adegboyega Ogunwale

Introduction

The global prison population is estimated at 10.7 million, either as pre-trial detainees/remand prisoners or having been convicted and sentenced (Stevenson, 2016; Public Radio International, 2018). Between 2000 and 2015, the number of women in prison increased by 50%, twice the rate of male prisoners (The Sentencing Project, 2018). This increase is huge in comparison with 20% for the male population, and is rising on all continents (United Nations Office on Drugs and Crime, 2020). This trend has also been observed across Africa, where women now constitute up to 6% of national prison populations (Ackermann, 2015). Approximately 7% of the world's prison population is women, with over 714,000 women and girls held in prisons and other closed settings. Many African countries have experienced a growth of over 200% in their women prison population in the last 20 years (Walmsley, 2017). Prisons in Sub-Saharan Africa (SSA) also have seen an increase of 22% in women prisoners in recent years (Global Prison Trends, 2016; Walmsley, 2006). Women constitute between 1 and 4% of the total SSA prison population (World Prison Brief, 2018). As of March 2013, there were 3380 incarcerated women in South African prisons, 2.2% of the total population. Of this figure, 988 are unsentenced and awaiting trial, and 2392 are sentenced (South African Institute of Race Relations, 2013). Similarly, the prison population in Nigeria is 63,322 with a female population of 1170, putting the proportion of female inmates at 2% as of 8 June 2020 (Nigerian Correctional Service, 2020). Of these, 924 (79%) females are awaiting trial (Nigerian Correctional Service, 2020).

The profile and background of women in prisons, and the reasons for which they are imprisoned, are different from those of men in the same situation (Coyle, 2009). Women admitted into prisons usually come from marginalized and disadvantaged backgrounds and they often have histories of violence and physical and sexual abuse (Stevenson, 2016). On the whole, women in prisons present specific challenges for correctional authorities despite, or perhaps because they constitute a very small proportion of the prison population. Due to the fact that there are few prisons for women, women tend to be imprisoned far from home; the distance separating them from their children, families and friends increases their isolation and can be a source of additional stress such as economic hardship and anxiety, for both the women concerned and their families.

Gender and criminality

The opportunity theory of female criminality propounded by Rita J. Simon in 1975 is one of the nuances of the opportunity theory. The theory dwells more on the descriptions of various forms of female criminality-nature, type and also the role of court and jails in this regard. Simon argues that there is no difference between females and males in terms of morality and that there is nothing particularly inherent in human biological sex that predisposes men or women towards crime. When succinct opportunities for criminal activities abound, both male and female are likely to perpetrate crime.

Crime opportunities are necessary prerequisites for crime to occur. Simon further contends that over time, males perpetrate more crimes than females because of their greater social opportunities, networking and competences. Gender gap in the extant opportunities is the cause of gender gap in crime rate. If female opportunity, social communication, efficiency and networking are increased, then the rate of female criminality will ultimately increase (Small, 2000). Simon (1975, p. 3) argues that:

> ... *when more women get access in labour market as skilled labour and possess highly specialized position in the job sector they commit more employment related property crime like men. Some women take the advantage of these opportunities, just as some men do before.*

Hence, the more women are emancipated politically, socially, culturally and economically, the more the opportunities to commit crime will abound and the more the female criminality will increase. Also, in most countries, boys are given greater leeway within and outside the family than girls, and this gives more opportunity to the boys to commit crime.

Notwithstanding this, women in prison face unique challenges. They typically come from backgrounds of disadvantage, including mental illness, trauma, abuse, neglect and domestic violence (Heard, 2017). In prison, they are vulnerable to mistreatment, including sexual assault. Because women make up a smaller percentage of the prison population than men, their specific needs are often neglected. And for the many women prisoners who are pregnant or primary caregivers, prison presents extreme challenges in health and childcare (Ackermann, 2015).

In some countries, many incarcerated women do not have access to health care services prior to incarceration (Mignon, 2016). This can be attributed to their low socio-economic status and problems such as substance use, lack of good nutrition and lack of preventive health care (Fearn & Parker, 2005). Lack of medical care prior to incarceration also can mean more serious health issues, including chronic health problems (Fearn & Parker, 2005). Historically, many female inmates with serious chronic physical illnesses failed to receive care while incarcerated (Wilper et al., 2009). The reproductive issues of women make the provision of health care more complicated for women than for men and are an additional challenge to health care services within prison walls. These include menstruation, pregnancy, childbirth, breastfeeding and menopause (International Committee of the Red Cross, 2009), which could all be complicated by mental and psychological challenges.

Offense profile of female prisoners

Female offenders represent a socially and criminally dissimilar group to that of male offenders. Both males and females are equally likely to be found guilty of criminal offenses, yet female involvement in crime is lower than that of males (Bartlett, 2006). Incarcerated females have become a cause for concern based on their increasing vulnerability (Johnson & Zlotnick, 2008), since the majority of female offenders suffer from lifetime victimization and illicit drug abuse (Moloney & Moller, 2009, p. 431). Many female offenders experience extensive childhood and adulthood abuse and report numerous traumatic experiences (Green, Miranda, Daroowalla, & Siddique, 2005, p. 134; Hatton & Fisher, 2008, p. 1305).

Two South African studies reported the biographical characteristics of female offenders. Authors reported that the majority of the female offenders they studied were younger than 35 years of age, not married, had secondary level of education and were employed before incarceration (Booyens & Steyn, 2013; Dastile, 2011). Another South African study (Nagdee et al., 2019) observed that the most prevalent offenses that led to court-referred forensic psychiatric evaluations were for violent index offense categories: offenses against life (e.g., attempted murder and murder) and against bodily integrity (e.g., assault and assault with intention to do grievous bodily harm). In fact, murder was the single most common index offense. Women who were first-time offenders were more likely to commit nonviolent index offenses, and those with a prior criminal history (of any kind) were more likely to engage in violent index offenses.

Another study conducted by the National Institute for Crime Prevention and the Reintegration of Offenders (NICRO) in South Africa among female prisoners reported that the most common offense committed by female prisoners was theft/attempted theft. The majority of the female prisoners were found to have abused children (aggressive offense). This could likely be due to the fact that women have more regular contact with children. Though male offenders accounted for majority of offenses referred to in the study, a significant percentage of females committed criminal acts of aggression. According to Van Dieten Jones and Rondon (2014, p. 2), the highest proportion of violent offenses committed by women occurs within the context of an intimate relationship. Unfortunately, South African data to support or refute this is not generally available. Identified violence risk factors for women include younger age, unemployment, low socioeconomic status, lack of social support and poverty. Sexual offense was found to be low among the female prisoners studied.

Mental disorders among female prisoners

Contextual factors

Mental disorders impose an enormous burden almost everywhere across the world (World Health Organization, 2016). It is one of the greatest challenges that the current and future generations will face (Halliwell et al., 2007). Globally, reported rates of psychiatric morbidity among prisoners vary widely. In addition to substance-use disorders, women in prison have alarmingly high rates of mental health problems, such as post-traumatic stress disorder, depression, anxiety, phobias, neurosis, self-mutilation and suicide. This is frequently a result of lifetime abuse and victimization (United Nation's Office on Drugs and Crime, 2009). Whether a woman's mental health improves or worsens during incarceration depends on several factors, including the prison structure, the treatment options, including the availability of trauma-responsive programming and the facilities and services provided to women (United Nation's Office on Drugs and Crime, 2009).

As a result of overcrowding due to high rates of pre-trial detention, poor infrastructure and weak health care delivery within the criminal justice systems, appalling psychological and physical conditions results. Additionally, prison environments that are characterized by staff and inmate physical and sexual abuse, food insecurity and inadequate sanitation as well as compromised access to health care services predispose or exacerbate mental disorders and physical illnesses including spread of infectious diseases such as human immunodeficiency virus (HIV) infection and tuberculosis (TB) in SSA prisons (Telisinghe et al., 2016; Todrys et al., 2011; Women in Prisons, 2018).

In the closed environment of prisons, women are especially vulnerable to sexual abuse, including rape by both male staff and other male prisoners. There are countries where women in prison are held in small facilities adjacent to or within prisons for men (United Nations Office on Drugs and Crime, 2008). In some prison facilities, there are no separate quarters for women and they may be supervised by male prison staff. They are also susceptible to sexual exploitation and may engage in sex in exchange for goods such as food, drugs, cigarettes and toiletries (Plugge et al., 2006).

Depression

Depression is a common, occasionally severe, but treatable mental disorder (Kumar et al., 2012). Out of people suffering from depression; 85% live in low- and middle-income countries that include SSA (World Health Organization, 2009). When compared to the general population, worldwide, prisoners were five to ten times more likely to develop depression (Beyen et al., 2017; Fazel & Danesh, 2002). According to studies conducted in different parts of Africa, 10.4% to 82.5% of prisoners are found to be depressed and the disorder is higher among females and young age groups (Naidoo & Mkize, 2012; Nwaopara &

Stanley, 2015; Ibrahim et al., 2014). A study conducted among female prisoners at Kirikiri maximum security in Lagos, Nigeria, found depression in 27.3% of convicted and 23.3% of remand female prisoners (Sakeeb, 2007) compared with about 3.1% in the general population (Gureje, Uwakewe, Oladeji, Makanjuola, & Esan, 2010). Incarceration is considered a highly stressful experience that has devastating effects on the well-being of offenders (Steyn & Hall, 2015). The environment and nature of correctional centers often produce psychological effects that are not conducive to the goals of rehabilitation and reducing re-offending. Instead, imprisonment negatively affects mental health and commonly produces symptoms of depression and anxiety (Steyn & Hall, 2015).

Substance-use disorders

Along with high rates of previous victimization and histories of abuse, many female offenders have a higher lifetime prevalence of drug abuse and substance use disorder (SUD) than the general population (Moloney & Moller, 2009). Studies indicate that women with substance abuse problems are more likely than men to have experienced physical and/or sexual abuse (United Nations Office on Drugs and Crime, 2004). A history of violent assault can increase the risk of substance use and post-traumatic stress disorder or other mental health problems. It has been reported that rates of post-traumatic stress disorder among women in substance abuse treatment range from 30 to 59% (cited in United Nations Office on Drugs and Crime, 2014). Some findings have indicated that the odds of women with coexisting psychiatric disabilities being returned to prison within 12 months of release were increased by 58% in comparison to women with only a substance addiction (compared to 40% in men) (Messina, Burdon, Hagopian & Prendergast, 2006 cited in United Nations Office on Drugs and Crime, 2014).

Drug-dependent former prisoners are also at a higher risk of death resulting from overdose, compared to the general population. For example, according to research carried out in the United Kingdom, in the week following release, prisoners were 40 times more likely to die than the general population. In this period, immediately after release, most of these deaths (over 90%) were associated with drug-related causes (United Nations Office on Drugs and Crime, 2014). In Australia, where former prisoners have death rates ten times that of the general population, with over half of these deaths being heroin related, women appear to be especially susceptible. Female ex-prisoners were 27 times more likely to die an unnatural death than their counterparts in the general population (United Nations Office on Drugs and Crime, 2014).

The increased rates of depression and SUD among female offenders have serious consequences, interfering with their ability to cope with stressors both inside and outside the correctional center. The poor mental health among female offenders has a number of negative consequences, including an impaired ability to follow rules, increased disciplinary problems, as well as self-mutilation and suicide attempts (Steyn & Hall, 2015). Psychological distress in the form of self-harm is higher among females than males, especially upon initial incarceration (Steyn-Hall, 2015).

Psychotic disorders

Psychotic disorders that include schizophrenia spectrum disorders as well as bipolar affective disorders are the leading contributors to disease burden globally (Mweslga et al., 2020). Psychotic disorders usually run a chronic course in the life of an individual. In empirical prison studies, female offenders have received little attention in comparison with male offenders, but the few South African studies that do exist have shown that women's pathways to imprisonment are characterized by prior sexual and physical victimization, parental neglect, stressful life events and mental health issues that include psychotic disorders (Artz et al., 2012).

A South African study by Nagdee et al. (2019) among female offenders referred for psychiatric evaluation in a mental health facility showed that a prior psychiatric history was documented in almost half (48.9%; n = 280) of the women. Also, in those whose previous psychiatric diagnosis was known, 12.2% were diagnosed with bipolar disorders, while 11.9% had psychotic disorders. In addition, 25.0% (n = 141) had a documented history of mental illness in a family member.

For the women who had been convicted of crimes against their own child or children (n = 116), 54.3% had disclosed a previous psychiatric illness. A closer analysis of this sub-sample revealed a relatively high number of psychotic disorders (11.2%) in comparison to the total sample and at the time of offending, the majority of the cases (33.6%) had active psychopathology. The most common form of psychopathology at the time of offending was psychosis (29.7%). Psychopathological factors were also significantly associated with violent index offending, cited in over one-third of the cases (Nagdee et al., 2019).

Anxiety disorders

Anxiety is a common experience in everyday life. Feeling anxious about certain things is normal and important for adaptation and survival. However, the degree of anxiety that some people feel is sometimes excessive, affects their functional capacity and can be debilitating. Anxiety disorders are diagnosed when anxiety is either persistent or persistently recurrent, and affects a person's ability to work, have relationships or interact with others in social situations (Dadi et al., 2016).

A cross-sectional survey conducted among male and female prisoners in North Ethiopia showed that more than one-third of the prisoners had an anxiety disorder (Dadi et al., 2016). It also reported that the odds of anxiety was 2.49 times higher among prisoners who reported to have had an unhappy life before they were imprisoned. This might be because their imprisonment might have added to their life stress that they have had or their anxiety symptoms may have been there for a long time (Dadi et al., 2016). Another study conducted exclusively among female prisoners in Nigeria reported anxiety disorder in 3.6% of convicted and 5.3% of remanded female inmates (Sakeeb, 2007). Most of the prisoners were in their productive years and were expected to contribute to their country upon their return from the prison. Moreover, the prison environment could offer the opportunity for various vocational training activities that could equip them with knowledge and skills for their future life. Such a positive outlook would be largely impeded by mental ill health such as anxiety disorder while in prison (Dadi et al., 2016).

Certain imprisonment conditions are likely to initiate or exacerbate anxiety. These include the loss of privacy, the strain experienced in adapting to communal life in prison and the lack of control over their bodies as a result of strip searches as well as the fear of losing interpersonal relationships with family and friends after incarceration. The separation of mother and child often intensifies the pain of imprisonment for women by creating an intense feeling of isolation that is accentuated by the frustration and guilt that these females experience as a result of the separation from their children and their inability to continue to care for them. Additionally, a significant number of incarcerated women were the sole breadwinners in their families before imprisonment. These feelings of despair are also aggravated by the non-cordial relationship that often exists between the female prisoners and the prison staff (Pogrebin & Dodge, 2006). All of these institutional factors could serve as drivers for the development or exacerbation of anxiety disorder in female prisoners.

Forensic consideration relevant to females in prison

The thin line between child discipline and abuse

Cultural relativity plays a role in determining what constitutes child discipline and consequently, child abuse. For example, the contemporary western viewpoint on child rearing is that corporal punishment is to be generally discouraged and where possible, statutorily criminalized. Virtually all African countries subscribe to the moral underpinnings of respect for the dignity of the child and have ratified the UN Convention on the Rights of the Child and (African Charter on the Rights and Welfare of the Child, 1990; Gose, 2002). However, in many African jurisdictions, corporal punishment is still regarded as a lawful and socially applauded approach to child discipline. For instance, the Nigerian Criminal Code Act permits corporal punishment as "a blow or other force, not in any case extending to a wound or grievous harm" and may be deployed for correcting a child (explicitly stated as being below 16 years). The additional caveat is that the child is capable of understanding the purpose for which the punishment is inflicted (Laws of the Federation of Nigeria, 2004; section 295). This presents a bit of complication for a child of 15 years who has intellectual disability. Another example is Ghana in which section 41 of the Criminal Offenses Act (2003) as well as article 13(2) of its Children's Act (1998) have been reported to sanction corporal punishment of children.

Against this backdrop, determinations of child abuse have been largely dependent on the evidence of physical injury (i.e., "wound" or "grievous harm"). Cases that have been prosecuted have included those in which children have been burnt, maimed or even accidentally fatally wounded in the process of discipline. Charges range from grievous bodily harm to manslaughter and murder. In many cases, the defendants have been females due to the traditional gender roles in African societies in which mothers are regarded as "keepers at home" and are primarily responsible for the discipline of children and wards within the extended family system. It is thus conceivable that when discipline transits to abuse, it is more likely that the perpetrator is the female who is saddled with the responsibility of the former.

Infanticide

Infanticide is defined as the killing of children under one year of age. Neonaticide is a specific form of infanticide in which a baby is killed within 24 hours of birth. In Nigerian law, for example, infanticide refers to an unlawful homicide, which is killing infants who are below 12 months of age by their mothers, through any willful act or omission due to disturbed balance of her mind by reason of having not recovered from the effect of giving birth to the child or by reason of the effect of lactation following the birth of the child (Lawrence, 2015). Conventionally, the offender is dealt with and punished as if she had been guilty of manslaughter of the child.

According to Section 306 of the Nigeria Criminal Code Act, "it is unlawful to kill any person unless such killing is authorized or justified or excused by law." Section 315 of Nigeria Criminal Code says any person who unlawfully kills another is guilty of an offense, which is called murder or manslaughter, according to the circumstances of the code. This law as such applies to women who commit the crime of infanticide in Nigeria.

Infanticide is the second most common reason women are in jail in Senegal after drug trafficking. Out of the countries' 283 female offenders in 2015, 19% were in prison for the crime of infanticide according to the UN Office for Human Rights in West Africa. Unlike in China and India where the practice stems from gender selection, in Senegal it was said to be as a result of immense stigma and social ostracization around unwanted pregnancies (Shryock & Gaestel, 2018).

In South Africa, research shows that 454 children under the age of five died due to homicide in 2009. More than half died within 28 days or younger, with the majority dying within the first six days of their lives. Tanzania has the highest reported rates of neonaticide. For every 100,000 births in the country, 27 babies are killed within the first 24 hours (Outwater et al., 2010). Another study in Ghana also reported that nearly 15% of deaths among children under three years could be linked to infanticide practices (Allotey & Reidpath, 2001). Child homicide is often not considered a priority against competing public health problems. Additionally, the statistics suggest that reproductive, mental health and social services are failing to identify and help vulnerable mothers in Africa (Abrahams, 2016) who may then fall through the service cracks and end up incarcerated after killing their infants. In a sense, such systemic inadequacies fail both the victims (the dead infants/children) and the perpetrators (homicidal mothers).

Domestic violence and "battered woman" syndrome as background factors in homicide offending

Numerous women experience domestic violence and abuse on a daily basis, and some retaliate and kill their intimate male partners. A World Health Organization (WHO) report on global and regional estimates of violence against women found that the global lifetime prevalence of Intimate Partner Violence (IPV) among ever-partnered women was 30%, and for Africa 37% (World Health Organization, 2013). Reports from the Nigerian national population commission estimated women's lifetime exposure to IPV from their current husband or partner at 19% for emotional IPV, 14% for physical IPV and 5% for sexual IPV (National Population-NPC/Nigeria and ICF International, 2014). Previous studies from Nigeria have shown the prevalence of IPV to range from 31 to 61% for psychological/emotional violence, 20 to 31% for sexual violence and 7 to 31% for physical violence (Mapayi et al., 2013). Studies have reported lifetime IPV prevalence rates of 52.8% in Congo, 42% in Kenya, 27% in Malawi, 32% in Rwanda, 48% in Zambia and 33% in Zimbabwe (Hindin et al., 2008). Males are more likely to abuse if they had grown up witnessing such abuse in the home and even more likely to abuse if they suffered paternal abuse (Redd, 2019). In a WHO multi-country study, women who had experienced IPV reported poorer health, more emotional distress and more suicidal thoughts and attempts than those who had not experienced IPV (García-Moreno et al., 2005). Two in three victims of intimate partner/family-related homicide are women (Hindin et al., 2008; World Health Organization, 2013). Abused women often experience negative psychological and physiological consequences of the abuse such as coping problems, a sense of inadequacy, anger and unpredictability which could result in murder (Pretorius & Botha, 2016). Battered women who kill their abusers in South Africa often face barriers to accessing criminal law defences to murder. According to the Department of Correctional Services, in 2004, 163 women were incarcerated in South African prisons for the murder of their partners (Department of Correctional Services, 2004).

Furthermore, according to Bester (2008), various factors may cause women to kill their intimate male partners. These factors include PTSD symptoms such as a state of hypervigilance and dissociation as well as coercive control by the abuser including needs deprivation and relationships marked by high levels of conflict. The use of substances on the part of both intimate partners may also play a significant role in fatal violence. Walker (1984) writes that women who kill their intimate partners may believe that their reports of the abuse were ignored or not seriously considered and, consequently, they have to protect themselves from current or future attacks. The intimate partners may, on occasion, also challenge the women to kill them. Some women may resort to murder in order to prevent their partners from gaining total control over their minds (Walker, 1984).

In the past, women were often blamed for any abuse that occurred, and the abuse itself was not considered a serious crime. Some people actually believed that women derived enjoyment from the abuse or felt a need to be punished (Walker & Browne, 1985). This view emanated partly from early psychoanalytic theories of violence in women that held that violent women were "masochistic, passive and personality-disordered" (Boonzaier & de la Rey, 2004, p. 444; Coolidge & Anderson, 2002; Walker, 1984). Early theories of abuse also held that sex role socialization was a factor associated with abuse. Such socialization was thought to result in a sense of learned helplessness that prevented the abuse from ending (Walker, 1984). One influential theory of violence that has been utilized in explaining the complex nature of spousal abuse is the Walker Cycle Theory of Violence (Walker, 1979, cited in Walker, 1984). According to this theory, abuse is cyclical and consists of three stages: "(1) tension building, (2) the acute battering incident, and (3) loving contrition" (Walker, 1984, p. 95). The theory seems to be in agreement with Martin Seligman's theory of learned helplessness. In the first stage, a buildup of tension occurs in which the abuser expresses disdain in verbally, emotionally or psychologically abusive ways. Moreover, in this stage, "minor" battering incidents may occur while the victim typically remains passive in an attempt to avoid greater violence. The second stage occurs when the tension between the abuser and the victim reaches a breaking point and an incident or series of incidents triggers extreme violence. Finally, the third stage, commonly called the "honeymoon phase," is when the abuser seeks forgiveness, perhaps promises not to repeat the same violent behavior and showers the victim with love, affection and/or gifts. As the tension and violence escalate, it becomes more difficult for the woman to end the abusive relationship (Frieze, 2005). Deciding to withdraw from an abusive relationship is an intricate process as leaving the relationship generally results in many changes and challenges such as relocation, financial concerns and disruption in social patterns.

Against this backdrop, battered woman syndrome (BWS) describes the behavioral effects of women who are the victims of repeated psychological, emotional and/or physical abuse, typically over an extended period of time at the hands of a dominant male partner. BWS is a subcategory of posttraumatic stress disorder (PTSD) as set forth in the *Diagnostic Statistical Manual of Mental Disorders, V*. PTSD manifests when a person has been "repeatedly and unpredictably exposed to a stressor and develop[s] certain psychological symptoms. A battered woman may have flashbacks, experience anger, be unable to concentrate, and experience sleep interruptions, similar to a person suffering from PTSD". Moreover, a woman with BWS may engage in conscious and unconscious efforts to avoid anything that reminds her of the violent relationship. Given the syndrome's connection to PTSD, expert testimony is often proffered in certain criminal and civil cases in order to provide an understanding of the person's conduct or testimony at trial.

In patriarchal African societies, females tend to enjoy more emotional and social support than males and, albeit it in a small way, this may act as a buffer against negative effects of strain on females. This type of emotional and social support comes from close relationships with family members and/or friends. Broidy and Agnew (1997, p. 284) argue that such relationships reduce stress. They maintain that "females who are more strongly invested in their intimate networks may try to avoid serious criminal behaviors that would threaten these ties." This line of reasoning is based on the fact that females desist from behavior, such as criminal and delinquent behavior, that may threaten or jeopardize their close relationships with others. Thus, these close relationships encourage females to access/utilize legitimate coping strategies to deal with the strain(s) that they may be experiencing. For example, they may speak to the people with whom they share these relationships about their problems. However, these interpersonal relationships are not devoid of their own unique strain which may result from the grave illness of a close friend or family member (Broidy & Agnew, 1997, p. 284).

Females participating in drug trafficking

According to Fleetwood (2015c), a drug mule can be defined as " … someone who carries drugs across international borders. They typically undertake this specific role only, working under the instructions of others. Mules carry drugs concealed in luggage, on their body or clothes, or swallowed in latex-wrapped capsules in order to avoid detection." The term *drug mule* is understood to refer to individuals specially selected or sought out by drug syndicates to carry drugs intentionally or unwittingly from one country to another (Tsotetsi, 2012).

More recently, however, female drug mules have emerged as key figures in the transportation of drugs. In November 2016, two South African women were arrested in the Ugandan capital of Kampala for cocaine smuggling (Bagala, 2016). A 2017 report by Interpol established that nearly 170 kg of drugs worth $10 million were seized after being found hidden in luggage, concealed in shoe heels and hair and/or swallowed by couriers in a sting operation code-named Folosa (Interpol, 2015). Operation Folosa targeted drug trafficking from Latin America to Europe via Africa. The operation's results are noteworthy specifically for the discovery of a methamphetamine trafficking route from Nigeria to South Africa. In 2016, for example, Tyrone Lee Coetzee was found guilty of smuggling drugs and handed a death sentence in Hanoi, Vietnam (Gous, 2018).

Singer et al. (2013) indicated that although many mules are men, the number of Nigerian women hired to carry drugs via air from Nigeria to Spain and England has increased. This could mean that women are making independent decisions regarding involvement in criminal activities as a study by Klein (2009) stipulates, and also that these women were aware of their culpability.

Fleetwood (2009, p. 20) asserts that women involved in this specific crime go against traditional views of femininity and states, "*Political and academic discourses emphasised women's victimhood and served to 'render them harmless', ergo translating the role of mules from deviant to 'inoffensive.'*" Similarly, female drug mules are portrayed as targets, hoodwinked into transporting drugs by drug syndicates, offering them "employment" (Tsotetsi, 2012, p. 1). Women who become drug mules are thus mainly portrayed as desperate individuals who are unemployed, in financial trouble or with minimal prior exposure to travel (Geldenhuys, 2016). For instance, as reported by Nokwazi Memela, a working mother of two, from Alexandra township in Johannesburg, was recruited by her "miracle-performing" Nigerian church pastors after being promised "a better life" in 2005 (Manala, 2017).

On the other hand, Hübschle (2014) reports that mules have little or no knowledge of the key players within drug networks because they are more often than not recruited by local men and women. An example of women perpetrating such exploitation is Angela Sanclemente, a former Colombian model known as the "cocaine queen"; and the doyen of an international drug smuggling operation, who used female models to drug mule (Fleetwood, 2015a). The case of Sheryl Cwele, ex-wife of Siyabonga Cwele, the former Minister of State Security in South Africa, sparked great interest in the country due to the high-profile characters involved. Sheryl Cwele was found guilty and sentenced to 20 years in prison for conspiring with a Nigerian counterpart to recruit two female drug mules to transport drugs to Brazil. Her sentence was reduced to 12 years on appeal, while the mule remained in jail in Brazil (Ramsayi, 2013). Overall, these cases support the view that research into female criminality has assumed that women commit crimes – such as being drug mules – due to "difficult life circumstances," which might not always be a valid assumption in the absence of other evidence (Bailey, 2013).

Unlu and Ekici (2012) report a 66% increase in female drug mules apprehended between 2006 and 2010. Being a drug mule carries a high risk, including harsh sentences when caught; often including the death penalty and/or death due to rupturing of the intestines and intoxication in cases where drugs were swallowed (appositely referred to "walking around with a belly full of death"). In addition, drug mules are often found murdered because they are viewed as expendable, and as posing a high risk of revealing their source to the authorities (Fleetwood, 2015a; Schemenauer, 2012; Unlu & Ekici, 2012).

Schemenauer (2012) posits that being a female drug mule is risky due to women being discriminated against by border control surveillance because they may be coming from low- or middle-income countries. This is because they are perceived as poor and foreign, which is a profile of a typical drug mule. This situation correlates with findings by Harris (2011a), who lists Jamaica, South Africa, Mexico, Nigeria and Ghana (countries considered to be the Third World) as the most common nationalities of drug mules in prisons in the United Kingdom. These perceptions are only substantiated by the nationalities of the typical drug mule arrested – for example, 30 Nigerian, and 19 South African mules arrested in Turkey between 2006 and 2010 (Unlu & Ekici, 2012).

Future directions: Practice and policy

Mental health is a positive sense of well-being, rather than just an absence of mental disability. In all cases, the emphasis of prison mental health care should be on promoting the mental well-being of all prisoners. As the WHO Consensus Statement on Mental Health Promotion in Prisons underlines, "[w]hile it may be difficult to contemplate the existence of positive mental health among prisoners, prisons should provide an opportunity for prisoners to be helped towards a sense of the opportunities available to them for personal development, without harming themselves or others" (United Nations Office on Drugs and Crime, 2014).

Once in prison, women's mental, psychological, social and physical health care needs will also be different. It follows that all facets of prison facilities, programs and services must be tailored to meet the particular needs of female offenders (United Nations Office on Drugs and Crime, 2008). Upon release, the stigma of imprisonment weighs more heavily on women than on men. In some countries, women are discriminated against and are unable to return to their communities once released from prison (United Nations Office on Drugs and Crime, 2008).

Due to the prevalence of mental health care needs among female offenders, the provision of adequate, gender-sensitive and interdisciplinary mental health care should be essential components of their rehabilitation program. Women's unique mental health care and psychological support needs should be recognized, including, among others, of those who demonstrate acute distress and depression due to isolation, separation from children, families and communities. Treatment should be individualized and aimed at addressing the reasons that provoke distress or depression, as well as other psychiatric conditions, based on an integrated approach of counseling, psychosocial support and medication, if necessary.

Currently, provisions of prison-based health care for incarcerated women in Sub-Saharan Africa appears inadequate, and fails to meet their distinct mental and psychosocial health care needs (African Commission on Human and Peoples' Rights, 2004). Fifteen Sub-Saharan African countries (Namibia, Uganda, Mozambique, Malawi, Cameroon, Botswana, Nigeria, Mali, Kenya, Benin, Zambia, Chad; South Central Somalia/Mogadishu, Ghana and Zimbabwe) reported on inadequate prison-based health services for women (African Commission on Human and Peoples' Right – Ethiopia, 2004; African Commission on Human and Peoples' Right – South Africa, 2004). Sub-standard and ill-equipped mental health and clinical services provisions were characterized by essential medicines stock outs, lack of trained health care personnel (or limited to restricted opening hours for women), lack of routine medical, mental and psychosocial checks for women and limited availability of equipment or lack of basic investigation equipment; for example, functioning sphygmomanometers, thermometers, absent or gender-insensitive prison health care policies and standard operating procedures (SOPs) for women (Wilper et al., 2009).

A lack of prison-based support for women's needs around menstruation was reported in prisons located in Namibia, Uganda, Mozambique, Malawi, Cameroon, Ethiopia, Zimbabwe, Zambia, Nigeria and South Africa (Hout & Mhlanga-gunda, 2018). This need is important as women are prone to irritability, anxiety and depression around or during their menstruation periods (pre-menstrual syndrome).

Pre-menstrual syndrome, a common cyclic disorder of young and middle-aged women, is characterized by emotional and physical symptoms that consistently occur during the luteal phase of the menstrual cycle (Dickerson et al., 2003). The Diagnostic and Statistical Manual of Mental Disorders, fourth edition (DSM-IV), provides criteria for Premenstrual Dysphoric Disorder (PMDD), which can be considered the most severe presentation on the PMS continuum (American Psychiatric Association, 2013). Premenstrual syndrome symptoms can create severe, debilitating psychological and physical problems. A study of female prisoners reported that almost half the prisoners had committed their crime during the pre-menstrual phase and 62% of crimes of violence by women had been committed during their pre-menstrual week (Yadukul et al., 2016). Prison staff could help female prisoners who suffer from PMS to cope with depression, anxiety and other symptoms through counselling, diet and stress management. The mental health team in the prison can assist in training prison staff to be able to identify these individuals early in order to allay suffering.

On a general level, a comprehensive program focused on promoting mental health in prisons, should include the provision of a varied and balanced prison regime, including access to education, vocational training, recreation, family contact, physical exercise, a balanced diet, opportunities to participate in arts, among others (United Nations Office on Drugs and Crime, 2014). Counseling and therapy should be offered as early as possible to those who appear to be at risk of developing mental disabilities. The mental health care needs of offenders whose offenses were known to be related to their mental disability, such as women who have killed their newborn babies due to post-natal depression, should be included in treatment provided.

Women with mental disabilities are at high risk of abuse in custodial settings. They should be protected, with adequate safeguards and supervision. These women are vulnerable to abuse particularly sexual abuse. Such treatment violates the international prohibition on torture, cruelty, inhuman or degrading treatment and punishment (United Nations, 2006).

The UN Standard Minimum Rules for the Treatment of Prisoners states that "men and women shall so far as possible be detained in separate institutions; in an institution which receives both men and women, the whole of the premises allocated to women shall be entirely separate" (United Nations, 2015; Coomaraswamy, 1999). Rule 53 (2) states that "no male member of the staff shall enter the part of the institution set aside for women unless accompanied by a woman officer." Further, paragraph 3 states, "women prisoners shall be attended and supervised only by women officers. This does not, however, preclude male members of the staff, particularly doctors and teachers, from carrying out their professional duties … " However, this provision, even when enforced in the past, has often been abandoned to provide equal employment opportunities for female and male prison staff (African Commission on Human and Peoples' Rights, 2004).

Conclusion

Overall, females represent a growing population in African prisons with a lot of unmet physical and mental health as well as other psychosocial needs. They remain vulnerable inmates within correctional settings that are male-biased in terms of service planning and delivery. While recognizing prevalent resource contraints in African correctional settings, better planned services that are gender-sensitive and culturally appropriate are likely to improve their incarceration experiences and offer greater chances of rehabilitation, recovery and re-integration.

References

Abrahams, N. (2016, May 8). *What lies behind child homicide in South Africa.* The Conversation. https://theconversation.com/what-lies-behind-child-homicide-in-south-africa-58900

Ackermann, M. (2015). Women in detention in Africa: A review of the literature. *Agenda, 29*(4), 80–91. doi: 10.1080/10130950.2015.1122345

Africa, A. (2015). Bad girls to good women – women offenders' narratives of redemption, *Agenda, 29*(4), 120–128. doi: 10.1080/10130950.2015.1124501

Artz, L., Hoffman-Wanderer, Y., & Moult, K. (2012). *Hard Time(s): Women's pathways to crime and incarceration.* Gender, Health and Justice Research Unit, University of Cape Town. www.ghjru.uct.ac.za

African Charter on the Rights and Welfare of the Child (1990). Retrieved from https://www.un.org/en/africa/osaa/pdf/au/afr_charter_rights_welfare_child_africa_1990.pdf

African Commission on Human and Peoples' Rights. (2004). *Ethiopia: Mission on Prisons and Conditions of Detention.* https://www.achpr.org/states/missionreport?id=62

African Commission on Human and Peoples' Rights. (2012). *Special Rapporteur on Prisons, Conditions of Detention and Policing in Africa.* https://www.achpr.org/specialmechanisms/detail?id=3

Allotey, P., & Reidpath, D. (2001). Establishing the causes of childhood mortality in Ghana: The 'spirit child'. *Social Science & Medicine, 52*(7), 1007–1012. https://doi.org/10.1016/s0277-9536(00)00207-0

American Psychiatric Association (2013). Diagnostic and Statistical Manual of Mental Disorders 5th ed. ISBN: 978-0-89042-556-5.

Bagala, A. (2016, November 24). *Uganda: Airport officials arrest south Africans over cocaine.* allAfrica.com. https://allafrica.com/stories/201611240629.html

Bailey, C. (2013). Exploring female motivations for drug smuggling on the island of Barbados. *Feminist Criminology, 8*(2), 117–141. https://doi.org/10.1177/1557085112474837

Bartlett, A. (2006). Female offenders. *Women's Health Medicine, 3*(2), 91–95. https://doi.org/10.1383/wohm.2006.3.2.91

Bester, M. C. (2008). *The psychological factors associated with women who kill an abusive intimate partner within cultural context.* Unpublished Master's dissertation, University of Johannesburg, Johannesburg, South Africa.

Beyen, T. K., Dadi, A. F., Dachew, B. A., Muluneh, N. Y., & Bisetegn, T. A. (2017). "More than eight in every nineteen inmates were living with depression at prisons of Northwest Amhara Regional State, Ethiopia, a cross sectional study design," *BMC Psychiatry, 17*(31), 1–9.

Boonzaier, F., & de la Rey, C. (2004). Women abuse: The construction of gender in women and men's narratives of violence. *South African Journal of Psychology*, *34*, 443–463.

Booyens, K., & Steyn, F. (2013). *A profile of short-term and medium-term adult female offenders*. Pretoria: University of Pretoria (Department of Social Work and Criminology).

Broidy, L., & Agnew, R. (1997.) Gender and crime: A general strain theory perspective. *Journal of Research in Crime and Delinquency*, *34*(3), 275–306.

The Children's Act. (1998). Act 560. Retrieved from http://www.unesco.org/education/edurights/media/docs/f7a7a002205e07fbf119bc00c8bd3208a438b37f.pdf

Coolidge, F. L., & Anderson, L. W. (2002). Personality profiles of women in multiple abusive relationships. *Journal of Family Violence*, *17*, 117–131.

Coomaraswamy R. (1999). Report of the mission to the United States of America on the issue of violence against women in state and federal prisons. UN Doc (E/CN.4/1999/68/Add.2).

Criminal Code Act. (2003). Act 29. Retrieved from https://www.ilo.org/dyn/natlex/docs/ELECTRONIC/88530/101255/F575989920/GHA88530.pdf

Coyle, A. (2009). *A human rights approach to prison management: Handbook for prison staff*. International Centre for Prison Studies.

Dadi, A. F., Dachew, B. A., Kisi, T., Yigzaw, N., & Azale, T. (2016). Anxiety and associated factors among prisoners in north west of Amhara regional state, Ethiopia. *BMC Psychiatry*, *31*, 76–83. https://doi.org/10.1186/s12888-016-0792-y

Dastile, N. P. (2011). *Female crime*. In C. Bezuidenhout (Ed.), A Southern African perspective on fundamental Criminology (pp. 288–304). Cape Town: Pearson Education (Heinemann).

Department of Correctional Services. (2004). 2003/04 annual report. Pretoria: Government Printer.

Dickerson, L.M., Mazyck, P.J., & Hunter, M.H. (2003). Premenstrual syndrome. *Am Fam Physician*, *15*, *67*(8), 1743–1752. PMID: 12725453.

Fazel, S., & Danesh, J. (2002). Serious mental disorder in 23 000 prisoners: A systematic review of 62 surveys. *The Lancet*, *359*(9306), 545–550. https://doi.org/10.1016/s0140-6736(02)07740-1

Fearn, N. E., & Parker, K. (2005). Health care for women inmates. *Californian Journal of Health Promotion*, *3*(2), 1–22. https://doi.org/10.32398/cjhp.v3i2.1760

Fleetwood, J. (2009). *Women in the international cocaine trade: Gender, choice and agency in context* [Unpublished doctoral dissertation]. University of Edinburg.

Fleetwood, J. (2015a). A narrative approach to women's lawbreaking. *Feminist Criminology*, *10*, 368–388.

Fleetwood, J. (2015b): Sentencing reform for drug trafficking in England and Wales. University of Leicester. Report. https://hdl.handle.net/2381/32011

Fleetwood, J. (2015c). Mafias, markets, mules: Gender stereotypes in discourses about drug trafficking. *Sociology Compass*, *9*(11), 962–976. https://doi.org/10.1111/soc4.12323

Frieze, I. H. (2005). *Hurting the one you love: Violence in relationships*. Belmont, CA: Wadsworth Publishing Company.

García-Moreno, C., Jansen, H., Ellsberg, M., Heise, L., et al. (2005). WHO multi-country study on women's health and domestic violence against women: Initial results on prevalence, health outcomes and women's responses. Geneva: WHO Press, World Health Organization. Retrieved from https://www.who.int/reproductivehealth/publications/violence/9241593512/en/

Geldenhuys, K. (2016). The tragic reality of drug mules. *Servamus Community-based Safety and Security Magazine*, *109*(2), 26–30.

Global Prison Trends. (2016). Penal Reform International. Retrieved from https://www.penalreform.org/resource/global-prison-trends-2016-2/

Gose, M. (2002). The African charter on rights and welfare of the child. *Community Law Centre*. ISBN 0-620-29420-5. Retrieved from https://dullahomarinstitute.org.za/childrens-rights/Publications/Other%20publications/The%20African%20Charter%20on%20the%20Rights%20and%20Welfare%20of%20the%20Child.pdf

Gous, N. (2018). South African drug mule sentenced to death in Vietnam. Retrieved from https://www.sowetanlive.co.za/news/south-africa/2018-08-28-south-african-drug-mule-sentenced-to-death-in-vietnam

Green, B. L., Miranda, J., Daroowalla, A., & Siddique, J. (2005). Trauma exposure, mental health functioning, and program needs of women in jail. *Crime and Delinquency*, *51*, 133–151.

Gureje, O., Uwakewe, R., Oladeji, B., Makanjuola, V. O., & Esan, O. (2010). Depression in adult Nigerians: Results from the Nigerian survey of mental health and well-being. *Journal of Affective Disorders*, *120*, 158–164.

Halliwell, E., Main, L., & Richardson, C. (2007). *The fundamental facts; The latest facts and figures on mental health*. Retrieved from https://www.mentalhealth.org.uk/sites/default/files/

Hatton, D. C., & Fisher, A. A. (2008). Incarceration and the new asylums: Consequences for the mental health of women prisoners. *Issues in Mental Health Nursing*, *29*, 1304–1307.

Harris, G. (2011a). TNI/IDPC – Sentencing council: Expert seminar on proportionality of sentencing for drug offences. Retrieved from http://dx.doi.org/10.2139/ssrn.2184341

Heard, C. (2017). Why are women prisoner numbers rising so rapidly?, PENAL REFORM INTERNATIONAL: UNEQUAL JUSTICE. https://www.penalreform.org/blog/why-are-women-prisoner-numbers-rising-so-rapidly/

Hindin, M. J., Kishor, S., & Ansara, D. L. (2008). Intimate partner violence among couples in 10 DHS countries: Predictors and health outcomes. Vol. No. 18, DHS Analytical Studies. Calverton, Maryland: Macro International Inc. Retrieved from https://dhsprogram.com/publications/publication-AS18-Analytical-Studies.cfm

Hout, M. C. Van., & Mhlanga-gunda, R. (2018). Contemporary women prisoners health experiences, unique prison health care needs and health care outcomes in sub Saharan Africa: A scoping review of extant literature. *BMC Int Health Hum Rights*, *18*, 31.

Hübschle, A. (2014). Of bogus hunters, queenpins and mules: The varied roles of women in transnational organized crime in Southern Africa. *Trends in Organized Crime*, *17*, 31–51.

Ibrahim, E. M., Halim, Z. A., Wahab, E. A., & Sabry, N. A. (2014). Psychiatric morbidity among prisoners in Egypt. *World Journal of Medical Sciences*, *11*(2), 228–232

Interpol. (2015). Operation targeting drug trafficking nets couriers in Latin America and Africa. Retrieved from https://www.interpol.int/en/News-and-Events/News/2015/Operation-targeting-drug-trafficking-nets-couriers-in-Latin-America-and-Africa.pdf

International Committee of the Red Cross. (2009). Health in prison: Looking after women in a man's world – ICRC [Internet]. ICRC website. 2009 [cited 2020 Jun 14]. Retrieved from https://www.icrc.org/en/doc/resources/documents/interview/women-health-prison-interview-020309.htm

Johnson, J. E., & Zlotnick, C. (2008). A pilot study of group interpersonal psychotherapy for depression in substance-abusing female prisoners. *Journal of Substance Abuse Treatment*, *34*, 317–377.

Klein, A. (2009). Mules or couriers: The role of Nigerian drug couriers in the international drug trade. In M. D. Childs, & F. Toyin (Eds.), *The changing worlds of Atlantic Africa: Essays in honor of Robin Law* (pp. 411–429). North Carolina: Carolina Academic Press.

Kumar, K. P. S., Srivastava, S., Paswan, S., & Dutta, A. S. (2012). Depression – symptoms, causes, medications and therapies. *The Pharmaceutical Journal*, *1*(3), 7–51.

Lawrence, E. O. (2015). Nigeria and the incidence of homicide. *American Journal of Social Science*, *4*(5), 103–114

Laws of the Federation of Nigeria. (2004). Childs Right Act, 2003. Retrieved from https://laws.lawnigeria.com/2018/04/26/index-lfn-laws-of-the-federation-of-nigeria/

Manala, L. (2017). Alex drug mule exposes church for her near-death ordeal in a foreign land. Retrieved from https://alexnews.co.za/101408/alex-drug-mule-exposes-church-for-her-near-death-ordeal-in-a-foreign-land/

Mapayi, B., Makanjuola, R. O. A., Mosaku, S. K., Adewuya, O. A., et al. (2013). Impact of intimate partner violence on anxiety and depression amongst women in Ile-Ife. *Nigeria. Arch Womens Ment Health*, *16*(1), 11–18. Retrieved from: https://www.researchgate.net/publication/230768882_Impact_of_intimate_partner_violence_on_a nxiety_ and_depression_amongst_women_in_Ile-Ife_Nigeria

Messina, N., Burdon, W., Hagopian, G., & Prendergast, M. (2006). Predictors of prison-based treatment outcomes: A comparison of men and women participants. *The American Journal of Drug and Alcohol Abuse*, *32*(1), 7–28. https://doi.org/10.1080/00952990500328463

Mignon, S. (2016). Health issues of incarcerated women in the United States. *Ciência & Saúde Coletiva*, *21*(7), 2051–2060. https://doi.org/10.1590/1413-81232015217.05302016

Moloney, K. P., & Moller, L. F. (2009). Good practice for mental health programming for women in prison: Reframing the parameters. *Public Health*, *123*, 431–433.

Mweslga, E. K., Nakasujja, N., Nakku, J., Nanyonga, A., et al. (2020). One year prevalence of psychotic disorders among first treatment contact patients at the National Psychiatric Referral and Teaching Hospital in Uganda. *PLoS ONE*, *15*(1), e0218843. https://doi.org/10.1371/journal.pone.0218843

Nagdee, M., Artz, L., Corral-Bulnes, C., et al. (2019). The psycho-social and clinical profile of women referred for psycho-legal evaluation to forensic mental health units in South Africa. *South African Journal of Psychiatry*, *5*(0), a1230. https://doi.org/10.4102/sajpsychiatry.v25i0.1230

Naidoo, S., & Mkize, D. L. (2012). Prevalence of mental disorders in a prison population in Durban, South Africa. *South African Journal of Psychiatry*, *15*(1), 30–35.

National Population- NPC/Nigeria and ICF International. (2014). Nigeria Demographic and Health Survey 2013 - Final Report. Abuja, Nigeria and Rockville, Maryland, USA: NPC/Nigeria and ICF International; 538. Retrieved from https://dhsprogram.com/publications/publication-fr293-dhsfinal-reports.cfm

Nigerian Correctional Service. (2020). Summary of inmate population by convict and awaiting trial persons as at 8th June, 2020. Nigerian Correctional Service website. Retrieved from http://www.corrections.gov.ng/statistics

Nwaopara, U., & Stanley, P. (2015). Prevalence of depression in Port Harcourt Prison. *South African Journal of Psychiatry*, *18*(6), 1000340.

Outwater, A. H., Mgaya, E., Jacqueline, C., Becker, S., et al. (2010). Homicide of children in Dar Es Salaam, Tanzania. East African Journal o Public Health, *7*(4), 345–349. doi: 10.4314/eajph.v7i4.64758

Plugge, E., Douglas, N., & Fitzpatrick, R. (2006). The health of women in prison study findings. Oxford. Retrieved from https://www.researchgate.net/publication/238730815_The_Health_of_Women_in_Prison_Stu

Pogrebin, M. R., & Dodge, M. (2006). Women's accounts of their prison experiences: A retrospective view of their subjective realities. In R. Tewksbury (Ed.) Behind bars: Readings on prison culture.New Jersey: Pearson, 28–46.

Public Radio International. (2018). There are more women in prison than ever before. https://interactive.pri.org/2018/04/unequal-justice/index.html

Pretorius, H. G., & Botha, S. A. (2016). The cycle of violence and abuse in women who kill an intimate male partner: A biological profile. *South African Journal of Psychology*, *39*(2), 242–252

Ramsayi, V. (2013). Drug dealer Cwele's sentence slashed. Retrieved from https://southcoastherald.co.za/7359/cweles-sentence-reduced-4

Redd, N. J. (2019). Learned helplessness and battered woman syndrome. The Encyclopaedia of Women and Crime. Retrieved from: http://doi.org/10.1002/9781118929803.ewac0323

Sakeeb, L. I. (2007). The prevalence of generalized anxiety disorder and major depression among female convicts in a Nigeria prison. Unpublished fellowship thesis submitted to West Africa College of Physicians.

Schemenauer, E. (2012). Victims and vamps, Madonnas and whores. *International Feminist Journal of Politics*, *14*(1), 83–102.

Simon, R. J. (1975). *Women and crime*. Lexington, MA: Lexington Books.

Singer, M., Tootle, W., & Messerschmidt, J. (2013). Living in an illegal economy: The small lives that create big bucks in the global drug trade. *SAIS Review of International Affairs*, *33*(1), 123–135. doi:10.1353/sais.2013.0010.

Skerker, M., Dickey, N., Schonberg, D., & Venters H. (2015). Improving antenatal care in prisons. *Bull World Health Organization*, *93*, 739–740.

Shryock, R., & Gaestel, A. (2018). Why infanticide is a problem in Senegal. Retrieved from: http://www.npr/section/goatsandsoda

Small, K. (2000). *Female crime in the United States (1963–1998): An Update.*Gender Issues, *Summer*, 75–90.

South African Institute of Race Relations. (2013). *South Africa Survey*, 831–833.

Steyn, F., & Hall, B. (2015). Depression, anxiety and stress among incarcerated female offenders. Acta Criminologica: Southern African Journal of Criminology Special Edition No 1/2015: Change in African Corrections: From incarceration to reintegration.

Stevenson, W. J. (2016). *World prison population list*. World Prison Brief – Institute for Criminal Policy Research. Retrieved from http://www.prisonstudies.org/

Telisinghe, L., Charalambous, S., Topp, S. M., Herce, M. E., et al. (2016). HIV and tuberculosis in prisons in sub-Saharan Africa. *The Lancet*, *388*, 1215–1227.

The Sentencing Project. (2018). Incarcerated women and girls. Retrieved from. Retrieved from https://www.sentencingproject.org/publications/incarcerated-women-and-girls/

Todrys, K. W., Amon, J. J., Malembeka, G., & Clayton, M. (2011). Imprisoned and imperiled: Access to HIV and TB prevention and treatment, and denial of human rights, in Zambian prisons. *Journal of International AIDS Society*, *14*, 8.

Tsotetsi, S. (2012). South African young people and drug trafficking. A knowledge brief for the National Youth Development Agency. Retrieved from http://www.nyda.gov.za/knowledgemanagement/Knowledge%20Briefs/South%20african%20young%20people%20and%20drug%20trafficking%20(3).pdf.

United Nations. (2006). Report of the Special Rapporteur on torture and other cruel, inhuman or degrading treatment or punishment. UN Doc E/CN.4, paragraphs 34-38.

United Nations. (2015). United Nations Standard Minimum Rules for the Treatment of Prisoners. A/Res/70/175.

United Nations Office on Drugs and Crime. (2004). *Drug abuse treatment toolkit, substance abuse treatment and care for women: Case studies and lessons learned* (p. 9). United Nations, New York: United Nations Publications.

United Nations Office on Drugs and Crime. (2008). Women and HIV in prison settings. Vienna; 1–6.

United Nation's Office on Drugs and Crime. (2009). World Health Organization Regional Office for Europe. Women's health in prison Correcting gender inequity in prison health. Copenhagen, Denmark: WHO Regional Office for Europe; 1–50.

United Nations Office on Drugs and Crime. (2014). Handbook of women and impriso-ment. 2nd edition, with reference to the United Nations Rules for the Treatement of Women Prisoners and Non-cusodial Measures for Women Offenders (The Bankok Rules). Retrieved from: http://.www.women_and_imprisonment_-_2nd_edition.pdf

United Nations Office on Drugs and Crime. (2020). Responding to the specific needs of women in prison. Retrieved from https://www.unodc.org/unodc/en/hiv-aids/women-in-prison.html

Unlu, A., & Ekici, B. (2012). The extent to which demographic characteristics determine international drug couriers' profiles: A cross-sectional study in Instanbul. *Trends in Organized Crime*, *15*, 296–312.

Van Dieten, M., Jones, J., & Rondon, M. (2014). Working with women who perpetrate violence: A practice guide. 10.

Vasques, B., Esteves-pereira, A. P., Sánchez, A. R., & Larouzé, B. (2016). Birth in prison: pregnancy and birth behind bars in Brazil. *Ciência & Saúde Coletiva*, *21*(7), 2061–2070.

Walker, L. E. (1984). *The battered woman syndrome*. New York: Springer Publishing Company.

Walker, L. E., & Browne, A. (1985). Gender and victimization by intimates. *Journal of Personality*, *53*, 179–195.

Walmsley, R. (2006). *World female imprisonment list*. London International Central Prison Study.

Walmsley, R. (2017). *World female imprisonment list*, Institute for Criminal Policy Research. http://www.prisonstudies.org/sites/default/files/resources/downloads/world_female_prison_4th_edn_v4_web.pdf

Wilper, A. P., Woolhandler, S., Boyd, J. W., Lasser, K. E., et al. (2009). The health and health care of US prisoners: Results of a nationwide survey. *American Journal of Public Health*, *99*(4), 666–672.

Women in prisons. (2018). Retrieved from https:// www.unodc.org/documents/hiv-aids/Women_in_prisons.pdf

World Health Organization. (2016). *Making Mental Health a Global Development Priority, To coincide with the World Bank Group/ IMF Spring Meeting*, Washington, DC, USA: World Health Organization. https://www.who.int/mental_health/WB_WHO_meeting_2016.pdf

World Health Organization. (2009). *ECOSOC meeting "Addressing noncommunicable diseases and mental health: major challenges to sustainable development in the 21st century" Discussing Paper "Mental health, poverty and development"*. Retrieved from https://www.who.int/nmh/publications/discussion_paper_en.pdf.

World Health Organization. (2013). *Global and regional estimates of violence against women Prevalence and health effects of intimate partner violence and nonpartner sexual violence*. Italy: World Health Organization. Retrieved from http://www.who.int/reproductivehealth/publications/violence/9789241564625/en/

World Prison Brief. (2018). World prison brief data. Retrieved from http://www.prisonstudies.org/world-prison-brief-data1

Yadukul, S., Sumangala, C. N., Parinitha, S., & Suresh, B. M. (2016). Pre-menstrual syndrome and crime: A study in Parappana Agrahara central jail, Bengaluru. *South India Medico-Legal Association*, *8*(1), 6–10.

Part IV

Conclusion

16 Future directions for forensic mental health in Africa

Adegboyega Ogunwale, Adegboyega Ogunlesi, Stephane Shepherd, Katrina I. Serpa, and Jay P. Singh

Introduction

Service development

Given the nascent state of forensic mental health services in Africa (Asare, 2012; El Hamaoui, Moussaoui, & Okasha, 2009; Njenga, 2006; Ogunlesi, Ogunwale, De Wet, Roos, & Kaliski, 2012) and the significant socio-economic challenges earlier highlighted across the different chapters of this book, a number of initiatives aimed at service development must be addressed. While some countries have been able to develop rudimentary secure forensic services of a particular level, many others still grapple with providing enough forensic beds within a broader context of inadequacies in mental health care delivery. In the latter category, correctional psychiatry appears to be the most pragmatic approach. This would involve the optimization of prison in-reach activities – improved staffing, broader inter-sectoral collaboration, training, etc. The integration of mental health care into the general medical care setting within prisons is also a practical model and this had been suggested by Ogunlesi and Ogunwale (2018). It seems Nigeria may be traveling towards this direction in the not-too-distant future. This approach is not only realistic but consistent with the ongoing debate in more developed climes as to the cost-effectiveness of specialist secure forensic services. It has also been argued that the rate of mental disorders is so high in prison settings that societies have a legal and moral duty to provide care within those systems (DiTomas et al., 2019; Niveau, 2007; United Nations, 2015).

Furthermore, it is important to stress that with shortages in human and financial resources, the current level of manpower may be spread thin across large geographical spaces and it may be unrealistic to expect meaningful service provision. In this connection, African countries will do well to explore the possibilities offered by information technology (IT) and leverage such contemporary approaches such as tele-psychiatry, which may provide the most realistic approach in some cases (Adjorlolo & Chan, 2015; Mars, Ramlall, & Kaliski, 2012). It may also not be far-fetched to consider private-sector participation in the setting up of correctional facilities as is obtainable in some Western countries as well as in South Africa (Harding, 1998; Roth, 2004; Sekhonyane, 2016). Many

African countries are reluctant to inject reasonable budgetary funds into the correctional system, thereby worsening the lot of vulnerable prisoners such as the mentally ill who are often incarcerated in unsanitary and overcrowded correctional facilities (Institute for Crime & Justice Policy Research, 2020; Obioha, 2011).

As noted above, the alternative to prison psychiatry remains the establishment of secure forensic facilities at regional levels within each country. Current experience in countries like South Africa suggests that the level of security in psychiatric facilities which currently handle involuntary admission and committed mentally ill offenders is quite unsatisfactory, thereby exposing mental health care professionals to both liability and injury (Janse van Rensburg, 2012). Such secure forensic psychiatric units (at different levels of security – low, medium and high) have been established and successfully run in countries like the UK and Canada which provide exemplars for the development of such services in African countries. It must be noted, however, that continuous considerations must be given to cost-effectiveness, ensuring the appropriate level of security for each individual and avoiding a warehousing effect in which forensic patients become "long stayers" in hospitals (Davoren et al., 2015; Duke et al., 2018).

To achieve any remarkable milestones in the development of prison/correctional psychiatry or secure forensic services, it is important to highlight the need for strong inter-sectoral collaborations involving the ministries of justice and health as well as those supervising police and correctional services in each country (Ogunlesi et al., 2012).

Contemporary changes to mental health legislation and criminal law

Existing research in different parts of the world and in particular, within Africa, has clearly shown that many countries either lack mental health legislation or have outdated ones (Ogunlesi et al., 2012; Ogunlesi & Ogunwale, 2012). This has significant implication for the care of the mentally ill either within non-secure settings or forensic contexts. In line with global standards (United Nations, 2009, 2015; World Health Organization, 1996, 2005), many aspects of the existing mental health laws have to be updated to reflect contemporary thinking and human rights recognition.

Clinical training in forensic psychiatry and related behavioral health fields

At the moment, there is no structured clinical training in forensic psychiatry in any part of the continent except a diploma certification in South Africa (El Hamaoui et al., 2009; Ogunlesi et al., 2012). Most practitioners became experts by field experience. In the same vein, there is hardly any certified training for psychologists, nurses or occupational therapists in the field of forensic mental health.

However, the West African College of Physicians has completed a review of its curriculum, whereby a fellowship certification in forensic psychiatry can be obtained when the curriculum is implemented. One pragmatic approach to developing structured training for other professionals apart from psychiatrists is to set up multi-disciplinary MSc and PhD programs in forensic mental health with a clinical component. This can be done after developing a faculty of trainers who have been trained in established centers in other parts of the world. Strategic training alliances with the global north are being developed in parts of the continent, as observed in Rwanda (Eytan, Ngirababyeyi, Nkubili, & Mahoro, 2018).

Development of research collaborations

There is a need to further develop research competencies in the forensic mental health field within the continent. This will provide the much-needed data to drive innovations in different aspects of forensic mental health practice and training. As with clinical/academic training, an effective "North–South" collaboration is key in which more established centers in other parts of the globe are able to provide the necessary training support and resources to improve research capabilities in Africa. One such collaboration is the Centre of Excellence in Forensic Psychiatry Research, which is a partnership between the University of Nottingham's Forensic Psychiatry and Applied Psychology division and Ain Shams University's faculty of medicine in Cairo, Egypt. The collaboration also involves the ministries of health, justice and social services in Egypt. The focus of the partnership is to develop guidelines on the management of forensic psychiatric patients and improve the outcome of long-stay forensic patients in Egypt (https://www.mhinnovation.net/organisations/centre-excellence-forensic-psychiatry-research; accessed: 18/7/2020). In addition to on-site training arrangements, such collaborations may leverage different IT platforms for facilitating training webinars as well as develop distance-learning online courses that may serve the need of African practitioners who may be unable to spend significant amount of time on training outside full employment.

Violence risk assessment/structured assessments in forensic settings

As highlighted in the chapter on violence risk assessment in forensic settings in Africa, it appears that most countries have systems that can provide the necessary opportunities for the development of violence risk assessment research and practice within a short time if the right impetus is generated. Organizing specific training programs in risk assessment is crucial and this can be done at both regional and national levels. Fortunately, virtual interactivity can be leveraged quite easily with the development of webinars on platforms such as Zoom, Googlemeet, etc. Additionally, in resource-limited African settings, there should be a preference for brief but valid simple-to-use instruments that will avoid mountains of paperwork foisted upon already stretched human resources (Roffey &

Kaliski, 2012; Tully, 2017). Innovative approaches such as automation of the risk assessment process by devising IT-enabled "risk calculators" should be given careful consideration (Fazel et al., 2016, 2017; Monahan et al., 2000). Furthermore, machine learning techniques have been developed with the aim of optimizing accuracy in violence risk assessment. However, criticisms have arisen as to the fairness of the underlying algorithms of these artificial intelligence-based techniques (Barabas, Dinakar, Ito, Virza, & Zittrain, 2018; Hamilton, Neuilly, Lee, & Barnoski, 2015; Menger, Spruit, van Est, Nap, & Scheepers, 2019; Tolan, Miron, Gómez, & Castillo, 2019) thereby highlighting the need for considering algorithmic transparency in order to ensure accuracy and fairness (https://scholar.harvard.edu/files/19-fat.pdf).

Overall, strategic objectives in developing violence risk assessment procedures in Africa countries should aim at psychometric evaluation of current Western-style assessment instruments in order to establish culturally appropriate norms, ensuring cost-effective research designs in violence risk assessment and instituting legislative change to reflect the contemporary role of violence risk assessment in implementing laws relating to the treatment of both mentally ill offenders and non-offenders.

Documentation

One of the key needs of the African continent in its quest for development in the forensic mental health arena is the culture of documentation. Based on anecdotal evidence, it would seem that there are genuine innovations in different countries which seek to develop and sustain services but these are not visible enough as a result of lack of documentation. Clinicians and academics must pursue increasing collaboration in ensuring that service or training innovations as well as novel research efforts are documented in book chapters, peer-reviewed journals, policy frameworks and practice guidelines, among others.

The need for practice guidelines as the field becomes more established across the continent

Based on some of the issues raised in the preceding chapters, it has become apparent that practice guidelines or professional codes of ethics specific to forensic mental health professions are lacking in many African jurisdictions. Although, it may be observed that general professional guidelines (e.g., the Medical and Dental Council of Nigeria Code of Medical Ethics) may exist and offer some level of guidance on practice broadly, they are insufficient in dealing with unique ethical and practical challenges that forensic practitioners would face. This is largely driven by the peculiarities of working in the interface between law and psychiatry which have been observed to follow different ethos. For instance, the Nigerian code of ethics for medical doctors only provides specific guidelines against contingency fees for expert testimony while allowing for reasonable payments for such services on a non-contingent basis. It offers no other guidance (Medical and Dental Council of Nigeria, 2008). Apart from the differences in the historical association between law and psychiatry across the globe, the variation in jurisdictional tendencies makes it substantially difficult to practice safely without professional standards. Guidelines relevant to different aspects of forensic mental health work will be helpful in standardizing practice. For instance, in 2012, the South African Society of Psychiatrists (SASOP) and its State Employed Special Interest Group (SESIG) released position statements on forensic psychiatric care in the public sector in South Africa (Janse van Rensburg, 2012). The statements essentially identified inadequacies in the level of security in psychiatric units that were meant to be secure and challenges of ensuring involuntary hospitalization in non-secure settings. They equally offered general guidance on the management of state patients and future directions for improving mental health care delivery in prisons. However, these position statements fell short of being practice guidelines per se.

Be that as it may, cues may be taken from some international professional bodies such as the World Psychiatric Association, Royal Australian and New Zealand College of Psychiatrists and the American Academy of Psychiatry and the Law who have issued ethical guidance for the practice of forensic psychiatry generally (American Academy of Psychiatry and the Law, 2005) and expert witness roles specifically (Janofsky, Hanson, Candilis, Myers, & Zonana, 2014; Mossman et al., 2007; Royal Australian and New Zealand College of Psychiatrists, 2015). In similar vein, the Royal College of Psychiatrists has issued ethical guidelines for the practice of psychiatry in general and the provision of expert opinions as well (Rix, Eastman, & Adshead, 2015; Royal College of Psychiatrists, 2014). These serve as models for African jurisdictions to follow but with the caveat that such guidelines must be both dynamic and flexible to provide practical utility (Buchanan & Norko, 201; Janofsky et al., 2014; Mossman et al., 2007; Howard Zonana, 2008).

The "battle of experts": An African position

Currently, in many African jurisdictions, only one expert is required to present a mental health–related opinion before the court. In jurisdictions where more than one is instructed, the two experts are expected to issue a joint report. This tactical avoidance of a battle of experts could be as a result of limited human resources in the mental health arena. Be that as it may, a judicial tendency in some jurisdictions like Nigeria is to reject an expert's opinion based on the independent assessment of the opinion by the trial judge. In this way, judges who are "lay" in the medical sense subject medical opinion to non-medical logic. While this guarantees the independence of the court as the final arbiter, it calls to question the technical validity of such decisions by the courts. Perhaps the most poignant of such scenarios is when a defendant raising the insanity defense has no other party to corroborate his/her claim. Nigerian courts have held that the evidence of insanity tendered by the defendant himself should be regarded as "suspect" and such defendants should not be "taken seriously" (Goubodia v State, 2004;

Onyekwe v State, 1998). This approach is considered unfair and might lead to miscarriage of justice since mental illness is largely a phenomenological experience with or without classical objective features. We consider it reasonable for the courts to dismiss solely subjective experience without any corroboration. However, where medical opinion corroborates the subjective state of distress, it would amount to the usurpation of the expert's technical know-how for the court to reject both the evidence of the accused and the opinion of the expert only because they are based on the accused person's subjective report alone. It would appear more equitable for there to be an opposing expert opinion in such cases so that the rejection of one expert opinion is *mutatis mutandis*, the acceptance of the other rather than the displacement of expert medical opinion by judicial wisdom. Apart from such cases, it might be an unnecessary waste of time and resources to engage multiple experts in adversarial fashion in African jurisdictions with human resource constraints.

Professional organization

Opportunities for international and inter-professional collaboration under the auspices of the African Association of Psychiatrists and Allied Professionals (AAPAP) should attract the attention of clinicians and academics in Africa spanning the fields of psychiatry, psychology, psychiatric nursing, social work and occupational therapy. Such a platform offers forensic mental health practitioners in different disciplines the basis for the formation of a forensic interest group within the association or an African association of forensic mental health practitioners as an offshoot of the AAPAP. As observed with other international organizations (e.g., the International Association of Forensic Mental Health Services, African Interest Group; http://iafmhs.org/African-Interest-Group; accessed 28/07/2020), such an African forensic network of professionals would provide an environment capable of improving research, training and service development in forensic mental health across the continent.

References

Adjorlolo, S., & Chan, H. C. (2015). Forensic assessment via videoconferencing: Issues and practice considerations. *Journal of Forensic Psychology Practice, 15*(3), 185–204.

American Academy of Psychiatry and the Law. (2005). *Ethics guidelines for the practice of forensic psychiatry*. Adopted May, 2005. http://aapl.org/ethics.htm

Asare, J. B. (2012). Comment: A historical survey of psychiatric practice in Ghana. *Ghana Medical Journal, 46*(3), 114–115.

Barabas, C., Dinakar, K., Ito, J., Virza, M., & Zittrain, J. (2018, July 14). Interventions over Predictions: Reframing the Ethical Debate for Actuarial Risk Assessment. *Proceedings of FAT Conference*. FAT Conference, New York. http://arxiv.org/abs/1712.08238

Buchanan, A., & Norko, M. (2011). *The psychiatric report: Principles and practice of forensic writing* (1st ed.). Cambridge University Press.

Davoren, M., Byrne, O., O'Connell, P., O'Neill, H., O'Reilly, K., & Kennedy, H. G. (2015). Factors affecting length of stay in forensic hospital setting: need for therapeutic security and course of admission. BMC Psychiatry, *15*(1), 1–15.

DiTomas, M., Bick, J., & Williams, B. (2019). Shackled at the end of life: we can do better. The American Journal of Bioethics, *19*(7), 61–63.

Duke, L. H., Furtado, V., Guo, B., & V"llm, B. A. (2018). Long-stay in forensic-psychiatric care in the UK. Social Psychiatry and Psychiatric Epidemiology, *53*(3), 313–321.

El Hamaoui, Y., Moussaoui, D., & Okasha, T. (2009). Forensic psychiatry in North Africa. *Current Opinion in Psychiatry*, *22*, 507–510.

Eytan, A., Ngirababyeyi, A., Nkubili, C., & Mahoro, P. N. (2018). Forensic psychiatry in Rwanda. *Global Health Action*, *11*(1), 1509933. https://doi.org/10.1080/16549716.2018.1509933

Fazel, S., Chang, Z., Fanshawe, T., Långström, N., Lichtenstein, P., Larsson, H., & Mallett, S. (2016). Prediction of violent reoffending on release from prison: Derivation and external validation of a scalable tool. *The Lancet Psychiatry*, *3*(6), 535–543. https://doi.org/10.1016/S2215-0366(16)00103-6

Fazel, S., Wolf, A., Larsson, H., Lichtenstein, P., Mallett, S., & Fanshawe, T. R. (2017). Identification of low risk of violent crime in severe mental illness with a clinical prediction tool (Oxford Mental Illness and Violence tool [OxMIV]): A derivation and validation study. *The Lancet Psychiatry*, *4*(6), 461–468. https://doi.org/10.1016/S2215-0366(17)30109-8

Goubodia v State (2004). 6 NWLR 360.

Hamilton, Z., Neuilly, M.-A., Lee, S., & Barnoski, R. (2015). Isolating modeling effects in offender risk assessment. *Journal of Experimental Criminology*, *11*(2), 299–318. https://doi.org/10.1007/s11292-014-9221-8

Harding, R. (1998). *Private prisons in Australia: The second phase*. Canberra, Australia: Australian Institute of Criminology.

Institute for Crime & Justice Policy Research. (2020). *World Prison Brief—Nigeria*. https://prisonstudies.org/country/nigeria

Janofsky, J. S., Hanson, A., Candilis, P. J., Myers, W. C., & Zonana, H. (2014). AAPL practice guideline for forensic psychiatric evaluation of defendants raising the insanity defence. *Journal of the American Academy of Psychiatry and the Law*, *42*(4), s3–s76.

Janse van Rensburg, B. (2012). The South African Society of Psychiatrists (SASOP) and SASOP State Employed Special Interest Group (SESIG) position statements on psychiatric care in the public sector. *South African Journal of Psychiatry*, *18*(3), 16. https://doi.org/10.4102/sajpsychiatry.v18i3.374

Mars, M., Ramlall, S., & Kaliski, S. (2012). Forensic telepsychiatry: A possible solution for South Africa? *African Journal of Psychiatry*, *15*(4), 244–247. https://doi.org/10.4314/ajpsy.v15i4.31

Medical and Dental Council of Nigeria. (2008). *The code of medical ethics in Nigeria*. Abuja: Medical and Dental Council of Nigeria.

Menger, V., Spruit, M., van Est, R., Nap, E., & Scheepers, F. (2019). Machine learning approach to inpatient violence risk assessment using routinely collected clinical notes in electronic health records. *JAMA Network Open*, *2*(7), e196709. https://doi.org/10.1001/jamanetworkopen.2019.6709

Monahan, J., Steadman, H. J., Appelbaum, P. S., Robbins, P. C., Mulvey, E. P., Silver, E., Roth, L. H., & Grisso, T. (2000). Developing a clinically useful actuarial tool for assessing violence risk. *British Journal of Psychiatry*, *176*, 312–319.

Mossman, D., Noffsinger, S. G., Ash, P., Frierson, R. L., Gerbasi, J., Hackett, M., Lewis, C. F., Pinals, D. A., Scott, C. L., Sieg, K. G., Wall, B. W., & Zonana, H. V. (2007). AAPL practice guideline for the forensic psychiatric evaluation of competence to stand trial. *Journal of the American Academy of Psychiatry and the Law, 35*(4), s3–s72.

Niveau, G. (2007). Relevance and limits of the principle of 'equivalence of care' in prison medicine. Journal of Medical Ethics, *33*(10), 610–613. doi: 10.1136/jme.2006.018077.

Njenga, F. (2006). Forensic psychiatry: The African experience. *World Psychiatry, 5*(2), 97.

Obioha, E. E. (2011). Challenges and reforms in the Nigerian prisons system. *Journal of Social Sciences, 27*(2), 95–109. https://doi.org/10.1080/09718923.2011.11892910

Ogunlesi, A., & Ogunwale, A. (2012). Mental health legislation in Nigeria: Current leanings and future yearnings. *International Psychiatry, 9*(3), 62–64. https://doi.org/10.1192/S1749367600003234

Ogunlesi, A., Ogunwale, A., De Wet, P., Roos, L., & Kaliski, S. (2012). Forensic psychiatry in Africa: Prospects and challenges. *African Journal of Psychiatry, 15*(1), 3–7. https://doi.org/10.4314/ajpsy.v15i1.1

Ogunlesi, A. O., & Ogunwale, A. (2018). Correctional psychiatry in Nigeria: Dynamics of mental healthcare in the most restrictive alternative. *BJPsych International, 15*(2), 35–38. https://doi.org/10.1192/bji.2017.13

Onyekwe v. State (1998). 1 NWLR 565.

Rix, K., Eastman, N., & Adshead, G. (2015). *Responsibilities of psychiatrists who provide expert opinion to courts and tribunals. College report CR193.* Royal College of Psychiatrists.

Roffey, M., & Kaliski, S. (2012). Forensic Forum: "To predict or not to predict – that is the question" An exploration of risk assessment in the context of South African forensic psychiatry. *African Journal of Psychiatry, 15*(4), 227–233. https://doi.org/10.4314/ajpsy.v15i4.29

Roth, L. (2004). *Privatisation of prisons.* NSW Parliamentary Library Research Service.

Royal Australian and New Zealand College of Psychiatrists. (2015). *Developing reports and conducting independent medical examinations in medico-legal settings.* Retrieved from https://www.ranzcp.org/Files/Resources/College_Statements/Practice_Guidelines/PPG-11-FFP-Developing-reports-and-conducting-indep.aspx. (Issue February, pp. 1–5).

Royal College of Psychiatrists. (2014). *Good psychiatric practice: Code of ethics. College report CR186.* Royal College of Psychiatrists. https://www.rcpsych.ac.uk/docs/default-source/improving-care/better-mh-policy/college-reports/college-report-cr186.pdf?sfvrsn=15f49e84_2

Sekhonyane, M. (2016). The pros and the cons: Public-private partnerships (PPP) in South African prisons. *South African Crime Quarterly, 3*, 33–36. https://doi.org/10.17159/2413-3108/2003/v0i3a1076

Tolan, S., Miron, M., Gómez, E., & Castillo, C. (2019). Why machine learning may lead to unfairness: Evidence from risk assessment for juvenile justice in Catalonia. *Proceedings of the Seventeenth International Conference on Artificial Intelligence and Law – ICAIL 19*, 83–92. https://doi.org/10.1145/3322640.3326705

Tully, J. (2017). HCR-20 shows poor field validity in clinical forensic psychiatry settings. *Evidence Based Mental Health, 20*(3), 95–96. https://doi.org/10.1136/eb-2017-102745

United Nations. (2009). *Handbook on prisoners with special needs.* United Nations: New York.

United Nations. (2015). *United Nations standard minimum rules for the treatment of prisoners (the Nelson Mandela rules) A/RES/70/175.* United Nations. https://cdn.penalreform.org/wp-content/uploads/1957/06/ENG.pdf

World Health Organization. (1996). *Mental health care law: Ten basic principles. Geneva: World Health Organization, Division of Mental Health and Prevention of Substance Abuse.* https://www.who.int/mental_health/media/en/75.pdf

World Health Organization (Ed.). (2005). *WHO resource book on mental health, human rights and legislation.* Geneva: World Health Organization.

Zonana, H. (2008). Commentary: When is a practice guideline only a guideline? *The Journal of the American Academy of Psychiatry and the Law, 36*, 302–305.

Index

Note: *Italicized* page numbers refer to figures, **bold** page numbers refer to tables

For Product Safety Concerns and Information please contact our EU
representative GPSR@taylorandfrancis.com
Taylor & Francis Verlag GmbH, Kaufingerstraße 24, 80331 München, Germany

www.ingramcontent.com/pod-product-compliance
Ingram Content Group UK Ltd.
Pitfield, Milton Keynes, MK11 3LW, UK
UKHW020145200926
475702UK00005B/926

* 9 7 8 0 3 6 7 4 5 6 1 0 8 *